Investigations in Paediatrics

Investigations in Paediatrics

Edited by
Douglas P Addy MB ChB FRCP DCH

Consultant Paediatrician
City Hospital
(formerly Dudley Road Hospital)
Birmingham, UK

WB Saunders Company Ltd
London   Philadelphia   Toronto
Sydney   Tokyo

W.B. Saunders Company Ltd	24–28 Oval Road London NW1 7DX, UK

Baillière Tindall

The Curtis Center
Independence Square West
Philadelphia, PA 19106–3399, USA

55 Horner Avenue
Toronto, Ontario, M8Z 4X6, Canada

Harcourt Brace & Company
(Australia) Pty Ltd
30–52 Smidmore Street
Marrickville, NSW 2204, Australia

Harcourt Brace (Japan)
Ichibancho Central Building
22–1 Ichibancho
Chiyoda-ku, Tokyo 102, Japan

A catalogue record for this book is available from the British Library

ISBN 0–7020–1737–X

This book is printed on acid-free paper

Typeset by Phoenix Photosetting, Chatham, Kent
Printed and bound in Great Britain by The Bath Press, Avon

Contents

Contributors

I W BOOTH   Institute of Child Health, Nuffield Building, Francis Road, Birmingham B16 8ET, UK

J T BROCKLEBANK   St James's University Hospital, Department of Paediatrics and Child Health, Clinical Science Building, Leeds LS9 7TF, UK

T J DAVID   Booth Hall Children's Hospital, Department of Child Health, Charlestown Road, Blackley, Manchester M9 2AA, UK

R DINWIDDIE   The Hospital for Sick Children, Great Ormond Street, London WC1N 3JH, UK

P A FARNDON   Birmingham Maternity Hospital, Clinical Genetics Unit, Edgbaston, Birmingham B15 2TH, UK

A R FIELDER   Birmingham and Midland Eye Hospital, Department of Ophthalmology, Church Street, Birmingham B3 2NS, UK

A GREEN   The Children's Hospital, Clinical Chemistry Department, Ladywood Middleway, Birmingham B16 8ET, UK

I M HANN   Hospitals for Sick Children, Haemophilia Center, Great Ormond Street, London WC1N 3JH, UK

R F HINCHLIFFE   Children's Hospital, Department of Paediatric Haematology, Western Bank, Sheffield S10 2TH, UK

C HOBBS   St James's University Hospital, Beckett Street, Leeds LS9 7TF, UK

D I JOHNSTON   University Hospital, Queen's Medical Centre, Nottingham NG7 2UH, UK

D A KELLY   The Children's Hospital, The Liver Unit, Ladywood Middleway, Birmingham B16 8ET, UK

I MCKINLAY   Royal Manchester Children's Hospital, Mackay-Gordon Centre, Pendlebury, Manchester M27 1HA, UK

D W MORGAN   Birmingham Heartlands, Department of ENT Surgery, Birmingham B9 5ST, UK

M G MOTT   Royal Hospital for Sick Children, Institute of Child Health, St Michael's Hill, Bristol BS2 8BJ, UK

K PEARMAN   Birmingham Heartlands, Department of ENT Surgery, Birmingham B9 5ST, UK

J W L PUNTIS   The General Infirmary at Leeds, Neonatal Unit, Clarendon Wing, Belmont Grove, Leeds LS2 9NS, UK

M L RIGBY   Royal Brompton National Heart and Lung Hospital, Sydney Street, London SW3 6NP, UK

C E SARTORI   Royal Hospital for Sick Children, St Michael's Hill, Bristol BS2 8BJ, UK

T R SOUTHWOOD   University of Birmingham Medical School, Childhood Arthritis Unit, Birmingham B15 2TJ, UK

G STEWART   Royal Alexandra Hospital, Paisley, PA2 9PN, UK

M J TARLOW   Birmingham Heartlands Hospital, East Birmingham Teaching Unit, Bordesley Green East, Birmingham B9 5SS, UK

T L TURNER   The Queen Mother's Hospital, Yorkhill, Glasgow G3 8SJ, UK

S J WALLACE   University Hospital of Wales, Department of Child Health, Heath Park, Cardiff CF4 4XW, UK

J E WRAITH   Royal Manchester Children's Hospital, Willink Biochemical Genetics Unit, Pendlebury, Manchester M27 1HA, UK

Foreword

A common answer to the examination question 'How would you investigate a child who presents with . . .' is 'I would start with a full history and examination'. However much this may irritate the examiner as a time wasting ploy, it is of course quite correct. The investigation of a child's medical problem starts in the mind of the doctor the moment the patient with his mother or other carer enters the consulting room, clinic, ward, or accident and emergency department. It is during the period of history taking and examination that decisons are taken about the nature of the problem, its immediate management, and whether further investigations are to be done. These may involve procedures which could be disturbing or painful for the child, using complex equipment which may not be readily available, and will nearly always require the expertise of other professionals. Even the simplest test costs time and money. It is clearly important therefore that every investigation is carefully planned and only embarked upon when a number of questions can be satisfactorily answered. Is the test really necessary? Will it help to establish, confirm, or refute a diagnosis which is clinically uncertain, or is it needed in order to monitor the progress of a disease or its treatment? Is it the most appropriate investigation for the required objective? Can the result be relied on to be accurate and will it be correctly interpreted by the doctor who ordered it?

Advances in medical knowledge and technology have resulted in a bewildering and ever increasing range of investigatory tools becoming available and it is inevitable – indeed, essential – that a doctor who is confronted with a patient whose problems can lie in any system of the body should have an up to date source of reference to consult. The format of most text-books requires at least a provisional diagnosis; there is plenty of information about each condition but this may not necessarily be useful if the initial choice of disease is wrong. It is rather like a guide book which is excellent on certain locations but provides no information on how to get to them. A route planner is likely to be better in this respect. Similarly a book which takes the presenting problem as the start point and puts investigations before disease identification should be particularly helpful. It should not be regarded as a competitor or substitute for standard works but as a means of ensuring that the right investigations are carried out and unnecessary ones avoided.

A final word about children. It may seem trite to reiterate that children are not small adults and that both the way in which investigations are performed and the interpretation of the results will vary according to the age and size of the child. Laboratories, however, the bulk of whose work may be concerned with adults, can run into difficulties when dealing with paediatric problems. A book which concentrates on investigations in paediatrics is thus of value not only to the clinician but to all those who contribute to the procedures involved in investigating and managing the sick child.

PROFESSOR JUNE K LLOYD DBE MB FRCP
Emeritus Professor of Child Health
University of London

Preface

As a general paediatrician I have often felt the need for expert guidance in choosing the appropriate investigations for difficult clinical problems. Therefore, when I was invited to edit this book, I immediately agreed. My aim has been to provide a text which will be used frequently on the wards, in out-patient clinics, and outside hospitals, wherever doctors see children, and which will provide "state of the art" answers to the questions, "Should I arrange investigation of this child and, if so, what investigations are appropriate?" and "At what stage should I refer to a specialist unit for further assessment and investigation?"

The emphasis is on those investigations which will usually be done at a District General Hospital. Nevertheless, it is important that general paediatricians should be aware of the investigations performed at tertiary referral centres and, therefore, these have been described.

I thank all the authors for their labours and Maria Khan of W.B. Saunders for her help and advice.

DOUGLAS P ADDY MB ChB FRCP DCH
Consultant Paediatrician
City Hospital
(formerly Dudley Road Hospital)
Birmingham, UK

1

Haematology

I M Hann

INTRODUCTION

The blood mirrors much of what goes on in the rest of the body and haematologists are as guilty as any of forgetting this simple fact. We are constantly having to remind ourselves of obvious points, for instance much of what we see is far more likely to be due to infection, poor nutrition or bleeding than to malignancy or rare disorders such as haemolytic anaemia. Those haematologists who are not used to dealing regularly with children may also lack a paediatric perspective and forget, for instance, that whereas iron deficiency in adults should lead to an immediate search for blood loss, in children the nutritional aspects are far more important.

Problems may also arise when clinicians forget to look in the other direction and rule out rare but important causes of a problem. Thankfully it is becoming less common to see a child who has persistent or excessive or unexplained bruising or bleeding who has not been investigated for a possible bleeding disorder (Hann 1991). Dentists are often astute at identifying such patients but all clinicians should be able to arrange the appropriate simple tests and interpret them. In this context an even more important point is the great importance of history and examination of the patient. So often coagulation tests are performed without looking carefully into the family history, which can often give the diagnosis or strong clues towards it. In this chapter the emphasis is on tests but it is important not to underestimate the importance of other aspects of management. Thus, if there is a strong family history of classical haemophilia A, a complex, time-consuming expensive and almost certainly irrelevant study of platelet function is clearly unnecessary in the initial investigation. As an example of the recommended approach the part of this chapter devoted to coagulation disorders is arranged in a practical three-phase manner.

Before starting to read the detail of this chapter, please consider some other pitfalls and intricacies which cannot possibly be covered in their entirety. One example would be the existence of a low platelet count. A patient with aplastic anaemia may present with thrombocytopenia or there may be minimal blood abnormalities and the condition is detected because of other features such as hypogonadism. In other cases there may be anaemia alone, leucopenia alone, or any combination of these findings. These features may also occur with other disorders such as toxic marrow suppression of any cause, leukaemia, hypersplenism, or tumour cells in the marrow. Patients can present with the serendipitous finding of, say, a low platelet count prior to surgery or the presentation could be with excessive bruising of unknown cause. Thus, the best way to proceed is to take the practical approach and to address the management of the child as he or she presents with "a problem", rather than detailing how one would have liked leukaemia, for example, to be investigated from the outset if one had know it were present.

BLEEDING AND/OR ABNORMAL CLOTTING TESTS

Children present in two main ways in relation to abnormalities of the coagulation system: abnormal bruising or bleeding; or an abnormal test result, possibly unexpected. Once again, it should be strongly emphasized that history and examination are critical in this context. The three-phase approach is outlined in Tables 1.1 to 1.3. The third phase (Table 1.3) is rarely required and entails considerable expense and usually large blood volumes for testing (usually carried out in the tertiary centre).

Table 1.1 Screening tests for bleeding disorders (phase I)

Prothrombin time*
Partial thromboplastin time*
Thrombin time*
Fibrinogen assay*
Fibrinogen degradation products
Bleeding time*
Platelet numbers
Platelet size and granulation
Neutrophil morphology
Renal and hepatic function tests

*Routine screening, e.g. for non-accidental injury.

Table 1.2 Interpretation of screening tests and further action

Indications	Further test (phase II)
Normal tests but history of bleeding	VIIIRag, VIIIVwF, VIIIc, VIIIRiCof
Normal tests but history of scarring and delayed bruising and cord separation	Factor XIII
BT long for level of platelet count	Platelet aggregation; factor VIIIc, VIIIRag VIIIVwF, VIIIRiCof
PT normal/PTT long/TT normal	Factor VIIIc, XI, XII, IX; contact factors; lupus anticoagulant
PT long/PTT long/TT normal	Factor II, V, IX, X
PT long/PTT normal/TT normal	Factor VII
PT long/PTT normal or long/TT long	FDP to detect DIC; reptilase to rule out heparin; fibrinogen

BT, bleeding time; PT, prothrombin time; PTT, partial thromboplastin time; Rag, related antigen; RiCof, ristocetin cofactor; TT, thrombin time; VwF, von Willebrand's factor.

Phase I

Careful Family History and Examination

This is absolutely essential and it is particularly important to ask about bleeding after operations, dental extractions and childbirth. Note that haemarthrosis (Figure 1.1) rarely occurs except in severe factor VIII or IX deficiency. Epistaxis and mucosal bleeding is suggestive

Table 1.3 Phase III clotting tests

Indications	Further tests
Abnormal platelet aggregation	Platelet storage and release nucleotides
Normal coagulation but strong bleeding history	Repeat all screen tests. Prothrombin consumption index. Factor VIIIc, IX, VIIIVwF. Euglobulin clot lysis. Consider Munchhausen-by-proxy
PT and PTT long and initial factor assays normal	Factors VII, VIII, IX, XI, XII and contact factors
If failure of production of platelets is a possibility	Bone marrow and chromosomes

PT, prothrombin time; PTT, partial thromboplastin time; VwF, von Willebrand's factor.

of a platelet disorder (Table 1.4) or von Willebrand's disease. Scarring and delayed bruising is typical of the blood vessel/connective tissue disorders (Table 1.5) and *if associated with delayed cord separation* suggests factor XIII deficiency. *Various dysmorphic features* are associated with Fanconi's anaemia (short stature, microcephaly, abnormal pigmentation, pointed chin, elf-like faces, hypoplasia of thenar and hypothenar eminences, malformed kidneys, strabismus, hypogonadism, cryptorchidism, hyperreflexia, mental retardation and deafness) and familial thrombocytopenias. Albinism is part of the *Hermansky–Pudlak and Chediak–Higashi* syndromes. Thrombocytopenia with absent radii (TAR) is also a well-described association. In general, bruising or bleeding early on in life is suggestive of a congenital cause as opposed to the often later onset of acquired disorders.

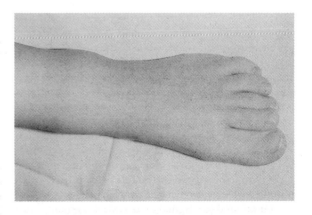

Figure 1.1 Haemophiliac haemarthrosis.

Table 1.4 Qualitative platelet disorders

Defective platelet → agonist interaction
(a) adrenalin
(b) collagen (glycoprotein la deficiencies)
(c) thromboxane A_2

Defective platelet → vessel wall adhesion
(a) von Willebrand's disease
(b) Bernard–Soulier syndrome (glycoproteins Ib, V and X deficiency)

Defective platelet → platelet aggregation
(a) Storage pool deficiency
(b) Glanzmann's thrombasthaenia (glycoprotein IIb/IIIa deficiency)
(c) Arachidonic acid pathway deficiencies
   (i) Cyclo-oxygenase deficiency
   (ii) Thromboxane synthetase deficiency
   (iii) Impaired release of arachidonate
(d) Secretion defects
   (i) Impaired calcium mobilization
   (ii) Defective phosphatidylinositol metabolism
   (iii) Defective myosin phosphorylation
(e) α-Granule deficiency (gray platelets)

Miscellaneous qualitative defects
(a) May–Hegglin anomaly
(b) Hermansky–Pudlak syndrome. Storage pool deficiencies
(c) Chediak–Higashi syndrome

Familial quantitative disorders
(a) Fanconi's syndrome
(b) Thrombocytopenia with absent radius (TAR) syndrome
(c) Wiskott–Aldrich syndrome
(d) Familial thrombocytopenias, e.g. Epstein's
(e) Amegakaryocytic

Table 1.5 Disorders of blood vessels and connective tissue

Hereditary haemorrhagic telangiectasia (Osler–Weber–Rendu disease)

Pseudoxanthoma elasticum

Marfan's syndrome

Osteogenesis imperfecta

Laboratory Tests (Tables 1.1 and 1.2)

Acquired abnormalities may be suggested by symptoms and signs of disease or by the results of liver and renal function studies. If hepatosplenomegaly is present then portal hypertension and marrow infiltrative disorders must be ruled out, the latter by marrow aspirate and trephine. The tables should be self-explanatory, but a few additional comments may be helpful.

The prothrombin time (PT), partial thromboplastin time (PTT), thrombin time (TT), fibrinogen and bleeding time comprise an excellent set of screening tests which is sufficient for medico-legal purposes (e.g. non-accidental injury), and preoperative screening for all major procedures and biopsies as well as the standard baseline investigation of a possible bleeding disorder. It is very rare for a significant bleeding disorder to exist in the face of a set of negative screening tests. Exceptions are very mild cases of von Willebrand's disease and of haemophilia, and factor XIII deficiency. There are a few details worth mentioning.

1. A prolonged PT and PTT may rarely signify factor X deficiency or very rare mixed inherited deficiencies, but much more frequently it is indicative of a hepatic or vitamin K defect.
2. Christmas disease (factor IXc deficiency) should never be diagnosed without confirming that the other vitamin-K-related factors (II, VII and X) and liver function tests are normal.
3. Isolated prolonged PTT usually indicates classical haemophilia A (low VIIIc), but it can reflect contact factor deficiency which may be the first indication of liver dysfunction, or very occasionally an inhibitor (especially the lupus anticoagulant).
4. The bleeding time is a difficult test because the times tend to be a little longer in normal children (95th percentile value 9 min) and the technique is crucial (Sanders et al 1990). It is essential to avoid superficial blood vessels, avoid low and high arm-cuff pressures and ensure capillary-effect blotting. The commonest cause of prolongation is poor technique followed (in the past and still occasionally) by aspirin ingestion and by platelet function disorders (Bellucci and Caen 1988) (Table 1.4).
5. It is much more difficult to differentiate liver problems from consumptive coagulopathy than is usually recognized. Fibrin degradation products rise in liver dysfunction due to failure of clearance. The only way to be sure is to assay factor VII (liver) and V or VIII (consumed) levels.

ABNORMAL BLOOD COUNT VALUES

As previously stated, a number of disorders can present with a low haemoglobin or platelets or white count or any

4   I M HANN

combination of the three, or with abnormally high counts. In order to prevent tedious repetition, the tables will be as comprehensive as possible, but the text will only deal with important examples and comment.

Pancytopenia

In everyday paediatric practice, the commonest cause of low haemoglobin, white cells, and platelets is toxic marrow suppression due to overwhelming infection or, occasionally, metabolic disorders. The diagnosis of aplastic anaemia is in fact made by excluding these causes, by demonstrating a failure of recovery of the counts and an "empty" bone marrow. The approach to investigation of a patient with pancytopenia or persistent low counts of any variety, which may be due to aplastic anaemia, is detailed in Tables 1.6 and 1.7. Points of importance to note are as follows.

1. Examination of the patient may reveal dysmorphic features of Fanconi's anaemia, the commonest of which are abnormal pigmentation, skeletal deformities (especially of the thumbs), stunted growth, microcephaly and renal and cardiac abnormalities (Evans 1992). Confirmation of the diagnosis is by *in*

Table 1.6   Causes of aplastic anaemia in childhood

Constitutional
Fanconi's anaemia:
● with other congenital defects (classical type)
● without other defects (Estren–Dameshek type)
● without chromosome changes

Dyskeratosis congenita

Shwachman's syndrome

Other rare types (radioulnar fusion, Scandinavian type, etc.)

Acquired
Idiopathic

Post-infectious:
● hepatitis
● other infections

Due to drugs:
● chemotherapy
● other drugs

Due to radiation

Due to chemicals and toxins

With paroxysmal nocturnal haemoglobinuria

Pre-leukaemia

From Evans (1992), by permission of Churchill Livingstone.

vitro demonstration of excess lymphocyte chromosome breaks.
2. Drugs and toxins very rarely cause aplastic anaemia in children and lists can be found in standard texts (Evans 1992).
3. In the younger child with hepatosplenomegaly, fevers and pancytopenia, one of the commoner causes is haemophagocytic lymphohistiocytosis (HLH) (Simpson 1992). This is a macrophage disorder which may

Table 1.7   Investigation of suspected bone marrow aplasia in children

Group I – aplasia suspected	Group II – aplasia confirmed
Full blood counts including:	*Tests for constitutional aplasias*
Haemoglobin and red cell count	Height and weight
Red cell indices	Head circumference
Reticulocytes	X-ray forearms and wrists for bone age and bone defects
Total white cell count and differential counts	Urine and plasma amino acids
Bone marrow aspiration	
Blood group and Rhesus type	*Tests for PNH*
Direct Coombs' test	Ham's acid serum test
	Sugar water test
Aplasia probable	Urine for haemosiderin
Bone marrow trephine biopsy	
Haemoglobin electrophoresis	*Test for Shwachman's syndrome*
HLA typing for potential marrow transplant donor	Faeces (trypsin and faecal fat)
Chromosome analysis (blood and bone marrow)	Fat loading test
Urea/creatinine	Pancreatic function tests/ duodenal intubation
Liver function tests	Urine sugar chromatography (galactose)
Immunoglobulins	
Hepatitis serology	
Virus isolation (throat, urine and faeces)	*Miscellaneous tests*
Urine (bilirubin, urobilin and urobilinogen, haemosiderin)	Leucocyte alkaline phosphatase
	Serum B_{12}
Family (full blood counts and HLA typing)	Red cell and serum folate
	Red cell antigens
Group I tests are desirable in all cases	CFU-bone marrow and blood
	Group II tests may help with specific diagnosis and should be selected for specific cases, in the tertiary referral centre

PNH, paroxysmal nocturnal haemoglobinuria.

occasionally be familial or follow a defined infection and has a very poor prognosis. It is notoriously difficult to diagnose unless there is a family history. The marrow aspirate and trephine and CSF may contain phagocytosing histiocytes and plasma triglyceride levels are usually elevated.

4. Always take a good travel history and do not forget leishmaniasis (serology and marrow aspirate), HIV infection, and (rarely) tuberculosis.
5. If the patient has a big spleen and none of the preceding causes then look for causes of hypersplenism, the commonest of which is portal hypertension following neonatal problems. Consider storage disorders (Hann et al 1990). (See Chapters 4 and 8.)
6. When "scraping the barrel" always remember autoimmune and immunoregulatory disorders such as systemic lupus. They frequently present with cytopenias.
7. Infiltration of the marrow by tumours such as Langerhan's cell histiocytosis (LCH), non-Hodgkins lymphoma (NHL), rhabdomyosarcoma and neuroblastoma can present with cytopenias and with a leucoerythroblastic anaemia (see below).

Leucoerythroblastic Anaemia

This means that the blood film contains left-shifted granulocytes (band forms, myelocytes, metamyelocytes, promyelocytes and very occasional myeloblasts) along with early erythroid forms including normoblasts. This type of picture is not absolutely specific for "infiltration" because it can occur in other situations where the marrow is stressed. Thus, one can often see such a picture in ill neonates, for instance those with respiratory distress syndrome or haemolytic disease of the newborn. Patients with myelodysplasia/myeloproliferation frequently present with leucoerythroblastic anaemia usually associated with dysplastic features and often a monocytosis and low platelet count.

In most cases the only way to reach a diagnosis is to perform a bone marrow aspirate and trephine, search for a tumour elsewhere if indicated, and remember to rule out osteopetrosis. Finally, it is necessary to consider the infections which can affect the marrow, especially leishmaniasis and tuberculosis.

Thrombocytopenia

There is a multitude of causes for a low platelet count (Tables 1.8 and 1.9). When considering the relevant tests it is important first to decide what is most likely in a particular context. For instance, in neonates isoimmune thrombocytopenia and maternal induced autoimmune causes are frequently seen where infection (including congenital infection) has been ruled out. In many cases a bone marrow test is required to determine whether this is one of the rare situations with reduced production and reduced marrow megakaryocytes. However, children presenting with a classical history of idiopathic thrombocytopenic purpura (ITP) do not need to have a marow test performed (Chessels and Chronic 1989) unless it is one of the rare cases where therapy is required. There are too many potential ways of investigating these patients for it to be possible to provide any other than an unnecessarily complex algorithm. Thus, it is necessary to observe a few points.

1. Transient falls in platelet count are common in relation to infection. There is often a consumptive element due to disseminated intravascular coagulation (DIC).
2. Hypersplenism usually presents with a platelet count in the $60-100 \times 10^9/l$ range and should be clinically obvious.
3. Drugs can (rarely) be causative and a careful history is essential. For lists see the standard texts (Lilleyman 1992).
4. If the patient does not have an infection and does not have hepatosplenomegaly then the most likely cause is ITP, especially if there is an acute onset with no other features in an otherwise well child. If in doubt, check the bone marrow and rule out autoimmune disorders. Wiskott–Aldrich syndrome is an extremely heterogeneous disorder described more fully in Chapter 12.

Table 1.8 Causes of thrombocytopenia due to reduced platelet life-span

Idiopathic thrombocytopenic purpura (ITP)
Neonatal isoimmune thrombocytopenia
Associated with infection
Drug-induced*
Associated with autoimmune disorders
Associated with malignant disease
Post-transfusion purpura
Disseminated intravascular coagulation (DIC)
Haemolytic uraemic syndrome (HUS)
Thrombotic thrombocytopenic purpura (TTP)
Haemangiomata (Kasabach–Merritt syndrome)
Cyanotic congenital heart disease (CCHD)
Liver disease
Intravascular prosthetics, e.g. valves/patches

From Lilleyman (1992), by permission of Churchill Livingstone.
*Can be immune- or non-immune-mediated.

Table 1.9   Causes of thrombocytopenia due to reduced production

Congenital	Acquired
Without megakaryocytes: *	*Aplastic anaemia/*
Thrombocytopenia/absent	*myelosuppression*
radius (TAR) syndrome	Idiopathic
Fanconi's anaemia	Drug induced
Other amegakaryocytic	Toxin induced
thrombocytopenia	Radiation induced
	Hepatitis associated
With megakaryocytes: *	
Wiskott–Aldrich syndrome	*Marrow replacement*
May–Hegglin anomaly	Leukaemia
Bernard–Soulier	Metastatic malignancy
syndrome	
Epstein's syndrome	*Megaloblastic anaemias*
Gray platelet syndrome	
Montreal syndrome	
Mediterranean	
thrombocytopenia	
Other hereditary	
thrombocytopenias	
Inherited megaloblastic	
anaemias	
Other metabolic disorders	

From Lilleyman (1992), by permission of Churchill Livingstone.
*The classification into "with" and "without" megakaryocytes is not absolute but is clinically useful.

Infection or skin problems or bleeding may be prominent. The bleeding disorder is related to thrombocytopenia. Platelet antibody testing is of dubious value except in the neonatal period.

5. Remember the simple things like family history and examination of platelet morphology. Chediak–Higashi and Bernard–Soulier syndromes should be diagnosed with this approach. Chediak–Higashi is an autosomal recessive trait with oculocutaneous albinism, fine light hair, susceptibility to infection and sometimes neurological problems and bleeding diathesis. The neutrophils, other white cells and other tissue cells show pyknotic nuclei and large irregular cytoplasmic granules. Bernard–Soulier syndrome is a disorder associated with giant platelets and autosomal recessive inheritance. The primary defect is a lack of platelet receptor sites for factor VIII associated protein.

6. Any of the disorders mentioned under the heading of pancytopenia can present with low platelet counts as the first manifestation of a more widespread marrow disorder. This should be clarified following clinical examination, blood film examination and bone marrow morphology.

7. Neonatal thrombocytopenia is often associated with autoimmune haemolysis (Evan's syndrome), and thus a simple direct Coombs test should be performed in all cases.

Thrombocytosis

High platelet counts are very common in children, and only extremely rarely are they associated with any serious consequence. By far the commonest cause is intercurrent infection or inflammatory disorders and, much less often (unlike adults), bleeding. A handful of cases of essential thrombocythaemia have been described in children and, very rarely, primary myeloproliferative disorders are associated with high platelet counts. It is rarely necessary to do more than a blood count, look for organomegaly and wait for the count to fall again. After splenectomy there is usually a raised platelet count which is associated with other blood film abnormalities such as Howell–Jolly bodies.

Anaemia

There is a potentially bewildering array of causes of anaemia, the vast majority of which will be irrelevant to the astute clinician. Rather than produce many long lists of highly unlikely causes which any doctor would find unhelpful, it is simply necessary to ask the following questions:

1. Is it bleeding?
2. Is it nutritional?
3. Is it isolated, i.e. what is the rest of the blood count?
4. Is it haemolysis?
5. Is there an underlying cause:
   (a) collagen/vascular,
   (b) other chronic disorders,
   (c) renal/hepatic, or
   (d) any other obvious predisposing cause?

So, the way to approach it is take a history, examine the patient and then look at the blood count and reticulocyte level (Table 1.10). The other points to note are as follows.

It is impractical to perform extensive investigations in every obvious case of iron deficiency with a proven nutritional deficit. It is, however, worth testing again after a 6-month course, to ensure compliance and response (check for thalassaemia trait and blood loss if the response is inadequate). If investigation is required, the best test is a ferritin level, along with transferrin saturation. This

Table 1.10 Investigation of anaemia

Indications	Further investigations
Phase I	
Low MCV, normal RBC	Iron studies. Nutritional assessment. FOBs. Look for blood loss if relevant
Low MCV, high RBC	Iron studies. Hb electrophoresis with A_2 and F estimations
Low Hb, high reticulocytes	Bilirubin. Urobilinogen. Direct Coombs test. If positive go on to phase II. Osmotic fragility test if spherocytes on film
Low Hb, low reticulocytes	Marrow for failure syndromes. CDAs. TEA. BDA. Parvovirus titres
Normal Hb, normal MCV	Search for chronic disorders. U&E, LFTs, etc.
Phase II (usually at a tertiary referral centre)	
Haemolysis	Haptoglobin level. Glycolytic enzymes and intermediates. H bodies. Red cell membrane studies
Haemoglobinopathy	Family studies. α-Haplotypes. Globin chain labelling
CDA	I/i red cell antigen titres. Ham's and sucrose-lysis tests. Electron microscopy of red cells
Marrow failure of pancytopenia	Marrow and trephines and *in vitro* culture. Chromosome breaks, etc.

BDA, blackfan diamond anaemia; CDA, congenital dyserythropoietic anaemia; FOBs, faecal occult bloods; I/i, blood group I/i antigen system; LFTs, liver function tests; MCV, mean corpuscular volume (fl); RBC, red blood cell count ($\times 10^{12}$/l); TEA, transient erythroid aplasia; U&E, Urea and electrolytes.

should detect patients with anaemia of chronic disorders (who should have normal iron saturation) and iron-deficient patients with a raised ferritin due to inflammatory or hepatic disorders (who will have a low transferrin saturation).

Ask yourself how to prove the existence of haemolysis. It is not always as easy as it sounds. Look for reticulocytosis, raised unconjugated bilirubin and low haptoglobin. If the Coombs test is negative, there are no microspherocytes on the blood film, and if the glucose-6-phosphate dehydrogenase and pyruvate kinase are normal, refer for special tests such as glycolytic intermediate levels, oxygen dissociation curves, and red cell membrane studies.

Neutropenia

The investigation is outlined in Table 1.11, but again it must be emphasized that the commonest cause is transient marrow suppression related to infection and further investigation is not necessarily required where there is an obvious predisposing cause and counts recover following its resolution. The most likely diagnosis in children with persistent neutropenia without a history of serious infections is chronic benign neutropenia, and severe neutropenia or Kostmann's syndrome is largely diagnosed on the evidence of recurrent infections along with the typical maturation arrest in the marrow granulocyte series.

Neutrophilia, Monocytosis and Eosinophilia

The most important point is to avoid overinvestigation of these normal reactions. There are very rarely any serious

Table 1.11 Investigation of neutropenia

Full blood counts with white cell differential, to document recovery or persistence or cyclical neutropenia

Blood film examination for white cell morphology – rule out leukaemia, myelokathexis (Zwelzer, 1970), other marrow infiltrations

Immunoglobulin levels, complement levels and T and B lymphocyte subsets to exclude immunological disorders, including reticular dysgenesis

Neutrophil antibodies and DNA binding and autoantibody screen to exclude isoimmune and autoimmune causes

Bone-marrow examination will identify agranulocytosis, maturation arrest of severe congenital neutropenia (Kostmann's syndrome), megaloblastosis of vitamin B_{12}/ folate deficiency, myelodysplasia and infiltrative disorders

Vitamin B_{12} and folate assays for megaloblastic anaemia

Exocrine pancreatic function for Shwachman's syndrome

Sucrose lysis and Ham's tests and urine haemosiderin for paroxysmal nocturnal haemoglobinuria

Blood chromosome breaks for Fanconi's anaemia and DNA repair defects

Skeletal survey for Fanconi's, cartilage hair hypoplasia, Shwachman's syndrome and dyskeratosis congenita (plus skin rashes and nail dysplasia)

Rebuck skin window for chemotactic defects

Plasma and urine amino acids to exclude organic acidaemia

causes for these abnormalities. Neutrophilia usually denotes an infectious or inflammatory aetiology, but is not specific for anything. Persistent extreme neutrophilia ($> 50 \times 10^9/l$) is extremely rarely associated with Philadelphia chromosome-positive leukaemia. Similarly, very rare causes of myeloproliferative disorder with eosinophilia occur. Otherwise, slight or moderate eosinophilia is found in association with allergic, parasitic and skin disorders. More rarely it is found with the primary hypereosinophilic syndrome (Alfaham et al 1987).

Leukaemia, Myeloproliferative and Leukaemoid Reactions

Leukaemia can present with any of the features of pancytopenia or even a normal blood count and the diagnosis may only be suggested by the presence of hepatosplenomegaly and/or lymphadenopathy (see below). More frequently, the white cell count is elevated, with primitive forms and low haemoglobin and platelets. The myeloproliferative disorders are also often associated with leucocytosis and blast cells, although dysplastic features such as reduced granularity of myeloid cells and abnormal nuclei may be more prominent. Investigation of these two sets of disorders is similar (Figure 1.2, Table 1.12) (Chessells 1992). Diagnostic subgroups are shown in Tables 1.13 and 1.14 (Eden 1992). Once the diagnosis is reasonably secure, usually following clinical examination and blood-film examination, referral to a tertiary centre is indicated for further investigation. The crucial tests nowadays are the bone-marrow morphology (Bennett 1981), cytogenetics and immunophenotyping. The term "leukaemoid" is not useful in practice, and in my opinion it should no longer be used.

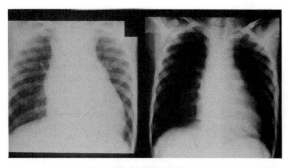

Figure 1.2   Chest X-ray of mediastinal mass in a case of T-cell non-Hodgkin's lymphoma.

Table 1.12   Investigation of leukaemia and myeloproliferative/myelodysplastic disorders (MDS)

Haemoglobin, red cell indices, WBC differential and film

Bone-marrow aspirate (plus trephine in MDS)

Bone-marrow cytochemistry, cytogenetics, immunophenotyping

Bone-marrow iron stain in MDS

HbF, neutrophil and platelet function in MDS

Bone-marrow colony culture assays in MDS

Urea and electrolytes, urate, calcium and phosphate for tumour lysis syndrome

Liver function tests

Coagulation tests and fibrin degradation products

Cerebrospinal fluid and cytospin for morphology

Chest X-ray for mediastinal mass (Figure 1.2)

MDS: Myelodysplasia = dysplastic changes of blood cells.

HEPATOSPLENOMEGALY AND LYMPHADENOPATHY (see also Chapters 5 and 8)

There are many potential causes of organomegaly, and clinical acumen is required in order to prevent over-investigation. An example would be the child who presents moderately unwell with sore throat, splenomegaly and lymphadenopathy. All that may be required is a simple blood count and monospot test. A blunderbuss approach with bone-marrow examination and so on would be unjustified.

Two very common presentations are cervical lymphadenopathy, with or without clinical evidence of a recent viral infection, and hepatosplenomegaly in an otherwise

Table 1.13   Diagnostic subgroups of myeloproliferative/myelodysplastic disorders

Philadelphia – positive chronic myeloid leukaemia
Philadelphia – negative chronic myeloid leukaemia
Juvenile chronic myeloid leukaemia
Infantile monosomy 7 syndrome
Chronic myelomonocytic leukaemia
Essential thrombocythaemia
Polycythaemia rubra vera
Myelofibrosis
Transient myeloproliferative disease of the newborn
Miscellaneous familial disorders
Refractory anaemia
Refractory anaemia with ringed sideroblasts
Refractory anaemia with excess blasts
Refractory anaemia with excess blasts in transformation

Table 1.14 Classification of acute leukaemias

Acute lymphoblastic		Acute myeloid	
L_1	"Microlymphoblastic"	M_1	Undifferentiated
L_2	"Macrolymphoblastic"	M_2	Differentiated
L_3	Usually mature B-cell surface membrane immunoglobulin-positive	M_3	Promyelocytic
		M_4	Myelomonocytic
		M_5	Monocytic
		M_6	Erythroid
		M_7	Megakaryoblastic

well child who has a history of neonatal problems including vascular catheterization. The approach to isolated lymphadenopathy in a well child with no blood count abnormality other than leucocytosis should be expectant. A chest X-ray should be checked and screening for viral and other infections carried out. If blood count abnormalities ensue then these should be appropriately investigated as already described. If the glands grow or appear abnormal in texture or fixation, then the only definitive test is biopsy and histological examination. However, this is often unnecessary if the blood counts are abnormal because a bone-marrow aspirate should provide the diagnosis. A suggested scheme of investigations is listed in Table 1.15 (Ladisch and Miller 1989) and a list of differential diagnoses is given in Table 1.16. There are a few final points of note.

1. Infants and babies with hepatosplenomegaly usually have a congenital or acquired infection, but if pancytopenia or less generalized low blood counts are present then the most likely diagnosis is haemophagocytic lymphohistiocytosis (HLH). This can be a tricky diagnosis to confirm, but excess phagocytosis in the marrow and/or CSF, raised triglycerides and persistent fever are all of value.
2. Most malignancies presenting with hepatosplenomegaly are best investigated by bone-marrow aspiration and trephine. It may occasionally be necessary to biopsy tissues such as pathologically enlarged lymph nodes. Details of staging schemes are complex (see Chapter 2).
3. Other tissues can sometimes be affected by haematological disorders. The skin may rarely be infiltrated by leukaemia in babies (Figure 1.3) and the gums, usually in monocytic leukaemias (Figure 1.4). Non-Hodgkin's lymphoma may also affect other sites, e.g. skin, lung parenchyma, bones and testes.

Occasionally, enlarged kidneys or testes are present at the outset of leukaemia.

(For blood disorders in the newborn, see Chapter 20.)

Table 1.15 Investigation of hepatosplenomegaly

Full blood count, film, differential and reticulocytes

Liver function tests. Unconjugated bilirubin. Urine urobilinogen

DNA binding. Autoantibody screen. ESR

Blood film for vacuolated lymphocytes* and malaria

Urine and blood for metabolic/organic acid screen

Infection screen (including TORCH in neonates)

Imaging for varices and liver/spleen texture

Direct antiglobulin test. Haptoglobin level

Bone-marrow aspirate and trephine for morphology, storage cells, phagocytosis, chromosomes, immunophenotyping

Plasma triglycerides (raised in HLH)

Urinary catecholamines for neuroblastoma

Chest X-ray for mediastinal mass

Abdominal CT Scan for staging of lymphoma

---

*Seen in mucopolysaccharidoses, sialidosis, etc.
CT, computed tomography; ESR, erythrocyte sedimentation rate; HLH, haemophagocytic lymphohistiocytosis; TORCH, toxoplasma, rubella, cytomegalovirus (CMV), herpes simplex.

Table 1.16 Causes of hepatosplenomegaly

Infection, e.g. malaria, *Leishmania*, CMV, EBV, TORCH, *Candida*

Portal hypertension

Haemophagocytic lymphohistiocytosis (HLH)

Storage disorders

Metabolic disorders

Lymphoma and leukaemia

Haemolytic anaemias

Autoimmune disorders

Kasabach–Merritt giant haemangioma of the spleen

Myelodysplasia/myeloproliferative disorders

Stage IV neuroblastoma. Rarely, other tumours

CMV, cytomegalovirus; EBV, Epstein–Barr virus; TORCH, toxoplasma, rubella, CMV, herpes simplex.

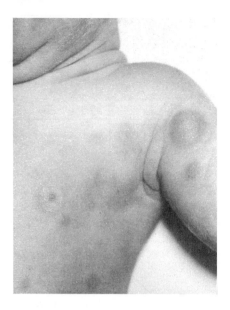

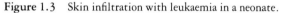

Figure 1.4   Gum infiltration in monocytic leukaemia.

Figure 1.3   Skin infiltration with leukaemia in a neonate.

REFERENCES

Alfaham MA, Ferguson SD, Shira B, Davies J (1987) The idiopathic hypereosinophilic syndrome. *Arch Dis Child* 62: 601–613.

Bellucci S, Caen JP (1988) Congenital platelet disorders. *Blood Rev* 2: 16–26.

Bennett JM, Catovsky D, Daniel MT et al (1981) The FAB cooperative group. The morphological classification of acute lymphoblastic leukaemia. *Br J Haematol* 47: 553–561.

Chessells JM (1989) Chronic ITP: Primum non nocere. *Arch Dis Child* 64: 1326–1328.

Chessells JM (1992) Chronic myeloid leukaemia, myeloproliferative disorders and myelodysplasia. In: Hann IM, Lilleyman JS (eds) *Paediatric Haematology*, pp. 59–82. Churchill Livingstone, Edinburgh.

Eden OB (1992) Malignant disorders of lymphocytes. In: Hann IM, Lilleyman JS (eds) *Paediatric Haematology*, pp. 329–366. Churchill Livingstone, Edinburgh.

Evans DIK (1992) Aplastic anaemia. In: Hann IM, Lilleyman JS (eds) *Paediatric Haematology*, pp. 23–57. Churchill Livingstone, Edinburgh.

Hann IM (1991) Inherited bleeding disorders. *Curr Paediatr* 1: 192–197.

Hann IM, Lake B, Pritchard J (1990) *Atlas of Paediatric Haematology*, 2nd edn. Oxford University Press, Oxford.

Ladisch S, Miller DR (1989) The spleen and disorders involving the monocyte-macrophage system. In: Miller R, Baehner RL (eds) *Blood Diseases of Infancy and Childhood*, 6th edn, pp. 727–732. Mosby. St Louis.

Lilleyman JS (1992) Disorders of platelets. I. Thrombocytopenia and thrombocytosis. In: Hann IM, Lilleyman JS (eds) *Paediatric Haematology*, pp. 129–166. Churchill Livingstone, Edinburgh.

Sanders JM, Holtkamp CA, Buchanan GR (1990) The bleeding time may be longer in children than adults. *Am J Pediatr Hematol/ Oncol* 72: 567–572.

Simpson E (1992) Non-haematological disorders with major effects on blood and bone marrow. In: Hann IM, Lilleyman JS (eds) *Paediatric Haematology*, pp. 457–481. Churchill Livingstone, Edinburgh.

Zwelzer WW (1970) Myelokathexis – new form of chronic granulocytopenia. *New Eng J Med* 282: 231–236.

Appendix: Reference Ranges

R F Hinchliffe

This Appendix contains childhood reference ranges for some of the more widely used haematological variables, the clinical uses of which are discussed in the preceding chapter.

Clinically important changes occur in many variables as children grow, especially in the first weeks and months of life, and must be borne in mind when interpreting laboratory data. Reference values can also be affected by other factors such as prematurity and race – for example, haemoglobin and neutrophil values may be lower in black children – and by the analytical methods used to produce the data. Ideally each laboratory should produce its own reference ranges, but this is rarely possible, and the data reproduced in this section, mostly obtained by current and widely used methods, should provide a satisfactory substitute.

Table A1.1   Normal blood count values in childhood

Age	Hb (g/dl)	RBC ($\times 10^{12}$/l)	Hct	MCV (fl)	WBC ($\times 10^9$/l)
Birth	14.9–23.7	3.7–6.5	0.47–0.75	100–135	10.0–26.0
2 weeks	13.4–19.8	3.9–5.9	0.41–0.65	88–120	6.0–21.0
2 months	9.4–13.0	3.1–4.3	0.28–0.42	84–105	6.0–18.0
6 months	11.1–14.1	3.9–5.5	0.31–0.41	68–82	6.0–17.5
1 year	11.3–14.1	4.1–5.3	0.33–0.41	71–85	6.0–17.5
2–6 years	11.5–13.5	3.9–5.3	0.34–0.40	75–87	5.0–17.0
6–12 years	11.5–15.5	4.0–5.2	0.35–0.45	77–95	4.5–14.5
12–18 years					
Female	12.0–16.0	4.1–5.1	0.36–0.46	78–95	4.5–13.0
Male	13.0–16.0	4.5–5.3	0.37–0.49	78–95	

Age	Neutrophils ($\times 10^9$/l)	Lymphocytes ($\times 10^9$/l)	Monocytes ($\times 10^9$/l)	Eosinophils ($\times 10^9$/l)	Platelets ($\times 10^9$/l)
Birth	2.7–14.4	2.0–7.3	0–1.9	0–0.84	150–450
2 weeks	1.8–5.4	2.8–9.1	0.1–1.7	0–0.84	at all
2 months	1.2–7.5	3.0–13.5	0.1–1.7	0.1–0.8	ages
6 months	1.0–8.5	4.9–13.5	0.2–1.2	0.3–0.8	
1 year	1.5–8.5	4.0–10.5	0.2–1.2	0.3–0.8	
2–6 years	1.5–8.5	1.5–9.5	0.2–1.2	0.3–0.8	
6–12 years	1.5–8.0	1.5–7.0	0.2–1.0	0.1–0.5	
12–18 years					
Female	1.8–8.0	1.2–6.5	0.2–0.8	<0.1–0.5	
Male					

Reproduced from Hinchliffe RF (1992) Reference ranges. In: Lilleyman JS, Hann IM (eds) *Paediatric Haematology*, pp. 1–22. Churchill Livingstone, Edinburgh, by permission of Churchill Livingstone.
Data given as approximate ranges, compiled from various sources.
Red cell values at birth derived from skin puncture blood, most other data from venous blood.

Table A1.2   Red cell values (mean ± 1 SD) on the first postnatal day from 24 weeks' gestational age

	Gestational age (weeks)							
	24–25 (n = 7)	26–27 (n = 11)	28–29 (n = 7)	30–31 (n = 35)	32–33 (n = 23)	34–35 (n = 23)	36–37 (n = 20)	Term (n = 19)
RBC (× 10^{12}/l)	4.65 ±0.43	4.73 ±0.45	4.62 ±9.75	4.79 ±0.74	5.0 ±0.76	5.09 ±0.5	5.27 ±0.68	5.14 ±0.7
Hb (g/dl)	19.4 ±1.5	19.0 ±2.5	19.3 ±1.8	19.1 ±2.2	18.5 ±2.0	19.6 ±2.1	19.2 ±1.7	19.3 ±2.2
Haematocrit	0.63 ±0.04	0.62 ±0.08	0.60 ±0.07	0.60 ±0.08	0.60 ±0.08	0.61 ±0.07	0.64 ±0.07	0.61 ±0.074
MCV (fl)	135 ±0.2	132 ±14.4	131 ±13.5	127 ±12.7	123 ±15.7	122 ±10.0	121 ±12.5	119 ±9.4
Reticulocytes (%)	6.0 ±0.5	9.6 ±3.2	7.5 ±2.5	5.8 ±2.0	5.0 ±1.9	3.9 ±1.6	4.2 ±1.8	3.2 ±1.4
Weight (g)	725 ±185	993 ±194	1174 ±128	1450 ±232	1816 ±192	1957 ±291	2245 ±213	

Reproduced from Zaizov R, Matoth Y (1976) Red cell values on the first postnatal day during the last 16 weeks of gestation. *Am J Hematol* **1**: 272–278, by permission of John Wiley & Sons Inc.
Counts performed on heel-prick blood using an electronic counter.

Table A1.3   Mean haematological values in the first 2 weeks of life in the term infant

	Cord Blood	Day 1	Day 3	Day 7	Day 14
Hb (g/dl)	16.8	18.4	17.8	17.0	16.8
Haematocrit	0.53	0.58	0.55	0.54	0.52
Red cells (× 10^{12}/l)	5.25	5.8	5.6	5.2	5.1
MCV (fl)	107	108	99.0	98.0	96.0
MCH (pg)	34	35	33	32.5	31.5
MCHC (%)	31.7	32.5	33	33	33
Reticulocytes (%)	3–7	3–7	1–3	0–1	0–1
Nuc.RBC (mm³)	500	200	0–5	0	0
Platelets (× 10^9/l)	290	192	213	248	252

Reproduced from Oski FA (1982) Normal blood values in the newborn period. In: Oski FA, Naiman JL (eds) *Hematologic Problems in the Newborn*, pp. 1–31. W B Saunders, Philadelphia, by permission of Dr F Oski and W B Saunders Co.
Nuc.RBC = Nucleated red blood cells or normoblasts.

Table A1.4 Normal Hb and RBC values in the first year of life

	Age (months)						
	0.5 ($n = 232$)	1 ($n = 240$)	2 ($n = 241$)	4 ($n = 52$)	6 ($n = 52$)	9 ($n = 56$)	12 ($n = 56$)
Hb (g/dl): mean	16.6	13.9	11.2	12.2	12.6	12.7	12.7
− 2 SD	13.4	10.7	9.4	10.3	11.1	11.4	11.3
Hct: mean	0.53	0.44	0.35	0.38	0.36	0.36	0.37
− 2 SD	41	33	28	32	31	32	33
RBC ($\times 10^{12}$/l): mean	4.9	4.3	3.7	4.3	4.7	4.7	4.7
− 2 SD + 2 SD	3.9–5.9	3.3–5.3	3.1–4.3	3.5–5.1	3.9–5.5	4.0–5.3	4.1–5.3
MCH (pg): mean	33.6	32.5	30.4	28.6	26.8	27.3	26.8
− 2 SD	30	29	27	25	24	25	24
MCV (fl): mean	105.3	101.3	94.8	86.7	76.3	77.7	77.7
− 2 SD	88	91	84	76	68	70	71
MCHC (g/dl): mean	31.4	31.8	31.8	32.7	35.0	34.9	34.3
− 2 SD	28.1	28.1	28.3	28.8	32.7	32.4	32.1

Reproduced from Saarinen UM, Siimes MA (1978) Developmental changes in red blood cell counts and indices of infants after exclusion of iron deficiency by laboratory criteria and continuous iron supplementation. *J Pediatr* **92**: 412–416, by permission of C.V. Mosby Co.
Values after the age of 2 months were obtained from an iron supplemented group in whom iron deficiency was excluded. Counts performed on venous blood.

Table A1.5 Hb values (median and 95% range) in the first 6 months of life in iron-sufficient (serum ferritin $\geq 10 \, \mu$g/l) preterm infants

		Birth weight (g)	
Age	n	1000–1500	1501–2000
2 weeks	17.39	16.3 (11.7–18.4)	14.8 (11.8–19.6)
1 month	15.42	10.9 (8.7–15.2)	11.5 (8.2–15.0)
2 months	17.47	8.8 (7.1–11.5)	9.4 (8.0–11.4)
3 months	16.41	9.8 (8.9–11.2)	10.2 (9.3–11.8)
4 months	13.37	11.3 (9.1–13.1)	11.3 (9.1–13.1)
5 months	8.21	11.6 (10.2–14.3)	11.8 (10.4–13.0)
6 months	9.21	12.0 (9.4–13.8)	11.8 (10.7–12.6)

Reproduced from Lundstrom U, Siimes MA, Dallman PR (1977) At what age does iron supplementation become necessary in low-birth-weight infants? *J Pediatr* **91**: 878–883, by permission of C.V. Mosby Co.
All had an uncomplicated course in the first 2 weeks of life and none received exchange transfusion. Counts obtained from venous and skin-puncture blood.

Table A1.6 The percentage of haemoglobin F in the first year of life

Age	n	Mean	2 SD	Range
1–7 days	10	74.7	5.4	61–79.6
2 weeks	13	74.9	5.7	66–88.5
1 month	11	60.2	6.3	45.7–67.3
2 months	10	45.6	10.1	29.4–60.8
3 months	10	26.6	14.5	14.8–55.9
4 months	10	17.7	6.1	9.4–28.5
5 months	10	10.4	6.7	2.3–22.4
6 months	15	6.5	3.0	2.7–13.0
8 months	11	5.1	3.6	2.3–11.9
10 months	10	2.1	0.7	1.5–3.5
12 months	10	2.6	1.5	1.3–5.0
1–14 years and adults	100	0.6	0.4	—

Reproduced from Hinchliffe (1992) Reference ranges. In: Lilleyman JS, Hann IM (eds) *Paediatric Haematology*, pp. 1–22. Churchill Livingstone, Edinburgh, by permission of Churchill Livingstone.
Data from Schröter W, Nafz C (1981) Diagnostic significance of hemoglobin F and A_2 levels in homo- and heterozygous β-thalassaemia during infancy. *Helv Paediat Acta* **36**: 519–525.
HbF measured by alkali denaturation.

Table A1.7   The percentage of haemoglobin A_2 in the first 2 years of life

Age (months)	A			B			
	n	Mean	SD	n	Mean	SD	Range
Birth	16	0.4	0.2				
1	6	0.8	0.3	5	0.8	0.4	0.4–1.3
2	7	1.3	0.7	9	1.3	0.5	0.4–1.9
3	8	1.7	0.3	8	2.2	0.6	1.0–3.0
4	9	2.1	0.3	3	2.4	0.4	2.0–2.8
5	8	2.3	0.2				
5–6				15	2.5	0.3	2.1–3.1
6	8	2.5	0.3				
7–8	6	2.5	0.4				
7–9				22	2.7	0.4	1.9–3.5
9–10	6	2.5	0.4				
10–12				14	2.7	0.4	2.0–3.3
12	5	2.5	0.3				
13–16				13	2.6	0.5	1.6–3.3
17–20				13	2.9	0.4	2.1–3.6
21–24				15	2.8	0.4	2.0–3.6

Data from two studies: (A) Galanello R, Melis MA, Ruggeri R, Cao A (1981) Prospective study of red blood cell indices, hemoglobin A_2 and hemoglobin F in infants heterozygous for β-thalassaemia. *J Pediatr* **99**: 105–108, measured by microcolumn chromatography; (B) Metaxotou-Mavromati AD, Antonopoulo HK, Laskari SS, Tsiarta HK, Ladis VA, Kattamis CA (1982) Developmental changes in Hemoglobin F levels during the first two years of life in normal and heterozygous β-thalassemia infants. *Pediatrics* **69**: 734–738, measured by elution following electrophoresis. Reproduced from Hinchliffe (1992), References ranges. In: Lilleyman JS, Hann IM (eds) Paediatric Haematology, pp. 1–22. Churchill Livingstone, Edinburgh, by permission of Churchill Livingstone.

Table A1.8   Values of serum iron (SI), total iron-binding capacity (TIBC) and transferrin saturation (S%) from a group of 47 infants

		Age (months)						
		0.5	1	2	4	6	9	12
SI (μmol/l)	Median	22	22	16	15	14	15	14
	95% range	11–36	10–31	3–29	3–29	5–24	6–24	6–28
SI (μg/dl)	Median	120	125	87	84	77	84	78
	95% range	63–201	58–172	15–159	18–164	28–135	35–155	
TIBC	μmol/l	34 ± 8	36 ± 8	44 ± 10	54 ± 7	58 ± 9	61 ± 7	64 ± 7
(mean ± SD)	μg/dl	191 ± 43	199 ± 43	246 ± 55	300 ± 39	321 ± 51	341 ± 42	358 ± 38
S%	Median	68	63	34	27	23	25	23
	95% range	30–99	35–94	21–63	7–53	10–43	10–39	10–47

Reproduced from Saarinen UM, Siimes MA (1977) Developmental changes in serum iron, total iron-binding capacity, and transferrin saturation in infancy. *J Pediatr* **91**: 875–877, by permission of C.V. Mosby Co.
Not all infants were tested on each occasion, and those with Hb < 11 g/dl, MCV < 71 fl or serum ferritin < 10 μg/l were excluded.

Table A1.9 Serum and red cell folate (µg/l, mean and range) and serum vitamin B_{12} (ng/l, range) levels in childhood

Age	Serum folate		Red cell folate		Serum vitamin B_{12}
	Term ($n = 24$)	Premature ($n = 20$)	Term ($n = 24$)	Premature ($n = 20$)	
Birth	24.5 (3–59)	19.2 (10–41)	315 (100–960)	689 (88–1291)	160–1300
2–3 months		4.8 (1–11)		164 (26–394)	
3–4 months	12.2 (5–30)		283 (110–489)		
6–8 months	7.7 (3.5–16)	8.9 (4.1–28)	247 (100–466)	299 (139–558)	
1 year	9.3 (3–35)		277 (74–995)		
>1 year	3–20		160–640		160–760

Data from Vanier TM, Tyas JF (1966) Folic acid status in newborn infants during the first year of life. *Arch Dis Child* **41**: 658–665; Vanier TM, Tyas JF (1967) Folic acid status in premature infants. *Arch Dis Child* **42**: 57–61 and Dacie JV, Lewis SM (1991) *Practical Haematology*, 7th edn. Churchill Livingstone, Edinburgh.

Table A1.10 Normal values for lymphocytes, monocytes and eosinophils ($\times 10^9$/l) from birth to 28 days of age based on a study of 393 infants

Cells	Percentile	Age (hours)		
		0.60	61–120	121–720
Lymphocytes	95	7.26	6.62	9.13
	50	4.19	8.66	5.62
	5	2.02	1.92	2.86
Monocytes	95	1.91	1.74	1.72
	50	0.6	0.53	0.67
	5	0	0	0.10
Eosinophils	95	0.84	0.81	0.84
	50	0.14	0.18	0.24
	5	0	0	0

Reproduced from Weinberg AG, Rosenfeld CR, Manroe BL, Browne R (1985) Neonatal blood cell count in health and disease. II. Values for lymphocytes, monocytes, and eosinophils. *J Pediatr* **106**: 462–466, by permission of C.V. Mosby Co.
Data based on 100-cell differential count.

Table A1.11   Values for neutrophils, band forms and lymphocytes (mean and range, $\times 10^9$/l) in African neonates

	Day 1	Day 7	Day 28
Neutrophils	5.67 (0.98–12.9)	2.01 (0.57–6.5)	1.67 (0.65–3.2)
Band forms	1.16 (0.16–2.3)	0.55 (0–1.5)	0.36 (0–0.39)
Lymphocytes	5.10 (1.4–8.0)	5.63 (2.2–15.5)	0.55 (3.2–9.9)

Summarized from Scott-Emuakpor AB, Okolo AA, Omene JA, Ukpe SI (1985b). Pattern of leukocytes in blood of healthy African neonates. *Acta Haematol* **74**: 104–107. Reproduced from Hinchliffe RF (1987), Reference ranges and normal findings. In Hinchliffe RF, Lilleyman JS (eds) *Practical Paediatric Haematology*, pp. 359–397. Wiley, Chichester, by permission of John Wiley & Sons Ltd.
Data based on 100-cell differential count.
The lower range of neutrophil values known to occur in blacks is evident in the neonatal period.

Table A1.12   Mean and 95% range of total leucocyte count ($\times 10^9$/l) and mean, 95% range and mean percentage values for neutrophils, lymphocytes, monocytes and eosinophils

Age	Total leucocytes		Neutrophils			Lymphocytes			Monocytes		Eosinophils	
	Mean	Range	Mean	Range	%	Mean	Range	%	Mean	%	Mean	%
1 month	10.8	5.0–19.5	3.8	1.0–9.0	35	6.0	2.5–16.5	56	0.7	7	0.3	3
6 months	11.9	6.0–17.5	3.8	1.0–8.5	32	7.3	4.0–13.5	61	0.6	5	0.3	3
1 year	11.4	6.0–17.5	3.5	1.5–8.5	31	7.0	4.0–10.5	61	0.6	5	0.3	3
2 years	10.6	6.0–17.0	3.5	1.5–8.5	33	6.3	3.0–9.5	59	0.5	5	0.3	3
4 years	9.1	5.5–15.5	3.8	1.5–8.5	42	4.5	2.0–8.0	50	0.5	5	0.3	3
6 years	8.5	5.0–14.5	4.3	1.5–8.0	51	3.5	1.5–7.0	42	0.4	5	0.2	3
8 years	8.3	4.5–13.5	4.4	1.5–8.0	53	3.3	1.5–6.8	39	0.4	4	0.2	2
10 years	8.1	4.5–13.5	4.4	1.8–8.0	54	3.1	1.5–6.5	38	0.4	4	0.2	2
16 years	7.8	4.5–13.0	4.4	1.8–8.0	57	2.8	1.2–5.2	35	0.4	5	0.2	3
21 years	7.4	4.5–11.0	4.4	1.8–7.7	59	2.5	1.0–4.8	34	0.3	4	0.2	3

Summarized from Dallman PR (1977) Blood and blood forming tissues. In: Rudolph AM (ed) *Pediatrics*, 16th edn, pp. 1109–1222. Appleton–Century–Crofts, New York, by permission of Appleton-Century-Crofts.
Data based on 100-cell differential count.

Table A1.13 Reference values for coagulation tests in the healthy full-term infant during the first 6 months of life

Test	Day 1 Mean ± SD	n	Day 5 Mean ± SD	n	Day 30 Mean ± SD	n
PT (s)	13.0 ± 1.43	61*	12.4 ± 1.46	77*	11.8 ± 1.25	67*†
APTT (s)	42.9 ± 5.80	61	42.6 ± 8.62	76	40.4 ± 7.42	67
TCT (s)	23.5 ± 2.38	58*	23.1 ± 3.07	64†	24.3 ± 2.44	53*
Fibrinogen (g/l)	2.83 ± 0.58	61*	3.12 ± 0.75	77*	2.70 ± 0.54	67*
II (u/ml)	0.48 ± 0.11	61	0.63 ± 0.15	76	0.68 ± 0.17	67
V (u/ml)	0.72 ± 0.18	61	0.95 ± 0.25	76	0.98 ± 0.18	67
VII (u/ml)	0.66 ± 0.19	60	0.89 ± 0.27	75	0.90 ± 0.24	67
VIII (u/ml)	1.00 ± 0.39	60*†	0.88 ± 0.33	75*†	0.91 ± 0.33	67*†
vWF (u/ml)	1.53 ± 0.67	40†	1.40 ± 0.57	43†	1.28 ± 0.59	40†
IX (u/ml)	0.53 ± 0.19	59	0.53 ± 0.19	75	0.51 ± 0.15	67
X (u/ml)	0.40 ± 0.14	60	0.49 ± 0.15	76	0.59 ± 0.14	67
XI (u/ml)	0.38 ± 0.14	60	0.55 ± 0.16	74	0.53 ± 0.13	67
XII (u/ml)	0.53 ± 0.20	60	0.47 ± 0.18	75	0.49 ± 0.16	67
PK (u/ml)	0.37 ± 0.16	45†	0.48 ± 0.14	51	0.57 ± 0.17	48
HMW-K (u/ml)	0.54 ± 0.24	47	0.74 ± 0.28	63	0.77 ± 0.22	50*
XIIIa (u/ml)	0.79 ± 0.26	44	0.94 ± 0.25	49*	0.93 ± 0.27	44*
XIIIb (u/ml)	0.76 ± 0.23	44	1.06 ± 0.37	47*	1.11 ± 0.36	45*
Plasminogen (CTA, u/ml)	1.95 ± 0.35	44	2.17 ± 0.38	60	1.98 ± 0.36	52

Test	Day 90 Mean ± SD	n	Day 180 Mean ± SD	n	Adult Mean ± SD	n
PT (s)	11.9 ± 1.15	62*	12.3 ± 0.79	47*	12.4 ± 0.78	29
APTT (s)	37.1 ± 6.52	62*	35.5 ± 3.71	47*	33.5 ± 3.44	29
TCT (s)	25.1 ± 2.32	52*	25.5 ± 2.86	41*	25.0 ± 2.66	19
Fibrinogen (g/l)	2.43 ± 0.68	60*†	2.51 ± 0.68	47*†	2.78 ± 0.61	29
II (u/ml)	0.75 ± 0.15	62	0.88 ± 0.14	47	1.08 ± 0.19	29
V (u/ml)	0.90 ± 0.21	62	0.91 ± 0.18	47	1.06 ± 0.22	29
VII (u/ml)	0.91 ± 0.26	62	0.87 ± 0.20	47	1.05 ± 0.19	29
VIII (u/ml)	0.79 ± 0.23	62*†	0.73 ± 0.18	47†	0.99 ± 0.25	29
vWF (u/ml)	1.18 ± 0.44	40†	1.07 ± 0.45	46†	0.92 ± 0.33	29†
IX (u/ml)	0.67 ± 0.23	62	0.86 ± 0.25	47	1.09 ± 0.27	29
X (u/ml)	0.71 ± 0.18	62	0.78 ± 0.20	47	1.06 ± 0.23	29
XI (u/ml)	0.69 ± 0.14	62	0.86 ± 0.24	47	0.97 ± 0.15	29
XII (u/ml)	0.67 ± 0.21	62	0.77 ± 0.19	47	1.08 ± 0.28	29
PK (u/ml)	0.73 ± 0.16	46	0.86 ± 0.15	43	1.12 ± 0.25	29
HMW-K (u/ml)	0.82 ± 0.32	46*	0.82 ± 0.23	48*	0.92 ± 0.22	29
XIIIa (u/ml)	1.04 ± 0.34	44*	1.04 ± 0.29	41*	1.05 ± 0.25	29
XIIIb (u/ml)	1.16 ± 0.34	44*	1.10 ± 0.30	41*	0.97 ± 0.20	29
Plasminogen (CTA, u/ml)	2.48 ± 0.37	44	3.01 ± 0.40	47	3.36 ± 0.44	29

Reproduced from Andrew M, Paes B, Milner R et al (1987) Development of the human coagulation system in the fullterm infant. *Blood* **70**: 165–172, by permission of Dr M Andrew and Grune and Stratton.

All factors except fibrinogen and plasminogen are expressed as units (u)/ml where pooled plasma contains 1.0 u/ml. Plasminogen units are those recommended by the Committee on Thrombolytic Agents (CTA). n, number studied.

*Values that do not differ statistically from the adult values.

†These measurements are skewed because of a disproportionate number of high values.

APTT, activated partial thromboplastin time; HMW-K, high molecular weight kininogen; PK, prekallikrein; PT, prothrombin time; TCT, thrombin clotting time; VWF, von Willebrand's factor.

Note: longer APTT and TCT values may be obtained in newborns and infants using reagent combinations other than those used in this study.

Table A1.14   Reference values for coagulation tests in healthy premature infants (30–36 weeks gestation) during first 6 months of life

	Day 1		Day 5		Day 30	
	Mean	Boundary	Mean	Boundary	Mean	Boundary
PT (s)	13.0	10.6–16.2*	12.5	10.0–15.3*†	11.8	10.0–13.6*
APTT (s)	53.6	27.5–79.4†	50.5	26.9–74.1†	44.7	26.9–62.5
TCT (s)	24.8	19.2–30.4*	24.1	18.8–29.4*	24.4	18.8–29.9*
Fibrinogen (g/l)	2.43	1.50–3.73*†	2.80	1.60–4.18*†§	2.54	1.50–4.14*†
II (u/ml)	0.45	0.20–0.77†	0.57	0.29–0.85†	0.57	0.36–0.95†§
V (u/ml)	0.88	0.41–1.44*†§	1.00	0.46–1.54	1.02	0.48–1.56
VII (u/ml)	0.67	0.21–1.13	0.84	0.30–1.38	0.83	0.21–1.45
VIII (u/ml)	1.11	0.50–2.13*†	1.15	0.53–2.05*†§	1.11	0.50–1.99*†§
vWF (u/ml)	1.36	0.78–2.10†	1.33	0.72–2.19†	1.36	0.66–2.16†
IX (u/ml)	0.35	0.19–0.65†§	0.42	0.14–0.74†§	0.44	0.13–0.80†
X (u/ml)	0.41	0.11–0.71	0.51	0.19–0.83	0.56	0.20–0.92
XI (u/ml)	0.30	0.08–0.52†§	0.41	0.13–0.69§	0.43	0.15–0.71§
XII (u/ml)	0.38	0.10–0.66§	0.39	0.09–0.69§	0.43	0.11–0.75
PK (u/ml)	0.33	0.09–0.57	0.45	0.28–0.75†	0.59	0.31–0.87
HMWK (u/ml)	0.49	0.09–0.89	0.62	0.24–1.00§	0.64	0.16–1.12§
XIIIa (u/ml)	0.70	0.32–1.08	1.01	0.57–1.45*	0.99	0.51–1.47*
XIIIb (u/ml)	0.81	0.35–1.27	1.10	0.68–1.58*	1.07	0.57–1.57*
Plasminogen (CTA, u/ml)	1.70	1.12–2.48†§	1.91	1.21–2.61§	1.81	1.09–2.53

	Day 90		Day 180		Adult	
	Mean	Boundary	Mean	Boundary	Mean	Boundary
PT (s)	12.3	10.0–14.6*	12.5	10.0–15.0*	12.4	10.8–13.9
APTT (s)	39.5	28.3–50.7	37.5	21.7–53.3*	33.5	26.6–40.3
TCT (s)	25.1	19.4–30.8*	25.2	18.9–31.5*	25.0	19.7–30.3
Fibrinogen (g/l)	2.46	1.50–3.52*†	2.28	1.50–3.60†	2.78	1.56–4.00
II (u/ml)	0.68	0.30–1.06	0.87	0.51–1.23	1.08	0.70–1.46
V (u/ml)	0.99	0.59–1.39	1.02	0.58–1.46	1.06	0.62–1.50
VII (u/ml)	0.87	0.31–1.43	0.99	0.47–1.51*	1.05	0.67–1.43
VIII (u/ml)	1.06	0.58–1.88*†§	0.99	0.50–1.87*†§	0.99	0.50–1.49
vWF (u/ml)	1.12	0.75–1.84*†	0.98	0.54–1.58*†	0.92	0.50–1.58
IX (u/ml)	0.59	0.25–0.93	0.81	0.50–1.20†	1.09	0.55–1.63
X (u/ml)	0.67	0.35–0.99	0.77	0.35–1.19	1.06	0.70–1.52
XI (u/ml)	0.59	0.25–0.93§	0.78	0.46–1.10	0.97	0.67–1.27
XII (u/ml)	0.61	0.15–1.07	0.82	0.22–1.42	1.08	0.52–1.64
PK (u/ml)	0.79	0.37–1.21	0.78	0.40–1.16	1.12	0.62–1.62
HMWK (u/ml)	0.78	0.32–1.24	0.83	0.41–1.25*	0.92	0.50–1.36
XIIIa (u/ml)	1.13	0.71–1.55*	1.13	0.65–1.61*	1.05	0.55–1.55
XIIIb (u/ml)	1.21	0.75–1.67	1.15	0.67–1.63	0.97	0.57–1.37
Plasminogen (CTA, u/ml)	2.38	1.58–3.18	2.75	1.91–3.59§	3.36	2.48–4.24

Reproduced from Andrew M, Paes B, Milner R et al (1988) Development of the coagulation system in the healthy premature infant. *Blood* **72**: 1651–1657, by permission of Dr M Andrew and Grune and Stratton.

All values are given as the mean followed by the lower and upper boundaries encompassing 95% of the population. Between 40 and 96 samples were assayed for each value for newborns.

*Values indistinguishable from those for adults.

†Measurements are skewed owing to a disproportionate number of high values. Lower limit which excludes the lower 2.5% of the population is given (B).

§Values different from those of full-term infants.

For abbreviations, see footnote to Table A1.14.

Table A1.15 Reference values for coagulation tests in healthy children aged 1–16 years compared with adults

	Age (years)							
	1–5		6–10		11–16		Adult	
Coagulation test	Mean	Boundary	Mean	Boundary	Mean	Boundary	Mean	Boundary
PT (s)	11	10.6–11.4	11.1	10.1–12.1	11.2	10.2–12.0	12	11.0–14.0
INR	1.0	0.96–1.04	1.01	0.91–1.11	1.02	0.93–1.10	1.10	1.0–1.3
APTT (s)	30	24–36	31	26–36	32	26–37	33	27–40
Fibrinogen (g/l)	2.76	1.70–4.05	2.79	1.57–4.0	3.0	1.54–4.48	2.78	1.56–4.0
Bleeding time (min)	6	2.5–10*	7	2.5–13*	5	3–8*	4	1–7
II (u/ml)	0.94	0.71–1.16*	0.88	0.67–1.07*	0.83	0.61–1.04*	1.08	0.70–1.46
V (u/ml)	1.03	0.79–1.27	0.90	0.63–1.16*	0.77	0.55–0.99*	1.06	0.62–1.50
VII (u/ml)	0.82	0.55–1.16*	0.85	0.52–1.20*	0.83	0.58–1.15*	1.05	0.67–1.43
VIII (u/ml)	0.90	0.50–1.42	0.95	0.58–1.32	0.92	0.53–1.31	0.99	0.50–1.49
vWF (u/ml)	0.82	0.60–1.20	0.95	0.44–1.44	1.00	0.46–1.53	0.92	0.50–1.58
IX (u/ml)	0.73	0.47–1.04*	0.75	0.63–0.89*	0.82	0.59–1.22*	1.09	0.55–1.63
X (u/ml)	0.88	0.58–1.16*	0.75	0.55–1.01*	0.79	0.50–1.17*	1.06	0.70–1.52
XI (u/ml)	0.97	0.56–1.50	0.86	0.52–1.20	0.74	0.50–0.97*	0.97	0.67–1.27
XII (u/ml)	0.93	0.64–1.20	0.92	0.60–1.40	0.81	0.34–1.37*	1.08	0.52–1.64
PK (u/ml)	0.95	0.65–1.30	0.99	0.66–1.31	0.99	0.53–1.45	1.12	0.62–1.62
HMWK (u/ml)	0.98	0.64–1.32	0.93	0.60–1.30	0.91	0.63–1.19	0.92	0.50–1.36
XIIIa (u/ml)	1.08	0.72–1.43*	1.09	0.65–1.51*	0.99	0.57–1.40	1.05	0.55–1.55
XIIIs (u/ml)	1.13	0.69–1.56*	1.16	0.77–1.54*	1.02	0.60–1.43	0.97	0.57–1.37

All factors except fibrinogen are expressed as units per millilitre, where pooled plasma contains 1.0 u/ml. All data are expressed as the mean, followed by the upper and lower boundary encompassing 95% of the population. Between 20 and 50 samples were assayed for each value for each age group. Some measurements were skewed due to a disproportionate number of high values. The lower limit, which excludes the lower 2.5% of the population, is given.

Bleeding time performed using a template technique with blood pressure cuff inflated to 40 mmHg, incision 3.5 mm long, 1 mm deep, made horizontally on forearm.

*Values that are significantly different from those of adults.

INR, international normalized ratio; for other abbreviations see Table A1.14.

Table A1.16 Bleeding time (min) in newborns

Subjects	No. tested	Sphygmomanometer pressure (mmHg)	Mean	Range
Term newborn	30	30	3.4	1.9–5.8
Pre-term newborn				
< 1000 g	6	20	3.3	2.6–4.0
1000–2000 g	15	25	3.9	2.0–5.6
> 2000 g	5	30	3.2	2.3–5.0

Summarized from Feusner JH (1980) Normal and abnormal bleeding times in neonates and young children using a fully standardised template technic. *Am J Clin Pathol* **74**: 73–77.

Bleeding time performed using a template technique, with incision 5 mm long, 0.5 mm deep. All subjects had normal platelet counts.

Table A1.17   Erythrocyte sedimentation rate (mm in 1 h) in healthy children

N	Age (years)	Mean	Range	% above 20 mm
Wintrobe method				
245	4–11	12.0	1–41	9
169	12–15	7.5	<1–34	7
Westergren method (read at 45 min)				
78	4–7	13	<1–55	
153	8–14	10.5	1–62	

Data from Hollinger N, Robinson SJ (1953) A study of the erythrocyte sedimentation rate for well children. *J Pediatr* **42**: 304–319; Osgood EE, Baker RL, Brownlee IE, Osgood MW, Ellis DM, Cohen W (1939a) Total, differential and absolute leukocyte counts and sedimentation rates of healthy children four to seven years of age. *Am J Dis Child* **58**: 61–70 and Osgood EE, Baker RL, Brownlee IE, Osgood MW, Ellis DM, Cohen W (1939b) Total, differential and absolute leukocyte counts and sedimentation rates of healthy children. Standards for children eight to fourteen years of age. *Am J Dis Child* **58**: 282–294. Reproduced from Hinchliffe (1992), by permission of Churchill Livingstone.

Table A1.18   Isohaemagglutinin titre in relation to age

Age	Isohaemagglutin titre (IHA)	
	Mean	Range
Cord blood	0*	
1–3 months	1:5†	0–1:10
4–6 months	1:10†	0–1:160
7–12 months	1:80‡	0–1:640
13–24 months	1:80‡	0–1:640
25–36 months	1:160§	1:10–1:640
3–5 years	1:80	1:5–1:640
6–8 years	1:80	1:5–1:640
9–11 years	1:160	1:20–1:640
12–16 years	1:160	1:10–1:320
Adult	1:160	1:10–1:640

Summarized from Ellis EF, Robbins JB (1978) In: Johnson TR, Moore WM (eds) *Children are Different: Developmental Physiology*. Ross Laboratories, Columbus, OH. Reproduced from Hinchliffe RF (1987) Reference ranges and normal findings. In: Hinchliffe RF, Lilleyman JS (eds) *Practical Paediatric Haematology*, pp. 359–397. Wiley, Chichester, by permission of John Wiley & Sons Ltd.
*IHA activity is rarely detectable in cord blood.
†50% of normal infants will not have IHA at this age.
‡10% of normal infants will not have IHA at this age.
§Beyond this age all normal individuals have IHA, with the exception of those of blood group AB.

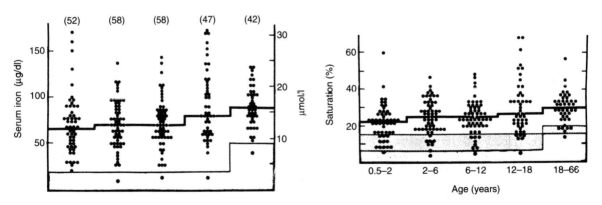

Figure A1.1   Normal values for serum iron and transferrin saturation in individuals with normal levels of Hb, MCV, serum ferritin and free erythrocyte porphyrin. The heavy horizontal lines indicate the median values, the lower lines the lower limit of the 95% range, and the stippled area an intermediate zone of overlap between iron-deficient and normal subjects. Numbers of subjects are given in parentheses. Reproduced from Koerper MA, Dallman PR (1977) Serum iron concentration and transferrin saturation in the diagnosis of iron deficiency in children: normal developmental changes. *J Pediatr* 91: 870–874, by permission of C.V. Mosby Co.

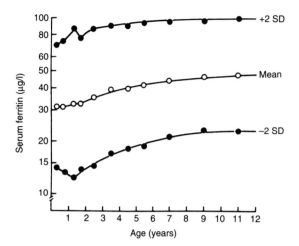

Figure A1.2 Serum ferritin concentration (mean ± 2 SD) in 3819 children aged 6 months to 12 years in whom there was no evidence of iron deficiency. Mean values for boys and girls were similar and there was no difference between whites, blacks and American Indians in age-matched samples. Reproduced from Deinard AS, Schwartz S, Yip R (1983) Developmental changes in serum ferritin and erythrocyte protoporphyrin in normal (non-anemic) children. *Am J Clin Nutr* **38**: 71–76, by permission of Dr AS Deinard and the American Society for Clinical Nutrition.

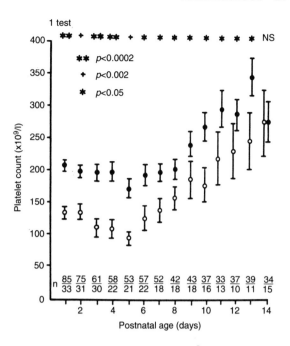

Figure A1.3 Platelet count ($\times 10^9$/l; bar indicates ± 1 SD) in the first 14 days of life in babies of appropriate weight for gestational age (●) and babies who were small for gestational age (○). Reproduced from McIntosh N, Kempson C, Tyler RM (1988) Blood counts in extremely low birthweight infants. *Arch Dis Child* **63**: 74–76, by permission of Professor N McIntosh and the editor of *Archives of Diseases in Childhood*.

2
Oncology

P C E Sartori and M G Mott

INTRODUCTION

The presenting symptoms of childhood neoplasia frequently overlap those of more common, non-neoplastic diseases. The aim of first-line clinical assessment and investigation is to identify those children who require further evaluation. The detailed evaluation of a child with neoplasia is designed to accomplish four goals (Fletcher and Pratt 1991, Nesbit 1993, Triche 1993, Parker and Moore 1993, Ortega and Siegel 1993).

1. A pathological diagnosis in almost every case.
2. An assessment of the extent of the primary lesion, to plan local treatment such as surgery or radiotherapy.
3. An assessment of the overall extent (stage) of the disease, both local and metastatic.
4. The establishment of baseline function for tissues at risk of therapy-induced damage.

It is best co-ordinated by a regional centre with a multidisciplinary team experienced in paediatric oncology, surgery, radiology and pathology. Further studies are required during and after treatment:

1. To assess the response of the tumour to treatment.
2. To screen for local recurrence and to detect the development of metastatic disease.
3. To monitor toxicity, both short term, such as myelotoxicity, and long term, such as growth and cardiac, renal, and endocrine function.

Because of the diversity of tissues and organs affected by neoplastic disease and its therapy, reference will frequently be made to other chapters.

ASSESSMENT OF THE PRIMARY TUMOUR
Tissue Diagnosis

A tissue diagnosis is required for most paediatric malignancies, although there are occasions where markers and imaging will suffice, for example pineal germ cell tumour can be diagnosed from characteristic computed tomography (CT) or magnetic resonance imaging (MRI) findings and an elevated α-fetoprotein (αFP).

Surgical Considerations

A biopsy must provide adequate tissue for all necessary studies without compromising later definitive surgery, for example biopsy of a bony lesion should not interfere with later limb salvage surgery. Such biopsies should therefore normally be performed by surgeons experienced in paediatric malignancy, and only after close consultation with paediatric oncologists, pathologists and radiologists.

Complete Excision

Initial surgery may be definitive, for example in the case of small localized tumours which can be resected without mutilation or compromise to other organs. In this case histological confirmation of the diagnosis will be obtained postoperatively. However, for most tumours, it is more common to defer definitive surgery, in order to allow preoperative shrinkage by chemotherapy. This also offers an opportunity to assess the effectiveness of the chemotherapy regimen. In this situation, biopsy is required for an accurate diagnosis to guide the choice of initial chemotherapy.

Type of Biopsy

There is a wide choice of method for biopsy; open incisional, closed needle core, and fine needle aspiration biopsy (FNAB) with or without ultrasound or radiological guidance (Silverman et al 1991, McGahey et al 1992). The choice will depend on the site and accessibility of the tumour, the general state of the patient and the suspected pathology. Delay or error in diagnosis due to inadequate tissue may have serious consequences, and for this reason alone open biopsy is recommended as the method of choice. It also ensures that additional material is available for biological studies and cryopreservation. At open biopsy it is advisable to obtain both peripheral and central samples, the latter often by needle. Needle biopsy is particularly appropriate for inaccessible sites and for the diagnosis of recurrence or metastasis. FNAB is particularly useful for unresectable tumours in sick patients who may pose a high anaesthetic risk, for example, extensive abdominal lymphoma. It can only be carried out if there is a safe route, good visualization and no bleeding tendency. Effective immediate processing by a skilled pathologist is necessary to assess the adequacy of the specimen and to determine the need for ancillary studies especially in small round blue cell tumours (SRBCT).

For all biopsies, prior consultation with a paediatric pathologist is essential, to ensure appropriate handling and storage of specimens. Portions of the specimen are usually preserved in a variety of different ways, including snap freezing in liquid nitrogen, primary culture for cytogenetics or inoculation into immune deprived mice.

Pathology

The aim of pathology studies is to establish a precise diagnosis and a pathological stage. It is vital, therefore, that specimens should be carefully prepared, and examined by a pathologist experienced in paediatric oncology. Far too many patients have inappropriate studies performed on suboptimal material, in situations where it may not be possible to remedy the situation subsequently, for example, if all the specimen is placed in formalin.

Light Microscopy

This is the standard technique for establishing a tissue diagnosis, and for many tumours will provide both diagnosis and subtype. In some tumours, different histological subtypes may have different aetiologies and may be associated with different outcomes; for example, embryonal rhabdomyosarcoma carries a better prognosis than alveolar rhabdomyosarcoma. In renal tumours, chemotherapy is determined by a combination of stage and histological subtype.

For many tumours, light microscopy is supplemented by ancillary studies, particularly that group of histologically homogenous tumours consisting of small, round, blue cells (SRBCT). This appearance may be found in Ewings' sarcoma, metastatic neuroblastoma, extranodal lymphoma, metastatic primitive alveolar rhabdomyosarcoma, small cell osteosarcoma and primitive neurectodermal tumour (PNET). These tumours may be differentiated by a variety of techniques, including immunocytochemistry, electron microscopy or cytogenetic and molecular studies.

Immunocytochemistry

This uses a panel of monoclonal antibodies which react specifically to antigens in tumour cells, which are then visualized by light microscopy (Mierau et al 1985). Examples are the cytoskeletal or intermediate filament proteins, neural markers such as neurone specific enolase, and lymphoid antigens. This technique is now well established in the routine processing of paediatric tumour biopsies.

Electron Microscopy

The technique can identify ultrastructual details which are characteristic of specific tissues. Preparation of specimens is critical and the technique is not universally available.

Cytogenetics

Specific chromosomal abnormalities are increasingly found in particular tumours, for example translocations between chromosome 8 and 2, 14 or 22 in B lymphoma, t(11;22) translocation in Ewings' sarcoma and PNET, t(2;13) translocation in alveolar rhabdomyosarcoma, deletions of 11p in Wilms' tumour, deletions of 13q in retinoblastoma, homogeneously staining regions (HSRs) and double minutes (DMs), associated with N-myc amplification, in neuroblastoma. Thus tumour cytogenetics may distinguish between different diagnostic possibilities. Tissue must be sent fresh to a specialized regional laboratory, so collaboration between the laboratory and clinicians is essential (Pearson et al 1988).

Molecular Studies

Molecular biology techniques have moved from the research into the routine laboratory. Examples include identification of submicroscopic deletions in chromosome 13q14 in retinoblastoma and in chromosome 11p13 in Wilms' tumour, and establishment of N-myc copy number in neuroblastoma, which is of major prognostic significance.

Research

Access to tumour material for research is important, not only to expand the field of knowledge but also because today's research techniques are tomorrow's routine methods. For example, fluorescent *in situ* hybridization (FISH) of chromosomes is currently a research tool, but it has the potential to become part of the routine assessment of childhood tumours, by allowing the rapid identification of a variety of common specific chromosomal abnormalities.

Markers

Some tumours synthesize large amounts of a protein, enzyme or hormone, which can be detected in blood, CSF or urine. Measurement of some of these biological markers may be helpful in arriving at a diagnosis.

Urinary Catecholamines

Most tumours of neural crest origin synthesize excess amounts of catecholamines. Vanillyl mandelic acid (VMA) and homovanillic acid (HVA) are metabolites of these catecholamines which are excreted in urine. Quantitative assays of VMA, HVA and dopamine have traditionally been performed on 24-h collections but this may not be practical in young children; shorter timed collections, or random specimens can now be used. When a random specimen is used, the HVA and VMA levels should be expressed in relation to the amount of urinary creatinine. The finding of elevated urinary catecholamines is specific to neural crest tumours, with more malignant, less well-differentiated tumours tending to produce the highest values. A high level may be diagnostic of neuroblastoma, for example if a biopsy of a primary tumour or bone marrow shows only small round blue cells. Urinary catecholamines should be measured in any child with a paravertebral or retroperitoneal tumour, and in children with evidence of non-haematological malignant infiltration of the bone marrow, as well as in children with the classical signs of neuroblastoma, including any child presenting with bizarre neurological signs suggesting opsomyoclonus.

α-Feto Protein (αFP)

Serum levels of αFP are very high in hepatoblastoma, hepatocellular carcinoma and yolk sac tumours, such as orchioblastoma. αFP should be assayed in any child presenting with a suspected tumour in the liver, ovary, testis, sacrococcygeal and presacral areas, or in the rarer sites for yolk sac tumours, including the retroperitoneum, mediastinum, pineal gland and vagina. The finding of an elevated αFP with a tumour in a characteristic position, for example pineal, may suggest a definitive diagnosis with no need for a biopsy.

β-Human Chorionic Gonadotrophin (βHCG)

This is elevated in 90% of non-germinomatous germ cell tumours, particularly embryonal carcinomas and choriocarcinomas. It should be assayed in any child presenting with a mass in the commoner sites for these tumours, namely testis, ovary, mediastinum and pineal gland.

Other Markers

Other biological markers have been described by researchers; few are specific enough to be used for diagnostic purposes but some appear to have important prognostic associations. Of particular importance are neurone specific enolase and ferritin in neuroblastoma; high levels of both markers have been associated with a poorer outcome.

Endocrine Tumours

Some childhood tumours may be detected through the investigation of various endocrine disorders. Craniopharyngioma may present with short stature and/or diabetes insipidus. Adrenal or ovarian tumours may present with Cushing's syndrome, precocious puberty or virilization and may produce characteristic patterns of steroid hormone metabolite production. (See Chapter 3.)

Imaging

Imaging fulfils two main functions:

1. Detection of a possible tumour in a child with suspicious symptoms.
2. Assessment of the extent of primary disease, in order to plan surgery or radiotherapy.

Plain radiographs may identify abnormalities, particularly in the abdomen, chest and limbs, and may be helpful in the initial screening of suspicious symptoms in these regions. Ultrasonography is particularly useful in assessing the abdomen and pelvis, but its use elsewhere is limited. CT is used for the detailed evaluation of most primary solid tumours, although MRI may provide images with finer definition, especially in the head, spine and limbs. Other imaging modalities play specific roles, although invasive procedures are now rarely used (Stanley 1986).

Abdomen and Pelvis

Plain Radiographs

Plain radiographs of the abdomen and pelvis may reveal direct evidence of a tumour, such as characteristic calcification in a neuroblastoma or displacement of bowel gas; or indirect effects such as intestinal obstruction or intussusception due to lymphoma.

Ultrasonography

A palpable abdominal mass is best assessed in the first instance by ultrasonography. It is quick, non-invasive, involves no radiation and can be performed without sedation in most children. Ultrasonography can distinguish solid from cystic masses and may identify a benign cause for an abdominal mass, such as hydronephrosis or polycystic kidney. It may identify the organ of origin of the tumour and indicate the extent of the mass and involvement of contiguous tissues, and is useful for obtaining tumour measurements. The aorta and inferior vena cava will be visualized in all children, although not in their entirety. Ultrasound is particularly good at demonstrating abnormalities in the bladder wall and the scrotum. Ultrasound is limited by interference from gas filled structures such as lungs or loops of bowel. The resolution of ultrasound images is rarely sufficiently high to provide all the necessary information and further more detailed images of most solid tumours are required.

CT Scanning

This is the method of choice for establishing the extent of disease in abdominal tumours. CT will demonstrate the organ of origin and extent of a tumour, it will identify retroperitoneal lymph node involvement and, will frequently demonstrate encroachment upon or compression of vascular structures. Loops of intestine can be identified by the use of oral contrast. Intravenous contrast will improve the delineation of hepatic, splenic, bladder, renal and adrenal masses. In Wilm's tumour, CT will demonstrate the extent of the tumour, the presence of disease in the contralateral kidney, local or regional lymph node involvement and, in most cases, involvement of the inferior vena cava. In neuroblastoma, CT will identify the origin and size of the tumour and calcification within the tumour. It will establish whether the tumour crosses the midline and if it involves adjacent organs, including the spinal canal and blood vessels. These features are important in the assessment of operability.

Contrast Radiology

This has largely been superseded by CT scanning apart from a few specific indications. Excretory urography may be used in some centres to demonstrate the relationship between an intra-renal tumour and the calyceal system, and to distinguish intrarenal from suprarenal tumours, as these distort the anatomy of the kidney primarily from outside. If contrast is injected via a pedal vein, the venous phase will demonstrate whether there is tumour involvement of the inferior vera cava, although this information may be obtained from CT or ultrasonography. Hepatic angiography should be used to assess the extent of liver tumours and their relationship to normal or variant vasculature prior to conservative surgery.

MRI Scanning

The role of MRI scanning in the assessment of intra-abdominal neoplasia is not yet clear. It can provide images of great clarity in a variety of planes, which may be of particular interest to surgeons, but it has not currently superseded CT scanning as the chosen mode of imaging.

Nuclear Studies

These may be helpful in limited circumstances, for example Meta Iodo Benzylguanidine (MIBG) scanning in neuroblastoma. MIBG is taken up by the majority of neural crest tumours; it is important to establish whether there is uptake if therapeutic use of MIBG is under consideration.

Limbs

Plain Radiographs

Soft tissue or bony tumours of the limbs may present with pain, swelling, limp or weakness. The initial investigation of such symptoms includes a plain radiograph. This may identify a benign lesion, such as an osteoid oestoma or a stress fracture; it may show a pathological fracture, or demonstrate features of a bony tumour, for example the characteristic bony destruction and spicular new bone formation of osteosarcoma, or the onion-skin appearance of periosteal new bone in Ewings' sarcoma. In this instance, a plain radiograph may suggest the diagnosis and show the site and extent of the tumour. However, in many cases a plain radiograph may show only non-specific abnormalities or no abnormality at all. It is important to proceed with further investigations, not only where the radiograph is abnormal but also where symptoms persist in spite of normal radiology.

Radioisotope Bone Scan

Abnormal areas of bone will show altered uptake on a radioisotope bone scan, although this appearance is non-specific; a bone scan will not distinguish between a primary bone tumour and osteomyelitis. Nevertheless, a bone scan is generally more sensitive than a plain film and will confirm the presence of an abnormality, even when plain radiology is normal.

MRI

Detailed assessment of a suspicious bony or soft tissue tumour is best done with an MRI scan. This will demonstrate the extent of the disease, soft tissue and bone marrow involvement, including skip lesions, and will delineate anatomical planes and neurovascular bundles. This is important when planning limb-sparing surgery. In addition to clarity of image, MRI offers the advantage of images in the sagittal and coronal as well as the axial planes (Figure 2.1).

CT Scanning

If MRI is unavailable, CT scanning will also demonstrate the extent of disease, including bone marrow and soft tissue involvement, although it is less sensitive than MRI.

Chest

Chest Radiograph

This is the simplest and most helpful first step in assessing a lesion in the thorax. It will demonstrate primary mediastinal lesions, rib lesions and pleural effusions; and may be helpful in assessing the degree of tracheobronchial compromise in primary mediastinal lesions.

CT Scanning

Further assessment of a chest lesion may be achieved with a CT scan. This will demonstrate hilar, mediastinal and paravertebral masses, and it will show the degree of chest wall involvement by intrathoracic tumours, and the involvement of the spinal canal in paravertebral tumours such as neuroblastoma.

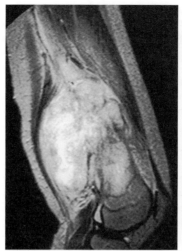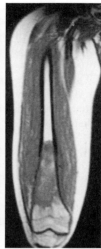

Figure 2.1   MRI scan of right upper leg of child with osteosarcoma. (A) A sagittal T2 weighted sequence showing a huge osteosarcoma involving the distal femur, with a substantial extraosseous component. The large posterior extension displaces and compresses the neurovascular bundle – the popliteal vessels may be recognized by their low signal intensity. (B) A coronal T1 weighted sequence showing the intramedullary extent of the tumour – the normal high signal intensity marrow fat has been replaced by intermediate signal intensity tumour. Scans such as these are invaluable for planning the extent of surgery and for designing prostheses. (In the case illustrated here, resection was clearly impossible, and an amputation was performed.)

Head, Neck and Spine

Plain Radiographs

Plain radiographs of the skull may demonstrate splaying of the sutures, intracranial calcification, enlargement of the optic foramina, or widening of the sella turcica, all of which suggest intracranial disease. They may also demonstrate soft tissue masses and bony erosion in extracranial tumours. However, plain radiographs are normal in up to half of all children with brain tumours. If a head and neck tumour is suspected, more detailed imaging is required. Plain radiographs of the spine may show bony erosion or enlargement of foramina, but a normal spinal radiograph will not exclude malignancy.

CT Scanning

This is the most commonly used modality for the initial assessment of head and neck tumours. A CT scan will usually display primary brain tumours and any associated hydrocephalus. The use of intravenous contrast will permit the differentiation of tumour from surrounding oedema. CT will also demonstrate soft tissue and bony abnormalities, such as those occurring in a rhabdomyosarcoma or bone tumour. The eye may be assessed by CT as this will demonstrate calcification, which is present in 90% of retinoblastomas but absent in benign conditions which may mimic retinoblastoma, such as persistent hyperplastic primary vitreous.

MRI

MRI scanning is the method of choice for assessing the brain and spinal cord. It is particularly useful for the posterior fossa, where bony artefacts may obscure CT images. Gadolinium Diethylene Pontacetic Acid (DTPA) enhanced images of brain tumours may be clearer than CT images, with better differentiation between tumour and surrounding oedema. MRI offers the advantage of scanning in different planes allowing better pre-operative assessment.

MRI is the preferred method for examining the spinal canal; producing clear longitudinal images which will identify spinal tumours and tumours extending into the spine, for example, neuroblastomas. This is achieved without any need for intrathecal contrast. If MRI is unavailable the spinal canal can be assessed by myelography and CT scanning.

STAGING

Staging includes assessment of the primary tumour and the search for metastatic disease. Staging is important for indicating prognosis, for comparison of different treatment regimens, and for determining the type of therapy to be given; for example, stage I Hodgkin's disease is treated with radiotherapy alone, whereas more extensive disease is treated with chemotherapy. Staging of the primary tumour includes preoperative assessment of the site and extent of the tumour, and, if primary resection is performed, radiological and pathological assessment of residual disease. The search for metastatic disease is determined by the type of tumour and its metastatic proclivities, and may include various modes of imaging and tissue examination.

Imaging

Chest

Lung metastases must be sought in most solid tumours apart from brain tumours and neuroblastoma. Metastases may be detected on plain radiographs but CT scanning is more sensitive as it can detect metastases as small as 2–3 mm in diameter, and it will image the peripheries of the lung fields which are difficult to assess on chest radiograph. It provides the most accurate assessment of the number, site and size of pulmonary metastases, which is of particular importance when planning their surgical removal.

Bone

Bony metastases may occur in patients with most types of solid tumour, particularly bone tumours, neuroblastoma, and rhabdomyosarcoma.

Isotope Bone Scan

The most sensitive method for detecting bony metastases is a radioisotope bone scan. Most metastases will show as hot spots on a scan before any abnormality is visible on plain X-rays.

Skeletal Survey

Some bony deposits, particularly from neuroblastoma, Langerhans' cell histiocytosis and leukaemia, may not produce an abnormality on a bone scan. These may be detected more easily on a survey of plain radiographs including the skull, spine, pelvis, abdomen, thorax and the long bones. Plain radiographs will give more detailed pictures of metastases detected by a bone scan, and can detect pathological fractures more easily. Both a radioisotope bone scan and a skeletal survey should be performed in a child with neuroblastoma.

Lymph Nodes

CT scans of the chest and abdomen are routinely used to detect involvement of thoracic or abdominal lymph nodes in Hodgkin's disease and non-Hodgkin's lymphoma, although CT cannot distinguish between lymph nodes enlarged by neoplastic disease and reactive enlarged nodes. MRI images will demonstrate both enlargement and architectural abnormalities in lymph nodes. Lymphangiography is now rarely used in children. Laparotomy and splenectomy are no longer routinely performed in staging Hodgkin's disease, although laparotomy and biopsy may occasionally be necessary to assess a suspicious area.

Liver

Hepatic metastases from intra-abdominal neoplasms are well demonstrated on ultrasound or CT; nuclear scans are less sensitive and are no longer used for this purpose.

Head

CT or MRI of the head should be performed in neuroblastoma if signs such as proptosis, orbital swelling, periorbital ecchymoses, or soft tissue mass suggest the presence of extradural or orbital deposits. Intracranial metastases are rarely seen from other solid tumours until the terminal stages, although they may occasionally be found in rhabdoid tumours. CT or MRI of the head should also be performed in non-Hodgkin's lymphoma affecting the central nervous system or nasopharynx.

Spinal Canal

Extradural spinal metastases (drop metastases) should be sought in medulloblastoma and PNET. MRI is the method of choice for examining the spinal cord and its coverings (Figure 2.2); it is sensitive and non-invasive, but if it is unavailable drop metastases may be demonstrated with CT scanning and myelography. Intraspinal extension of paravertebral neuroblastoma may be detected on CT scanning, but myelography or MRI scanning may be required if results are ambiguous. The spinal canal should also be imaged in CNS lymphoma.

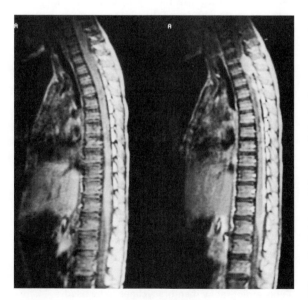

Figure 2.2 Sagittal MRI scan of the spine in a child with medulloblastoma. The left hand side of the figure shows a T2 weighted sequence with no contrast highlighting irregularity in the outline and signal intensity of the spinal cord and the right hand side depicts a gadolinium enhanced T2 weighted image and clearly shows numerous "drop" metastases throughout the length of the spinal canal.

Tissue
Bone Marrow

Bone marrow aspiration may reveal involvement in lymphoma and neuroblastoma, but in many tumours this will only be revealed by a trephine biopsy. Trephine biopsies should be performed in any solid tumour apart from brain tumours. In neuroblastoma and lymphoma, both aspirates and biopsies from multiple sites are usually obtained because of patchy involvement of the bone marrow. In neuroblastoma and lymphoma, a positive bone marrow aspirate may avoid the need for biopsy of the primary tumour.

Cerebrospinal Fluid (CSF)

CSF may be examined for the presence of parameningeal disease in head and neck tumours (including brain, bone and soft tissue tumours), in paravertebral tumours and distant tumours which may metastasize to the CNS, particularly lymphoma. If there is no raised intracranial pressure, lumbar puncture is a simple and safe procedure. In children with raised intracranial pressure due to intracranial tumours, CSF may be obtained at the time of inserting a shunt.

Biopsy of Suspicious Lesions

Where the diagnosis of metastatic disease is entirely based on a single ambiguous abnormality, biopsy of the lesion is necessary. This is particularly important if such information alters the management of the patient. An example is Hodgkin's lymphoma, where an isolated lung lesion on a chest radiograph or diffuse enlargement of the liver on ultrasound are considered suspicious but not diagnostic of metastatic disease.

ASSESSMENT OF THERAPEUTIC EFFECT

Repeated assessment of the primary tumour and metastatic disease is needed both to monitor response to therapy and to detect recurrence.

Imaging of Primary

Repeated imaging of the primary tumour is necessary to assess tumour shrinkage following chemotherapy or radiotherapy, to plan the timing of surgery and to detect residual or recurrent disease postoperatively. The preferred modality will depend on the site of the tumour and practicality. MRI scanning is preferred for the follow-up of brain tumours, particularly postoperatively. CT scanning is used for the reassessment of the majority of solid tumours. Abdominal ultrasound may be used for interim assessments of abdominal tumours. Chest radiographs are an easy way to follow thoracic pathology such as mediastinal masses, although again, definitive reassessment will require CT scanning. Gallium scanning is currently a research tool, but it may have a role in detecting minimal residual mediastinal disease in Hodgkin's lymphoma. Reassessment is usually undertaken after 2–3 courses of chemotherapy to assess the tumour response, before surgery to assess operability, postoperatively to assess residual disease, and at the end of treatment. Further assessment after the end of treatment should be considered where there is residual unresected primary disease, and in tumours with a tendency to local relapse, for example rhabdomyosarcoma.

Monitoring of Markers

The response of certain tumours to treatment may be followed by monitoring the levels of specific serum or urinary markers. Following resection of liver and germ cell tumours, αFP levels will slowly fall towards normal with a half-life of 5 days. A predictive rate of fall can be drawn on a graph; failure to follow this line, or to reach normal levels may indicate the presence of residual disease.

In neuroblastoma, urinary catecholamines and serum ferritin and neurone specific enolase often return to normal after therapy, although this is not prognostic of prolonged survival.

Markers may also be monitored after the end of treatment to detect early recurrence. Urinary catecholamines can be used to monitor neuroblastoma; if elevated levels develop, MIBG scanning may be helpful in locating the site of recurrence. In sacrococcygeal teratoma, monitoring of serum αFP will detect recurrence of a malignant component of the tumour at a stage when curative therapy is still possible.

Screening for Metastatic Disease

In children presenting with metastatic tumours, the response of metastases to therapy can be assessed by repetition of bone scans and skeletal X-rays for bony deposits, and CT scanning for lung metastases. Children presenting with localized tumours, particularly bone tumours, rhabdomyosarcoma and Wilms' tumour may relapse with metastatic disease and should be monitored for the development of lung metastases by regular CXRs. Although this is less sensitive than CT, it is simple,

quick and ideal for repeated examinations. Surveillance for lung metastases in bone tumours should continue for at least 5 years after the end of treatment.

Biopsy of Suspected Recurrences

Although much recurrent or metastatic disease will produce characteristic signs on imaging, in other cases, routine surveillance will reveal lesions of a suspicious but uncertain nature, particularly following surgery or radiotherapy, where inflammatory reaction and scarring may mimic recurrence. In the absence of specific markers for most tumours, the only route to a definite diagnosis is to biopsy the suspicious lesion. This situation may provide a particularly useful role for FNAB, as less tissue will be required to confirm a recurrence than to fully classify a newly presenting tumour.

INVESTIGATIONS OF TOXICITY

The therapy of childhood tumours produces toxic effects on many organ systems; the exact pattern of toxicity depends on the chemotherapeutic agents used and on the site and dose of radiotherapy. Baseline values should be established at diagnosis for any organ system likely to be involved in toxicity (see Table 2.1).

Table 2.1 Baseline investigations at diagnosis

Anthropomorphic measurements: height, weight, surface area and assessment of nutrition (weight for height, mid-upper-arm circumference)

Full blood count, differential and platelet count

Serology for common viral infections which pursue a particularly serious course in immunosuppression, i.e. varicella zoster virus, herpes simplex virus, measles (particularly in tumours with prolonged therapy, such as NHL)

Immunoglobulins

Electrolytes including calcium and phosphate, urea and creatinine, liver function tests

Urinalysis

Echocardiography if anthracyclines to be used

Chromium EDTA clearance if nephrotoxic agents to be used

Audiometry if protocol includes cis-platinum

Pulmonary function tests if busulphan or bleomycin included in treatment

Myelotoxicity

Blood Counts

Many chemotherapeutic agents produce predictable myelotoxicity. Monitoring of blood counts after each course of chemotherapy is necessary in order to identify the need for transfusion of blood products, to indicate periods when the child is at risk for febrile neutropenia, to determine the timing of the next course of chemotherapy after count recovery and to determine whether dose reductions are necessary for subsequent courses.

Investigation of Neutropenic Fever

Cultures

Neutropenic fever is defined as a single temperature recording of 38.5°C or over, or a sustained temperature of 38°C when the neutrophil count is below $1.0 \times 10^9/l$. (The majority of episodes occur when the neutrophil count is below $0.5 \times 10^9/l$). Any episode should be treated as a presumed septicaemia. Urine, blood and throat swabs should be taken for culture before starting the child on intravenous broad-spectrum antibiotics. If a central venous catheter (CVL) is *in situ* blood cultures should be taken from the line; additional peripheral cultures may not add any additional information and are no longer routinely performed in many units. Fungal as well as bacterial pathogens should be sought, particularly following use of broad-spectrum antibiotics for persistent fever (beyond 72 h). In the majority of episodes, no pathogens will be identified.

Imaging

The routine use of chest radiographs at the initial assessment of a febrile neutropenic episode has a low yield of positive findings. Chest radiographs should therefore only be obtained if there is a clinical indication or if there is prolonged fever. Echocardiography may occasionally be required in a child with persistent fever and an *in situ* CVL, particularly if there are features suggestive of embolic episodes, as these may be caused by thrombus on the end of the catheter.

Bronchoscopy

This may be indicated if there is a persistent abnormality on chest radiographs, and may detect bacterial, fungal, viral or pneumocystis infections.

Cardiac

Anthracyclines produce both acute myocardial damage, which is partially reversible, and chronic damage which is proportional to the total cumulative dose received. Dysfunction will usually develop during treatment or during the first year after treatment finishes. It is therefore important to monitor cardiac function during and after therapy which includes these agents. Deteriorating function during therapy may be an indication to modify or withdraw anthracycline therapy (Steinherz et al 1992).

Electrocardiography

Specific electrocardiographic changes occur late, often after considerable myocardial damage has occurred. It is, therefore, not a useful technique for detecting early changes.

Echocardiography

This is the method of choice for monitoring cardiac function in oncology. It is non-invasive and rarely requires sedation. Fractional shortening (FS) measures myocardial contractility; a decline in FS has been shown to be predictive of myocardial damage. This is assessed before the start of treatment, before alternative courses until the cumulative dose is 300 mg/m², then before each course. Cardiac function will be considered to be impaired if the fractional shortening index is less than 30%, or if there has been an absolute decrease of 10% or more from baseline values.

Endomyocardial Biopsy

This is the definitive diagnostic tool in distinguishing different causes of persistent abnormal myocardial function, but is rarely indicated in children.

Renal

Renal function may be compromised by certain chemotherapeutic agents, particularly *cis*-platinum, ifosfamide and high dose methotrexate; and by other nephrotoxic agents such as aminoglycosides and amphotericin.

Glomerular Function

In the absence of specific nephrotoxic drugs, glomerular function is adequately monitored by measuring serum creatinine. If toxic drugs are used a regular assessment of glomerular filtration rate is necessary. The preferred method is chromium EDTA clearance. This is usually performed at the start of treatment, after alternate courses of chemotherapy and at the end of treatment. Persistently low glomerular filtration rate may be an indication to stop *cis*-platinum; this is defined as more than two standard deviations below the age-appropriate mean; for children over 2 years of age this is below 70–80 ml/min per $1.73\,m^2$. Further examinations after the end of treatment may be necessary if there has been any deterioration in function.

Tubular Function

Electrolytes

Tubular damage may produce loss of electrolytes and amino acids in urine and nephrogenic diabetes insipidus. During and after therapy with tubular toxic drugs (including ifosfamide, *cis*-platinum and amphotericin), serum electrolytes should be monitored regularly in order to determine the need for supplements, particularly sodium, potassium, magnesium and calcium.

Fractional Excretion and Electrolytes

Fractional excretion of electrolytes can be calculated from timed urine specimens and concurrent serum measurements.

Markers of Tubular Damage

The degree of tubular damage can be inferred from the degree of leakage of small proteins, of which the most commonly measured are β_2-microglobulin and retinol binding protein.

Fractional excretions and markers of tubular damage should be measured after every 2–3 courses of ifosfamide and at the end of therapy.

Growth and Endocrine

Growth

Linear growth should be monitored in all children with a malignancy until adult height is attained. Children at particular risk of growth failure are those who have received cranial or spinal irradiation, particularly combined with chemotherapy. Spinal irradiation affects truncal height, producing a disproportion between sitting and standing height centiles. Cranial irradiation can cause growth hormone deficiency, for example in children treated for brain tumours and nasopharyngeal rhabdomyosarcomas and children who have received "prophylactic" cranial irradiation as part of the treatment for non-Hodgkin's lymphoma. Other pituitary hormones may also be disturbed, resulting in precocious or delayed

puberty, for example. In any child who shows signs of growth deceleration or abnormal pubertal development, full pituitary assessment including growth hormone, follicle stimulating hormone (FSH) and luteinizing hormone (LH), oestrogen or testosterone, should be considered, in consultation with a paediatric endocrinologist (see Chapter 3).

Gonadal Damage

Boys may sustain gonadal damage from chemotherapy, and should therefore be assessed for testicular failure if puberty is unexpectedly delayed. Infertility will need to be considered in adulthood. Ovarian failure is less common following chemotherapy alone, but is almost universal following pelvic irradiation.

Thyroid Gland

Irradiation of the neck, commonest in localized Hodgkin's disease, may result in delayed hypothyroidism. Thyroid function should be measured yearly in patients who have undergone this treatment. Any nodules found on routine annual palpation of the thyroid should be promptly investigated for secondary malignancy. This may include ultrasonography, radionucleotide scanning and biopsy.

Lung Toxicity

Pulmonary function abnormalities may be detected in up to half of long-term survivors, particularly those who have received bleomycin, busulphan, cyclophosphamide and lung irradiation (Miller et al 1986). Lung function is assessed with chest radiographs, diffusion capacity and spirometry. These should be performed regularly during and after treatment with these agents.

Neurosensory

Various neurosensory toxicities may be evoked by particular agents, for example peripheral neuropathies with vincristine, high tone sensorineural deafness with *cis*-platinum. Audiometry should be performed after alternate courses of *cis*-platinum and at the end of therapy. Symptomatic hearing loss may be an indication to stop therapy with *cis*-platinum.

Psychological and Intellectual Function

Intellectual function may be affected by intracranial tumours and CNS directed therapy, particularly radiotherapy. Prompt assessment is required in any child presenting with new schooling difficulties. Psychological late effects are frequently found in survivors of childhood cancer, when they are assessed by a variety of experimental investigations. Although there are no tests used routinely for this purpose, the assessment of psychological well being is an important part of long-term follow-up.

SCREENING

Screening for paediatric cancer is not of value in most circumstances, as paediatric cancers are very rare. However targeted screening and surveillance of groups at high risk may be more worthwhile.

Neuroblastoma

Screening of infants for neuroblastoma is possible through the collection of urine specimens for catecholamine determination. A national screening programme for 6-month-old infants was developed in Japan in the hope of detecting neuroblastoma at an early curable stage. Unfortunately, recent studies suggest that those tumours detected by screening may be those with a more benign natural history and a tendency to spontaneous maturation, whereas disseminated aggressive lesions, occurring after the first year of life, may occur in children found to be negative by screening at 6 months (Kaneko et al 1990). The role of such screening in reducing the mortality from this tumour remains uncertain.

High-risk Populations

There are a number of conditions that are associated with an increased risk of developing childhood tumours (see Table 2.2). Children suffering from these disorders need

Table 2.2 Cancer-predisposing conditions and their associated cancers

Disease	Associated cancer
Chromosome instability disorders	
Xeroderma pigmentosum	*Basal cell carcinoma, melanoma*
Fanconi anaemia	*Leukaemia, hepatoma*
Ataxia telangiectasia	*Lymphoma, tumours of brain, ovary and GI tract*
Bloom syndrome	*Acute leukaemia, GI tract tumours*

Disease	Associated cancer
Immunodeficiency	
Bruton's agammaglobulinaemia, SCID, Wiskott–Aldrich syndrome, common variable immunodeficiency, IgA deficiency	*Leukaemia and lymphoma*
Constitutional chromosomal abnormalities	
11p deletion	*Wilms' tumour, aniridia, genital malformations, mental retardation*
13q21 deletion	*Familial retinoblastoma*
Turners' syndrome	*Gonadoblastoma*
Down's syndrome	*Leukaemia*
Congenital abnormality syndromes associated with childhood tumours	
Beckwith–Wiedemann syndrome, hemihypertrophy	*Wilms' tumour adrenocortical tumours, hepatoblastoma*
Neurocutaneous syndromes	
Neurofibromatosis	*Schwannoma, optic glioma, rhabdomyosarcoma*
von Hippel Lindau, Sturge–Weber, tuberous sclerosis	*Brain tumours*
Naevoid basal cell carcinoma syndrome	*Basal cell carinoma, medulloblastoma*
Polypoid gastrointestinal disorders	
Polyposis coli, Gardner's	*Colonic carcinoma*
Multiple endocrine adenomatosis syndromes	*Tumours of parathyroid, pituitary, pancreatic islet cell and adrenal gland, carcinoid tumours, schwannoma medullary thyroid carcinoma, phaeochromocytoma*
Dysplastic skeletal disease	
Multiple exostoses, enchondromatosis Fibro-osseous dysplasias	*Osteosarcoma, chondrosarcoma*
Metabolic liver disease	
Glycogen storage disease type IV, hereditary tyrosinaemia, hypermethionaemia, galactosaemia α-antitrypsin deficiency	*Liver tumours*
Li–Fraumeni syndrome	*Sarcomas* in children, *carcinomas* in young adults

GI, gastrointestinal.

to be identified and then screened appropriately. Identification may arise through clinical findings; for example, neurofibromatosis or aniridia may be readily recognized; or through a family history, for example in familial polyposis coli or familial retinoblastoma. Additional studies may help to identify which of these children are actually at risk of developing a neoplasm; cytogenetic or molecular studies may show if a child has inherited the 13q21 deletion which predisposes to retinoblastoma; molecular studies will show whether the 11p13 deletion at the aniridia locus includes the WT1 gene, which would predispose to the development of Wilms' tumour. These techniques are currently research tools but their clinical implications are obvious.

Having identified a child to be at risk for a particular neoplasm, regular and practicable surveillance should be instituted. Examples include regular ophthalmological follow-up for children with familial retinoblastoma, and regular renal, hepatic and adrenal ultrasonography and αFP measurements in Beckwith–Wiedemann syndrome. Current recommendations suggest the latter should be carried out at 3-month intervals up to the age of 5 years, then at 6-month intervals until adolescence.

Survivors of Previous Neoplasm

There is a small but significant risk of second neoplasms in survivors of childhood cancer, who therefore require a higher index of suspicion when presenting with new symptoms. Myeloid leukaemias are the most common secondary malignancy in children previously treated with chemotherapy. Secondary solid tumours may arise in the radiation fields of previous tumours, for example gliomas in children who received cranial irradiation as treatment for leukaemia, or osteosarcoma in irradiated bones.

REFERENCES

Fletcher BD, Pratt CB (1991) Evaluation of the child with a suspected malignant tumour. *Pediat Clin N Am* 38: 223–248.

Kaneko Y, Kanda N, Maseki N, Nakachi K, Takedo T, Okabe I, Sakurai M (1990) Current urinary mass screening for catecholamine metabolites at 6 months of age may be detecting only a small portion of high risk neuroblastomas: a chromosome and N-*myc* amplification study. *J Clin Oncol* 8: 2005–2013.

McGahey BE, Moriarty AT, Nelson WA, Hull MT (1992) Fine needle aspiration biopsy of small round blue cell tumours of childhood. *Cancer* 69: 1067–1073.

Mierau GW, Berry PJ, Orsini EN (1985) Small round cell neoplasms: can electron microscopy and immunohistochemical studies accurately classify them? *Ultrastruct Pathol* 9: 99–111.

Miller RW, Fusner JE, Fink RJ, Murphy TM, Getson PR, Votjova JA, Reaman GH (1986) Pulmonary function abnormalities in long-term survivors of childhood cancer. *Med Pediatr Oncol* 14: 202–207.

Nesbit ME (1993) Clinical assessment and differential diagnosis of the child with suspected cancer. In: Pizzo PA, Poplack DG (eds) *Principles and Practice of Pediatric Oncology*, 2nd edn. JB Lippincott, Philadelphia.

Ortega JA, Siegel SE (1993) Biological markers in pediatric solid tumors. In: Pizzo PA, Poplack DG (eds) *Principles and Practice of Pediatric Oncology*, 2nd edn. JB Lippincott, Philadelphia.

Parker BR, Moore SG (1993) Imaging studies in the diagnosis of pediatric malignancies. In: Pizzo PA, Poplack DG (eds) *Principles and Practice of Pediatric Oncology*, 2nd edn. JB Lippincott, Philadelphia.

Pearson ADJ, Reid MM, Davison EV, Bown N, Malcolm AJ, Craft AW (1988) Cytogenetic investigations of solid tumours of children. *Arch Dis Child* 63: 1012–1015.

Silverman JF, Gurley AM, Holbrook T, Joshi VV (1991) Pediatric fine needle aspiration biopsy. *Am J Clin Pathol* 95: 653–659.

Stanley P (1986) Advances in pediatric tumour imaging. *Cancer* 58: 414–420.

Steinherz LJ, Graham T, Sondheimer HM, Schwartz RG, Shaffer EM, Sandor G, Benson L, Williams R (1992) Guidelines for cardiac monitoring during and after anthracycline therapy: report of the cardiology committee of the children's cancer study group. *Pediatrics* 89: 942–949.

Triche TJ (1993) Pathology of pediatric malignancies. In: Pizzo PA, Poplack DG (eds) *Principles and Practice of Pediatric Oncology*, 2nd edn. JB Lippincott, Philadelphia.

3
Endocrinology

D I Johnston

GROWTH

Growth failure is the cumulative result of a subnormal growth rate, and presents either as failure to thrive in infancy, as as short stature in childhood or adolescence. There are no simple definitions for either of these presentations, and it requires a comprehensive assessment of the child, family and environment before deciding on the degree of growth deviation that justifies full investigation.

The growth curve reflects the superimposition of three phases: infancy, childhood and puberty (Table 3.1). Although control mechanisms overlap, it is useful to consider the major determinants in each period.

Infancy growth is gradual deceleration of fetal growth through to approximately 24–36 months. Nutrition, rather than the classical endocrine system, is the dominant influence.

Childhood growth emerges from age 6 months and reflects the increasing control exercised by polygenic inheritance (parental heights) and the endocrine system, notably growth hormone (GH) secretion.

Pubertal growth is a phase of acceleration superimposed on decelerating childhood growth. This increased tempo is linked to sexual development (growth hormone (GH) and sex steroids). Polygenic inheritance determines the rate of maturation. Constitutional delay of growth and puberty (CDGP) may be familial or non-familial, and manifests as a low childhood growth rate before delayed puberty.

In the absence of a simple definition of pathological short stature it is helpful to calculate the height standard deviation score (ht SDS)

$$ht\ SDS = \frac{\text{Child's height} - \text{Mean height appropriate for population, age and sex}}{\text{Height SD}}$$

In the majority of children presenting with heights above −3 SD, full history and examination will either

Table 3.1 Causes of growth failure

Infancy growth failure
Antenatal
  Chromosomal and genetic
    Autosomal chromosome disorders, e.g. trisomies, deletions
    Sex chromosome disorders, e.g. 45XO and variants
  Syndromic IUGR, e.g. Russell–Silver, Prader–Willi
  Congenital infections
  Skeletal disorders
  Uteroplacental disorders
  Maternal disorders
Postnatal
  Organ and systemic disorders
  Malnutrition

Childhood growth failure
Familial short stature
Social and environmental problems
Organ and systemic disorders
  Conspicuous, e.g. severe asthma
  Inconspicuous, e.g. chronic inflammatory bowel disease
Endocrine disorders

Pubertal growth failure
CDGP
Hypogonadism

CDGP, Constitutional delay of growth and puberty.

establish that she or he has normal variant stature or will provide clues to the underlying diagnosis and the direction of investigation. In the absence of a diagnosis, the growth rate should be monitored at 3- to 6-month intervals. A presenting height less than −3 SD and/or a subnormal growth rate merit investigation. There may be clinical clues to GH deficiency, for example micropenis, infantile facies, delayed dentition or relative obesity.

Children who are inappropriately short for their genetic background or who have low growth rates need formal assessment.

Initial Investigations

Blood
- Full blood count (FBC), erythrocyte sedimentation rate (ESR).
- Electrolytes, urea, creatinine, calcium, phosphate, liver function test (LFT).
- Thyroxine (T4), thyroid stimulating hormone (TSH).
- Cortisol (after exercise).
- Gliadin antibodies.
- Karyotype in girls.

Urine
- Microscopy, pH, concentration and culture.

Imaging
- Left hand and wrist bone age.
- Pituitary fossa X-ray.

Optional Investigations

Blood
- Insulin-like growth factor-1 (IGF-1), IGF-binding protein-3 (IGFBP-3).

Urine
- Early morning urine osmolality to detect diabetes insipidus.
- Urinary GH.

Dynamic hormone tests
- Exercise test for GH and cortisol response.
- Short synacthen test to assess cortisol response.

Imaging
- Skeletal survey for evidence of dysplasia.
- Pituitary area computerized tomography (CT)/ magnetic resonance imaging (MRI).
- Pelvic ultrasound scan (USS) to assess ovarian maturation or detect gonadal dysgenesis

Tissue
- Intestinal biopsy

Interpretation

Growth hormone deficiency is relatively easily diagnosed when it is familial, severe, part of multiple pituitary deficiency, or associated with structural disorders of the hypothalamic–pituitary axis (Table 3.2). In practice, a large proportion of the short children who may benefit from human growth hormone (HGH) therapy have partial, isolated GH deficiency and are not clearly demarcated from their peers with normal variant short stature. The bone age is invariably delayed and approximates to height age. Plain skull X-rays are seldom diagnostic but it is important to detect a craniopharyngioma. High

Table 3.2 Causes of GH deficiency

Congenital
Familial, e.g. gene deletion
Idiopathic GHRH deficiency
Isolated pituitary hypoplasia
Complex, e.g. septo-optic dyplasia

Acquired
Tumours of hypothalamic-pituitary axis
Tumours of adjacent structures, e.g. optic nerve glioma
Irradiation
Trauma
Infection

GH receptor defects
  e.g. Laron syndrome

IGF receptor defects

resolution pituitary imaging may establish structural anomalies such as disruption of the pituitary stalk; such anatomical findings make multiple pituitary hormone deficiency more likely.

The investigation of potential GH deficiency should focus on:

- Excluding other causes of growth failure.
- Identifying multiple pituitary deficiency.
- Identifying pituitary area structural anomalies.

Dynamic tests of GH secretory capacity may confirm hypopituitarism, but they do not reliably differentiate partial GH deficiency from normal. A child with low stimulated GH levels, and no other systemic or endocrine problem, is likely to respond to HGH treatment. Borderline GH responses are less useful in predicting response to therapy. The traditional approach has been to base the diagnosis of GH deficiency on subnormal responses to at least two standard tests. However, many authorities now accept that if the clinical and investigative findings are compatible with growth restraint due to GH insufficiency, and if the child faces height handicap sufficient to merit intervention, then there may be a case for a therapeutic trial of HGH with or without formal tests of GH secretion. Urinary GH measurement may prove to be a useful screening procedure but is not yet routinely available. IGF-1 levels have been promoted for screening but reflect age and nutrition as well as GH status. IGFBP-3 measurement shows promise as a better index of spontaneous GH secretory status.

Options for GH Measurement

- *GH and pituitary hormone measurement during fast-induced hypoglycaemia.* Neonates and infants with multiple pituitary hormone deficiency are liable to fasting hypoglycaemia and should not be exposed to additional provocation.

- *Exercise testing*
  Purpose: Outpatient screen for GH deficiency; helps to assess adrenal status.
  Condition: Fasting optional.
  Method: 50% maximum working capacity for 10 min.
  Sample: Plasma for GH at 20 min after exercise.
  Normal: GH > 15 mu/l (30% of normal children do not reach this level).

- *Glucagon test – suitable for young children (under age 3–5 years)*
  Purpose: Guide to GH and ACTH/cortisol reserve.
  Condition: Overnight fast; observe closely for delayed hypoglycaemia after test, and do not allow home until adequate meal or snacks retained.
  Dose and route: Glucagon 15 mcg/kg body weight/ intravenous
  Samples: Plasma for GH, cortisol at baseline, 30, 60, 90, 120 and 180 min.
  Normal: GH > 15 mu/l.
  Cortisol increase > 150 nmol/l and/or peak > 500 nmol/l.
  Deficiency: GH < 7 mu/l.

- *Clonidine test – suitable for older children (over age 3–5 years)*
  Purpose: Guide to GH reserve, thyrotropin releasing hormone (TRH) and luteinizing hormone releasing hormone (LHRH) tests can be incorporated.
  Condition: Overnight fast; monitor for drowsiness and hypotension.
  Dose and route: Clonidine 150 mcg/m^2 SA (25 mcg tablets) orally.
  Samples: Plasma for GH at baseline, 30, 60, 90 and 120 min.
  Normal: GH > 20 mu/l.

- *Arginine test – suitable for older children (over age 3–5 years)*
  Purpose: Guide to GH reserve, TRH and LHRH tests can be incorporated.
  Condition: Overnight fast.
  Dose and route: 0.5 g/kg BW as IV infusion of 10% arginine HCl in normal saline over 30 min.

  Samples: Plasma for GH at baseline, 15, 30, 45, 60, 90 and 120 min after infusion.
  Normal: GH > 20 mu/l

Problems with GH Stimulation Tests

- GH levels above 15–20 mu/l exclude deficiency, and levels below 7–10 mu/l are suggestive of deficiency. However, intermediate levels are common and need to be interpreted in the light of the child's height velocity and other investigations.
- Interpretation is difficult in early pubertal children because of so-called physiological GH deficiency. Sex steroid priming is recommended (stilboestrol 1 mg twice daily for 3 days) but does not always correct physiological deficiency.
- There are problems of GH assay standardization and quality control.
- The tests are potentially hazardous (insulin-induced hypoglycaemia has been excluded from routine paediatric practice).
- They are unpleasant for children.

Tests Suitable for Research rather than Routine Use

- Overnight or 24-h serial 20 min blood sampling for GH pulse analysis.
- GH releasing hormone (GHRH) test.

Multiple Pituitary Hormone Deficiency

Congenital Hypopituitarism

This may be suspected because of mid-line facial anomalies or because of blindness (septo-optic dysplasia). Other presentations include:
- Micropenis and cryptorchidism (GH and luteinizing hormone (LH) deficiency).
- Hypoglycaemia (GH and adrenocorticotrophic hormone (ACTH) deficiency).
- Prolonged neonatal jaundice (T4 and ACTH deficiency).
- Early failure to thrive (T4, ACTH and antidiuretic hormone (ADH) deficiency).
- Hypernatraemia (ADH deficiency).

Initial Investigations

Blood
- Glucose, electrolytes, osmolality.
- T4. TSH.

- Fasting or hypoglycaemia related cortisol, ACTH and GH.
- LH, testosterone/oestradiol.

Urine
- Osmolality.

Imaging
- Cranial USS or CT.

Other
- Ophthalmic assessment.

Interpretation

Spontaneous or fast-induced hypoglycaemia provides an opportunity to evaluate pituitary function. Deficiencies may be partial and evolving so that regular review is essential. Confirmation of GH status may be left until growth failure reveals itself, but some infants require early HGH therapy to control recurrent hypoglycaemia.

Hypothyroidism and cortisol deficiency are more readily confirmed but diabetes insipidus is sometimes overlooked in infancy.

Acquired Hypopituitarism

This usually evolves insidiously with one or more of the following:
- Growth failure (GH and T4 deficiency).
- Delayed puberty (LH and follicular stimulating hormone (FSH) deficiency).
- Less specific features sometimes precipitated by coincidental illness (ACTH deficiency).
- Thirst and polyuria (ADH deficiency).

Pituitary area tumours, such as craniopharyngioma, more commonly present with visual impairment or neurological signs. Such children require specialist investigation and endocrine management during surgery or cranial irradiation. Successful treatment programmes for brain tumours and acute leukaemia have increased the childhood population susceptible to irradiation induced disorders of the hypothalamic–pituitary axis, thyroid and gonads. These patients require regular monitoring of growth and sexual maturation as they are susceptible to growth failure associated with either precocious or delayed puberty.

Initial Investigations

Blood
- Electrolytes, osmolality.
- T4, TSH.
- Fasting glucose, cortisol, ACTH.
- LH, FSH, testosterone/oestradiol, prolactin.

Imaging
- Bone age.
- Skull X-ray.
- Cranial CT, MRI.

Further Investigation

This will be determined by the nature of the pituitary area lesion and its management.
Urine
- GH.

Dynamic tests
- Combined pituitary provocation test: clonidine + TRH + LHRH.
- Synacthen test.

Interpretation

Hypothyroidism is diagnosed by measuring T4 (TSH will remain low or subnormal). Thyroxine therapy may precipitate adrenal insufficiency, and therefore symptoms, erect blood pressure and morning cortisol levels need to be checked during its introduction. ACTH deficiency does not necessarily require cortisol replacement and, if therapy is required, the dose should be limited to that which allows a normal life-style. Families should be warned of the need to introduce and increase cortisol dosage during illness or trauma.

Diabetes insipidus may only become manifest after the start of cortisol treatment. Thirst sensation is vital to body fluid homeostasis but may be lost as the result of hypothalamic disease or surgery.

Raised intracranial pressure or threatened vision demand urgent cranial imaging and neurosurgery. Detailed endocrine investigation is inappropriate other than to take a baseline sample to detect hypothyroidism, cortisol status and electrolyte disturbance. High dosage dexamethasone is frequently part of perioperative management. The management of postoperative problems such as acute diabetes insipidus requires specialist resources.

Other Pituitary Function Tests

- *TRH stimulation*

Purpose:	To assess pituitary–thyroid axis.
Condition:	Fasting optional, may be included in combined pituitary function test.
Dose and route:	TRH 7 mcg/kg BW to a maximum 200 mcg IV.
Samples:	Plasma for T4, TSH, prolactin at baseline.

plasma for TSH at 30, 60, (90, 120) min.

Normal: TSH increase > 2 mU/l to peak at 30 min. > 3.4 mU/l.

- *LHRH stimulation*

Purpose: To assess pituitary–gonadal axis.

Condition: Fasting optional, may be included in combined pituitary function test.

Dose and route: LHRH 2.5 mcg/kg BW to a maximum 100 mcg IV.

Samples: Plasma for LH, FSH, testosterone/oestradiol at baseline.
Plasma for LH, FSH at 30, 60, (90, 120) min.

Normal: LH, FSH levels relate to pubertal stage.
Prepubertal peak LH 3–4 U/l, FSH 2–3 U/l, but an absent response does not establish pituitary deficiency.

- *IGF-1*

Check laboratory age-dependent normal range: prepubertal 20–180 mcg/l; pubertal 75–580 mcg/l.

Treatment Note: Monitoring Replacement Therapy in Hypopituitarism

GH therapy: dose range 12–15 U/m^2 SA/week
- Height velocity.
- Annual bone age.
- Height SDS calculated for chronological and bone age.
- Checks for evolution of multiple hormone deficiency.

Thyroxine therapy: dose range 2–3 mcg/kg BW/day or 100 mcg/m^2 SA/day
- Energy and school performance.
- T4 level, aiming for upper normal adult range.

Cortisol therapy: dose range 10–12 mg/m^2 SA/day
- Symptomatic assessment, cortisol measurement of limited value.
- Ensure that hydrocortisone is increased during illness, etc.

Desmopressin (DDAVP): dose range 2.5–20 mcg/day
- Regular home weighing.
- Guidelines for daily fluid intake if impaired thirst sensation.
- Interval plasma sodium, osmolality.

Sex steroid therapy
- Graduated escalation of testosterone depot injections (50–250 mg/month) from male bone age 12 years.
- Graduated escalation of ethinyloestradiol (5–20 mcg/day) from female bone age 10 years.

- Norethisterone or a combined oestrogen–progestogen formulation introduced to avoid irregular breakthrough bleeding.

Tall Stature

The great majority of tall children are healthy and appropriate for their above-average-stature parents. Clinical assessment, including exact measurement, pubertal grading and a bone age, is sufficient to reassure most of these youngsters. Factors that alert concern include:
- Abnormally high growth rates.
- Disproportionate tall stature.
- Dysmorphic features, e.g. arachnodactyly, joint laxity, cardiac and eye defects.
- Advanced sexual development.
- Other endocrine features, e.g. goitre, proptosis.
- Visual field defects.

Initial Investigations

Blood
- T4, TSH.
- LH, FSH, prolactin, testosterone/oestradiol.

Imaging
- Bone age.
- Skull X-ray.
- Pelvic USS.

Optional Investigations

Blood
- Karyotype.
- IGF-1.

Urine
- GH.

Dynamic tests
- Glucose load for GH suppression.
- Serial 20 min GH sampling for pulse analysis.

Imaging
- Pituitary area CT, MRI.

Interpretation

Pituitary gigantism is a rare disorder that requires referral to an experienced endocrine unit for diagnosis and therapy. Normal pubertal IGF-1 and GH levels may be difficult to distinguish from those seen in early gigantism.

Hyperthyroidism (see p. 55).
Sexual precocity (see p. 45).

Obesity

Obesity is a common cause for referral but seldom has an endocrine basis. Nutritional obesity is likely if parents are also obese, there is a long established pattern of obesity, and the child has normal or above average height. Pathological obesity should be considered when there are height growth failure, asymmetrical obesity (trunk but not limb involvement), or features of a syndrome (see Table 3.3). Investigation should be guided by the additional clinical features of, for example, growth failure, suspected hypothyroidism or glucocorticoid excess.

Table 3.3 Causes of obesity

Nutritional/familial

Endocrine
Hypopituitarism
Post-craniopharyngioma surgery
Hypothyroidism
Adrenal glucocorticoid excess
Pseudohypoparathyroidism

Syndromatic
Turner
Prader–Willi
Laurence–Moon

Iatrogenic
Corticosteroid therapy
Excessive insulin dosage (especially in adolescent girls)
Sodium valproate

DIABETES INSIPIDUS AND HYPERNATRAEMIC DEHYDRATION

Diabetes insipidus in children with intact thirst sensation presents with polyuria and polydipsia. Dependent infants and older children with defective thirst are unable to compensate, become dehydrated and develop irritability, fever and failure to thrive. Functional polydipsia can usually be recognized in an otherwise healthy child because of the variability of thirst, and the day rather than night-time drinking habit.

Differential Diagnosis

Defective thirst sensation (hypodipsia-hypernatraemia syndrome)
- Hypothalamic disorder.

ADH deficiency (central diabetes insipidus)
- Primary: Idiopathic
                Familial
                DIDMOAD or Wolfram syndrome (autosomal dominant disorder comprising diabetes insipidus, diabetes mellitus, optic atrophy and deafness).
- Secondary: Often with multiple pituitary hormone deficiency.

ADH unresponsiveness (nephrogenic diabetes insipidus)
- Primary: Idiopathic
                X-linked recessive.
- Secondary: Renal tubular damage.

Initial Investigations

Blood
- Random sodium, osmolality.
- Glucose, calcium, potassium, urea, creatinine.
- Fasting morning sodium, osmolality.

Urine
- Measured urine volume.
- Fasting morning osmolality.

Interpretation

An overnight fast is useful in confirming behavioural polydipsia with retention of normal plasma osmolality and urine osmolality exceeding 400 mOsm/kg.

Diabetes insipidus typically results in elevated plasma sodium and osmolality levels, with impaired urine concentration (under 300 mOsm/kg). However, urine osmolality has to be judged against the matching plasma osmolality as there may be an increased threshold for ADH release rather than total deficiency. Fasting and water deprivation are contraindicated if a random plasma osmolality exceeds 305 mOsm/kg or sodium exceeds 148 mmol/l.

Suspected ADH deficiency in a child with known hypopituitarism or an established disorder of the hypothalamus does not have to be confirmed by water deprivation. Cortisol and thyroxine deficiency mask diabetes insipidus so that polyuria or hypernatraemia may emerge only after the start of pituitary replacement therapy.

Optional Investigations

Blood
- 08.00 h cortisol, T4, TSH.
- ADH autoantibody titre.

Imaging
- Cranial CT/MRI.

Dynamic test – water deprivation
Depending on age, compliance and suspected severity, start test at 20.00 h or 08.00 h.

- Start: body weight; empty bladder.
- 08.00 h: weight; plasma osmolality and sodium; urine volume and osmolality.
- Hourly: weight; urine volume and osmolality.
- End: weight; plasma osmolality and sodium; urine volume and osmolality.

Optional test – plasma ADH levels
Continue water deprivation until:

- Urine osmolality > 850 mOsm/kg or > 500 mOsm/kg in infants under 3 months.
- Weight loss ⩾ 5%.
- Urine osmolality fails to increase over a 3-h period after duration of more than 4 h.
- Plasma osmolality ⩾ 305 mOsm/kg, sodium ⩾ 148 mmol/l.

Dynamic test – trial of desmopressin nasal spray
- Dose: age over 1 year, 10–20 mcg; under 1 year; 5–10 mcg.
- Urine volume and osmolality are monitored at 2 to 4-h intervals for next 12 h; the child is allowed food and a fluid volume equivalent to urine output.

Interpretation

ADH deficiency (central diabetes insipidus) is confirmed by failure to achieve osmolality above 850 mOsm/kg during water deprivation followed by a greater than 50% increase after desmopressin. Deprivation testing may be difficult to perform or produce equivocal results. An option is to commence a trial of gradually escalating intranasal desmopressin (DDAVP) therapy with monitoring of weight, plasma osmolality and sodium to avoid water overload.

ADH unresponsiveness (nephrogenic diabetes insipidus) is likely if neither acute nor prolonged ADH therapy reduces polyuria, and urine osmolality remains below 300 mOsm/kg.

Diabetes Insipidus Reference Values

See Table 3.4.

Table 3.4 Diabetes insipidus reference values: blood

		Comments
Plasma osmolality	285–295 mOsm/kg	
ADH random	2.5–7.5 pmol/l	Levels need to be interpreted against plasma osmolality

SEXUAL DEVELOPMENT
Ambiguous Genitalia

This complex problem is best approached by considering the elements of gender determination:

- Genetic: XX, XY or mixed karyotypes.
- Gonadal: ovary, testis or mixed.
- Internal genitalia: Müllerian or mesonephric duct derivatives.
- External genitalia: phallic size; urethral, vaginal or urogenital openings.

Priorities are to:

- Reach a specific diagnosis.
- Determine the appropriate functional gender for the infant.
- Anticipate and prevent life-threatening complications.
- Consider genetic implications.

Classification of Ambiguous Genitalia

- *Female pseudohermaphroditism (no palpable gonads).* Virilized female: XX karyotype, normal ovaries and Müllerian derivatives.
- *Male hermaphroditism (gonads may or may not be palpable).* Undermasculinized male: XY karyotype but potential disorders of testes or androgen responsive tissues.
- *True pseudohermaphrodite.* Varied karyotypes with malformed, streak or mixed gonads.
- *Malformation syndromes* – associated with gonadal and genital anomalies.

Initial Investigations

Blood
- Karyotype.
- Birth and day-2 17-hydroxyprogesterone.
- Store plasma for other hormone assays.

Imaging
- Pelvic and abdominal USS.

Interpretation

A normal female karyotype indicates that the infant is inappropriately virilized due to either endogenous or transplacental androgens.

Congenital adrenal hyperplasia (Table 3.5) caused by 21-hydroxylase deficiency accounts for 90% of female pseudo-

Table 3.5 Congenital adrenal hyperplasia – clinical features and investigation

Enzyme defect		Ambiguous genitalia	Early virilization	Salt loss	Elevated BP	Plasma steroids	Urinary steroids
21α-Hydroxylase salt losing	F	+	+	+	0	17OHProg ↑ ↑ Δ⁴-A ↑ ↑	Pregnanetriol ↑ ↑
	M	0	+	+	0	T ↑	
21α-Hydroxylase simple virilizing	F	+	+	0	0	as above	as above
	M	0	+	0	0		
11β-Hydroxylase	F	+	+	0	+	17OHProg ↑ Δ⁴-A ↑ ↑	Tetrahydro-S ↑ tetrahydrodeoxycortisol ↑
	M	0	+	0	+	T ↑ 11-Deoxycortisol ↑	
3β-Hydroxysteroid dehydrogenase	F	+	+ Mild variant	+	0	17OHProg n/ ↑ Ratio 17OHPreg/	Ratio Δ⁵/Δ⁴ steroids ↑
	M	+	0	+	0	17OHProg ↑	

17OHProg, 17-hydroxyprogesterone; 17OHPreg, 17-hydroxypregnenolone; Δ⁴-A, androstenedione; T, testosterone.
↑, increased; ↑ ↑, greatly increased.
+, present; 0, absent.

hermaphroditism. 17-Hydroxyprogesterone levels are abnormally elevated (usually above 100 nmol/l) and urinary steroid analysis confirms elevated pregnanetriol excretion. The compensatory increase in ACTH secretion generates normal cortisol levels so that hypoglycaemia is a rare presenting problem. Pelvic imaging confirms the presence of a uterus.

The next stage is to anticipate and treat mineralocorticoid deficiency by reviewing feeding pattern, weight gain and measuring:

- Serial plasma electrolytes watching for hyperkalaemia.
- Urinary sodium.

Optional Investigation

- Plasma renin activity and aldosterone level.

Potential salt loss is anticipated by rising plasma potassium. Plasma renin activity is increased and aldosterone levels are low.

Treatment Note: Monitoring of Glucocorticoid Therapy in Congenital Adrenal Hyperplasia Caused by 21α-Hydroxylase Deficiency

- Height growth.
- Annual bone age.
- Hydrocortisone dose in usual range 15–20 mg/m² SA per day.

- Interval plasma androgen (androstenedione) or testosterone (not in pubertal boys).
- Interval saliva or capillary blood 17-hydroxyprogesterone profiles.

Treatment Note: Monitoring of Mineralocorticoid Therapy in Congenital Adrenal Hyperplasia Caused by 21α-Hydroxylase Deficiency

- Blood pressure.
- Occasional plasma electrolytes (unnecessary if stable).
- Fludrocortisone dose in usual range 50–200 mcg/day.
- Plasma renin activity.

Female Pseudohermaphroditism

Differential Diagnosis

Congenital adrenal hyperplasia (relative prevalence)
- 21α-Hydroxylase deficiency (90%)
    simple virilizing (40%)
    salt-losing (60%).
- 11β-Hydroxylase deficiency (5%).
- 3β-Hydroxysteroid dehydrogenase deficiency (< 5%).

Other fetal adrenal disorders
- Adrenal adenoma.
- Nodular adrenal hyperplasia.

Transplacental androgen excess
- Maternal adrenal or ovarian tumour.
- Maternal virilizing adrenal hyperplasia.
- Maternal androgen therapy.

Further Investigations

Further investigation of female pseudohermaphroditism if initial pattern is not diagnostic of 21α-hydroxylase deficiency:

Blood
- Testosterone and adrenal steroids (11-deoxycortisol).
- ACTH.
- HLA and gene probe.

Dynamic test
- Short synacthen test measuring 17-hydroxyprogesterone, adrenal steroids and testosterone.

Urine
- Adrenal steroid profile.

Imaging
- Pelvic sinogram.
- Fibre-optic endoscopy.

Interpretation

11β-Hydroxylase deficiency in females produces virilization at birth. Characteristically it subsequently leads to salt-retention and hypertension, although there may be an initial salt-losing phase. Basal 17-hydroxyprogesterone levels are low by comparison with 21-hyroxylase deficiency. Elevated plasma 11-deoxycortisol levels (> 1000 nmol/l) and urinary 6-hydroxytetrahydro-11-deoxycortisol and tetrahydro-S are confirmatory.

3β-Hydroxysteroid dehydrogenase deficiency causes virilization of females but incomplete masculinization of males. The enzyme block leads to a severe deficiency of both glucocorticoid and mineralocorticoid secretion so that infants present with life-threatening adrenal failure as well as ambiguous genitalia. An elevated ratio of plasma 17-hydroxypregnenolone to 17-hydroxyprogesterone localizes the defect.

True hermaphroditism is usually linked to 46XX but with variable gonadal differentiation. Detailed imaging of internal genitalia is essential.

Male Pseudohermaphroditism

These disorders exhibit a wide spectrum extending from hypospadias, cryptorchidism and minimal ambiguity to an apparently female phenotype.

Differential Diagnosis

Disorders of testicular differentiation
- Leydig cell hypoplasia (gonadotrophin unresponsiveness).
- Mixed gonadal dysgenesis.
- Pure gonadal dysgenesis.
- Drash anomalad (associated glomerulonephritis and Wilms' tumour).

Disorders of testicular function
- Enzyme defects in corticosteroid and testosterone synthesis – 20,22-desmolase (cholesterol side-chain cleavage); 3β-hydroxysteroid dehydrogenase; 17α-hydroxylase.
- Enzyme defects in testosterone synthesis – 17,20-desmolase; 17β-hydroxysteroid dehydrogenase.
- Defects in Müllerian inhibitory factor synthesis.

Disorders of androgen dependent target tissues
- Enzyme defect in testosterone metabolism – 5α-reductase.
- Androgen receptor defects – partial or incomplete testicular feminization; complete testicular feminization.

Initial Investigations

Blood
- Karyotype.
- Testosterone (save plasma for dihydrotestosterone).
- Adrenal steroids (save plasma).
- LH, FSH.

Dynamic tests
- LHRH.
- hCG stimulation.

Urine
- Adrenal steroid profile.

Imaging
- Pelvic sinogram.
- Fibreoptic endoscopy.
- Abdominal and pelvic USS.
- Adrenal/gonadal CT/MRI.

Tissue
- Exploratory laparotomy or laparoscopy with gonadal histology.

Interpretation

Testosterone levels need to be evaluated with reference to the developmental stage of the child. The newborn period is a phase of Leydig cell stimulation and relatively high testosterone levels. High basal levels avoid the need for dynamic tests. Low basal and hCG stimulated testosterone levels point to disorders of testicular differentiation or function.

Leydig cell hypoplasia produces elevated LH, FSH but low testosterone levels; hCG stimulation fails to generate a response. Müllerian tube regression is complete because MIF production by Sertoli cells is intact.

Bilateral dysgenetic gonads differ by having persistent Müllerian derivatives indicative of both Leydig and Sertoli cell failure.

Mixed gonadal dysgenesis is suggested when a single palpable gonad is accompanied by asymmetry of internal genital differentiation. The functioning testis will secrete normal levels of testosterone. There may be 45X/46XY mosaicism.

Male Pseudohermaphroditism due to Enzymatic Blocks

This is suggested by presence of testes, hypoplastic Wolffian ducts and absence of Müllerian derivatives together with a specific precursor metabolite pattern:
- 20,22-Desmolase def. – low levels of all adrenal steroids.
- 3β-Hydroxysteroid dehydrogenase def. – elevated plasma 17-hydroxypregnenolone, DHEA and urinary pregnanetriol.
- 17α-Hydroxylase def. – elevated plasma progestrone and urinary corticosterone.
- 17,20-Desmolase def. – elevated plasma 17-hydroxyprogesterone, 17-hydroxypregnenolone and urinary pregnanetriolone.
- 17β-Hydroxysteroid dehydrogenase def. – elevated androstenedione/testosterone ratio.

Disorders of Androgen-dependent Target Tissues

These result in increased basal or hCG stimulated testosterone levels confirming intact Leydig cell capacity. Absent Müllerian derivatives establish that MIF production is also intact. These disorders account for the majority of male pseudohermaphroditism.

Further Investigations

Further investigation of suspected disorders of androgen-dependent target tissues

Blood
- Testosterone and dihydrotestosterone levels.
- Gene probe studies.

Urine
- Steroid profile: 5β/5α ratio (aetiocholanolone to androsterone).

Dynamic test
- Basal and hCG stimulated testosterone and dihydrotestosterone levels.
- Phallic growth response to exogenous testosterone (or DHT).

An important practical test in all potential males with micropenis (< 2.5 cm length) is to measure response to testosterone depot 25–50 mg/month for 3 months. Mean normal penile growth response is reported as 2.0 ± 0.6 (SD) cm. The test needs to be performed early in infancy if gender assignment remains an issue after preliminary investigation. Short-term testosterone treatment can also be given later in childhood to boys with persisting micropenis.

Tissue
- Fibroblast 5α-reductase activity.
- Receptor analyses.

Interpretation

5α-Reductase deficiency is confirmed by an elevated T/DHT ratio matched by urinary derivatives.

Partial androgen receptor defects are suggested by elevated testosterone levels and a normal T/DHT ratio. There is no phallic growth in response to exogenous testosterone. Tissue receptor studies may show either quantitative or qualitative androgen binding defects.

Micropenis with or without Cryptorchidism

The presence of a small but anatomically complete penis suggests qualitatively intact but quantitatively deficient pathways of testosterone synthesis and response. Intact pituitary function is important for penile growth and testicular descent. Hypopituitarism must therefore be considered especially if the infant also presents with hypoglycaemia, prolonged jaundice or failure to thrive.

Differential Diagnosis

Hypothalamic-pituitary disorders
- Hypogonadotrophic hypogonadism – isolated LH deficiency; multiple pituitary deficiencies; associated syndrome (Kallmann, Prader–Willi, Septo-optic dysplasia).
- Isolated GH deficiency.

Disorders of testicular function

Disorders of androgen dependent target tissues

Sex chromosome disorders
- X-chromosome polysomies (XXY, XXXY, etc.).

Other dysmorphic syndromes associated with micropenis
- Noonan, Down, William, Smith–Lemli–Opitz.

Initial Investigations

Blood
- Blood glucose monitoring 6–12 hourly from birth until normoglycaemia maintained and infant tolerating full feeds.
- Karyotype.
- Testosterone.
- LH, FSH.

Dynamic tests
- LHRH.
- hCG stimulation.

Imaging
- Pelvic and abdominal USS.
- Cranial USS.

Interpretation

Isolated LH deficiency may be easier to confirm in early infancy when there is normally a surge of LH release paralleled by increased (low adult range) testosterone levels.

Precocious Puberty

The definition of precocious puberty is generally accepted as "sexual development appearing in a girl before age 6 to 8 years, and in a boy before 9 years", but it is more important to consider the nature of the puberty and its impact on the child and family. Reviewing the growth rate and skeletal maturation are vital to this assessment.

The endocrine axis responsible for sexual maturation is established in fetal life. Transient surges of gonadotrophin and sex steroid secretion occur after birth and during early infancy. The axis is then suppressed through childhood, although it is recognized that gradual reactivation occurs from as early as 6–8 years. The mechanisms responsible for childhood suppression are ill-understood but a range of cerebral insults can provoke early puberty. In females, the LHRH pulse generator is more prone to early reactivation, and commonly the cause is either unexplained or familial. In the minority with organic brain disease there are usually neurological or visual signs, but there has to be a low threshold for cranial imaging. The early puberty may be transient, show a fluctuating evolution, or progress towards maturity with growth acceleration and bone age advance. Pelvic ultrasound provides a useful tool for confirming and monitoring ovarian maturation. Symmetrical ovarian maturation suggests activity of the pituitary–gonadal axis.

In the male, complete precocious puberty is more indicative of serious intracranial pathology, and cranial imaging is essential. Bilateral testicular enlargement readily confirms that puberty is complete.

Differential Diagnosis

Isosexual precocity
- Complete isosexual precocious puberty (LHRH pulse generator dependent):
  Constitutional.
  Organic brain disease; tumours, trauma, post-infectious, irradiation.
  Late treated congenital adrenal hyperplasia.
- Incomplete isosexual precocious puberty (LHRH pulse generator independent):
  Girls – Ovarian cysts and tumours.
      Adrenal oestrogen producing tumours.
  Boys – hCG secreting tumours: intracranial and visceral.
      Congenital adrenal hyperplasia (21α-hydroxylase deficiency, 11β-hydroxylase deficiency).
      Adrenal tumours.
      Leydig cell tumours.
      Familial testotoxicosis (see below, p. 47).
  Both sexes – McCune–Albright syndrome.
      Hypothyroidism.
      Exogenous sex steroid exposure.
- Partial forms of precocious puberty:
  Premature thelarche.
  Premature adrenarche.
  Premature isolated menarche.

Contra- or hetero-sexual precocity
- Congenital adrenal hyperplasia.
- Adrenal tumours.
- Gonadal tumours.
- Exogenous sex steroid exposure.

Partial Precocious Puberty

Breast Development (Isolated Thelarche)

Isolated, usually self-limiting and often asymmetrical breast development is relatively common in young girls, especially under 2 and seldom after 4 years. Investigation is unwarranted if height growth is appropriate and there is no other sexual development. There may be transient elevations of FSH and oestradiol paralleled by ovarian cyst formation.

Pubic and Axillary Hair (Isolated Adrenarche)

This is relatively common, especially in girls, from age 6 years. It is accompanied by mild height and bone age acceleration. It usually reflects accentuation of the normal onset of adrenal sex steroid production.

Initial Investigations

Blood
● Androstenedione, 17-hydroxyprogesterone, testosterone.

Imaging
● Bone age.
● Pelvic USS.

Interpretation

Androstenedione levels are in the pubertal range and ovarian maturation is appropriate to age. Serial observation confirms normal progression of the remainder of puberty. A minority with more pronounced hair and skin changes are heterozygotes for 21α-hydroxlase deficiency, confirmed by ACTH stimulation with 17-hydroxyprogesterone measurement.

Breast Development Accompanied by Height Acceleration

This (p. 39) merits investigation aimed at assessing the cause, and the likelihood of unacceptable early menses or reduced final height. A normal, although premature, progression of sexual maturation with breast formation, enlargement of labia minora and vaginal mucosal maturation favours activation of pituitary–gonadal axis. Disordered progression with excessive sexual hair or virilization without breast development raises the possibility of adrenal pathology.

Initial Investigations

Blood
● Basal oestradiol, LH, FSH, hCG.
● T4, TSH, prolactin.

Imaging
● Bone age.
● Skull X-ray.
● Pelvic ultrasound.

Optional Investigations

Blood
● 17-Hydroxyprogesterone, testosterone.

Dynamic tests
● LHRH test (usually adds little to information available from pelvic USS).
● Serial LH and FSH levels over 12–24 h.

Imaging
● Cranial CT, MRI.
● Abdominal CT.
● Skeletal X-rays: polyostotic fibrous dysplasia in McCune–Albright syndrome.

Interpretation

Complete isosexual precocity is supported by elevated LH, FSH and oestradiol levels together with multicystic ovaries and uterine growth. An unacceptable puberty may be suppressed by using gonadorelin analogues (LHRH superagonists). Subcutaneous depot preparations such as goserelin or leuprorelin are more effective than nasally applied buserelin but such therapy requires detailed monitoring of pubertal staging, growth and pelvic ultrasound.

Autonomous ovarian follicular cysts may manifest as a mass, or as abdominal pain, or may produce transient or recurrent breast development and vaginal bleeds. Follicles in excess of 10 mm diameter are outside the range expected in normal girls. Although they may originate following short-lived surges of gonadotrophin secretion, they become autonomous often with fluctuating size and oestradiol release. They are also refractory to therapy with LHRH superagonists.

Ovarian tumours are very rare and should be recognized with modern imaging procedures.

Precocious Puberty with Symmetrical Testicular Enlargement

Initial Investigations

Blood
● Basal testosterone, LH, FSH, hCG, AFP.
● T4, TSH, prolactin.

Imaging
● Bone age.
● Skull X-ray.
● Cranial CT, MRI.

Optional Investigation

● Chest or abdominal CT MRI.

Interpretation

True precocious puberty is strongly associated with hypothalamic hamartomas and other neoplasms. The former act as ectopic LHRH pulse generators, and basal or stimulated LH levels are increased.

Chorionic gonadotrophin-secreting tumours result in elevated hCG but not LH, and the LHRH test is prepubertal.

Sources of hCG include teratomas, chorioepitheliomas and germinomas of hypothalamus, pineal area, mediastinum, retroperitoneum and gonads. Hepatomas or hepatoblastomas are other important neoplasms. Elevated AFP may be a marker.

Familial testotoxicosis is an autosomal dominant disorder of testicular autonomy producing elevated testosterone levels despite prepubertal LH and FSH secretion.

Precocious puberty without testicular enlargement may be due to congenital adrenal hyperplasia or adrenal carcinoma/adenoma.

Precocious puberty with asymmetrical testicular enlargement suggests either an interstitial cell tumour or an enlarging adrenal rest associated with congenital adrenal hyperplasia.

Delayed Puberty

Ninety-five percent of 12-year-old girls and 14-year old boys have entered puberty. The majority of healthy children who enter puberty late have constitutional delay. The family history is an important guide, and it is usually evident from growth records that the child has had a slow tempo of maturation. Boys, in particular, complain because of low height growth, and this will be accentuated if there is a combination of familial short stature with delay.

An interrupted or unusually prolonged (over 5 years) puberty may reflect underlying problems.

Differential Diagnosis

Constitutional delay of growth and puberty (CDGP)
- Familial, non-familial.

Hypogonadotrophic hypogonadism (defective LHRH pulse generator)
- Isolated gonadotrophin deficiency (± hyposmia).
- Multiple pituitary hormone deficiency.
- CNS disorders, e.g. congenital, tumours, irradiation.
- Syndromatic, e.g. Prader–Willi.
- Chronic systemic disease and malnutrition.
- Anorexia nervosa, exercise amenorrhoea.

Hypergonadotrophic hypogonadism (defective gonads)
Females:
- Gonadal dysgenesis including Turner syndrome.
- Ovarian damage, e.g. irradiation, chemotherapy.
- Autoimmune oophoritis.

Males:
- Seminiferous tubular dysgenesis including Klinefelter syndrome.
- Noonan syndrome.

- Testicular damage, e.g. irradiation, chemotherapy, surgery.
- Anorchia.

Initial Investigations

These have to be selected after comprehensive evaluation including body proportions, dysmorphic features, smell, and size of penis and testes. Features of systemic illness with growth restraint or multiple hormone deficiency require fuller investigation.

Blood
- Testosterone, oestradiol.
- LH, FSH.
- T4, TSH, prolactin.
- Karyotype.

Imaging
- Bone age.
- Skull X-ray.
- Pelvic USS.

Optional Investigation

Dynamic tests
- Serial LH, FSH levels over 12–24 h.

Imaging
- Cranial CT, MRI.

Interpretation

CDGP and isolated gonadotrophin deficiency cannot be differentiated on the basis of low sex hormone, LH and FSH levels alone. Various tests have been proposed but none consistently discriminates between the two diagnoses or replaces the value of family history and long-term observation.

Kallmann syndrome (isolated gonadotrophin deficiency with hyposmia) is commoner in boys, and more severe cases present with micropenis and cryptorchidism. The early infancy surge of testosterone cannot be detected. MRI may demonstrate hypoplastic olfactory bulbs.

Gonadal dysgenesis with abnormal karyotypes are readily identified. Abnormally elevated LH and FSH levels with normal karyotypes require careful anatomical definition of the gonads by detailed imaging, laparoscopy and biopsy.

Gonadal reference values

See Table 3.6.

Table 3.6 Gonadal reference values: blood

		Comments
LH (iu/l)		In paediatric
Prepubertal	< 1	endocrinology,
Adult male	1–10	an immunoradio-
Adult female:		metric assay
follicular/luteal	1–15	(IMRA) is
mid-cycle	15–80	recommended to
		provide high
		sensitivity
FSH (iu/l)		IMRA
Prepubertal	< 4	
Adult male	1–10	
Adult female:		
follicular/luteal	1–8	
mid-cycle	8–22	
Testosterone (nmol/l)		
Male infants 1–8 weeks	1.8–12	
Prepubertal	< 0.7	
Adult male	8–27	
Adult female:	< 3.0	
Dihydrotestosterone nmol/l	< 0.5	
Oestradiol (pmol/l)		
Prepubertal	< 50	
Adult male	< 220	
Adult female:		
follicular	< 220	
mid-cycle	400–1400	
luteal	200–1000	

Gonadal dynamic tests

- LHRH test (p. 39).

- hCG test:

Purpose:	To assess Leydig cell functional reserve or testosterone biosynthesis.
Condition:	None.
Dose and route:	Short version hCG 1000 units daily for 3 days IM. Long version hCG 2000 units twice weekly for 3 weeks IM.
Samples:	Plasma at baseline and 24–48 h after last injection.
Normal:	Infant boys: testosterone increases by greater than 2–3 fold. Prepubertal boys: testosterone increases by 5–10 fold (peak > 2 nmol/l).

Pubertal boys have a higher baseline and lower increment.
Ratios of androstenedione, testosterone and dihydrotestosterone can be studied.

ADRENAL DISORDERS

Adrenal Failure in Infancy

Adrenal failure is rare but must be considered in infants with poor weight gain and vomiting or vascular collapse associated with hypoglycaemia, hyponatraemia and hyperkalaemia.

Differential diagnosis

Adrenal
- Congenital adrenal hyperplasia.
- Congenital adrenal hypoplasia:
  Sporadic in association with pituitary hypoplasia
  Autosomal recessive
  X-linked cytomegalic form
  X-linked with glycerol kinase deficiency.
- Familial glucocorticoid deficiency (with achalasia and alacrima).
- Infarction.

Pituitary
- Panhypopituitarism.

Hypothalamus

Initial Investigations

Blood
- Glucose.
- Electrolytes, urea.
- Cortisol, ACTH*.
- 17-Hydroxyprogesterone.
- Store frozen plasma.

Urine
- Store for steroid measurement.

Imaging
- Cranial ultrasound.
- Adrenal area ultrasound.

Interpretation

Laboratory diagnosis of adrenal insufficiency in infancy is usually based on finding a low plasma cortisol during

*Here and throughout, an asterisk denotes that a sample requires special handling.

physiological stress such as hypoglycaemia or electrolyte imbalance. Ideally, at least two paired cortisol and ACTH measurements should be performed. Correction of suspected adrenal failure must not be delayed after collecting initial samples.

Congenital adrenal hyperplasia rarely presents with symptoms of cortisol deficiency. Hypoglycaemia is a greater threat after the treatment regimen has commenced (see pp. 42 and 58).

Congenital adrenal hypoplasia may present abruptly after birth with vascular collapse and convulsions. Some present with growth failure and increasing pigmentation.

Familial glucocorticoid deficiency has been linked to mutations of the ACTH receptor gene. ACTH levels are elevated but cortisol production is deficient.

Hypopituitarism is usually accompanied by other manifestations of intracranial or ocular disease, or by additional pituitary hormone deficiency (pp. 37–39).

Optional Investigations

Blood
- Androstenedione and other adrenal steroids.

Dynamic test
- Short synacthen test.

Urine
- Adrenal steroid profile.

Imaging
- Cranial CT/MRI.
- Adrenal CT/MRI.

Adrenal Failure in Childhood

Childhood adrenal failure may present as a medical emergency with abdominal pain, vomiting, dehydration, shock and biochemical findings of hypoglycaemia, hyponatraemia, hyperkalaemia, azotaemia, and hypercalcaemia. A greater diagnostic challenge is an insidious onset with growth failure, lethargy, and ill-defined nausea and abdominal pain. Important clues may be provided by a family history of autoimmune disease or by finding vitiligo, alopecia, and skin or mucosal hyperpigmentation. In the list that follows hypopituitarism is more frequent than primary adrenal disease.

Differential Diagnosis

Adrenal
- Autoimmune:
  Isolated

Polyglandular type 1 – hypoparathyroidism, mucocutaneous candidiasis;
Polyglandular type 2 – thyroid disease, IDDM.
- Adrenoleucodystrophies.
- Infarction, haemorrhage.
- Infective – tuberculosis, fungal, AIDS related.
- Infiltrative – lymphoma.
- Drug induced.

Pituitary
- Panhypopituitarism.
- Isolated ACTH deficiency.

Hypothalamic
- Cranial irradiation.
- Cerebral infiltration.

Initial Investigations

Blood
- Glucose.
- Electrolytes, urea.
- Cortisol, ACTH*.
- 17-Hydroxyprogesterone.
- Store frozen plasma.
- Adrenal autoantibodies.

Urine
- Store for steroid measurement.

Imaging
- Adrenal area ultrasound.

Interpretation

The laboratory diagnosis of acute adrenal insufficiency is often based on finding a low plasma cortisol during physiological stress, hypoglycaemia or electrolyte imbalance. However, an elevated cortisol level does not rule out adrenal failure in a severely stressed patient. Hyponatraemia can occur with severe cortisol deficiency due to either primary or secondary adrenal insufficiency. Hyperkalaemia indicates mineralocorticoid deficiency and therefore primary adrenal disease. Ideally, at least two paired cortisol and ACTH samples should be collected. Correction of clinically apparent adrenal failure should not be delayed, and the child must be promptly resuscitated with intravenous normal saline and dextrose together with corticosteroids. Initial intravenous dexamethasone therapy has the potential advantage of permitting measurement of plasma cortisol levels if a short synacthen test is subsequently judged appropriate. Hydrocortisone therapy interferes with cortisol assay but it is still possible to confirm adrenal failure at a later date. Mineralocorticoid therapy is not required in initial treatment.

In less acute presentations a short synacthen test is valuable in confirming reduced adrenal function. ACTH levels, adrenal autoantibodies and imaging studies usually make the distinction between primary and secondary or tertiary adrenal failure. It is seldom necessary to have to resort to a prolonged synacthen test.

Optional Investigations

Blood
- Androstenedione and other adrenal steroids.
- Renin activity, aldosterone*.
- Very long chain fatty acid (VLCFA) levels and phytanic acid.

Dynamic tests
- Short synacthen test.
- Prolonged synacthen test.
- Corticotrophin releasing factor (CRF) test.

Urine
- Adrenal steroids.

Imaging
- Cranial CT/MRI.
- Adrenal CT/MRI.

Interpretation

Autoimmune adrenalitis is the most common cause of primary adrenal failure. Diagnostic problems arise because of slow and insidious evolution of either cortisol or aldosterone deficiency before the other becomes apparent.

Adrenoleucodystrophies are inherited peroxisomal disorders with X-linkage. Elevated VLCFA and phytanic acid levels provide biochemical confirmation.

Treatment Note: Monitoring Glucocorticoid Therapy (Primary and Secondary Adrenal Failure)

- Relief of symptoms.
- Growth rate.
- Appropriate dose hydrocortisone 15–20 mg/m^2 SA per day.
- Morning plasma ACTH* between 4 and 18 pmol/l (optional parameter).

Treatment Note: Monitoring Mineralocorticoid Therapy (Primary Adrenal Failure)

- Blood pressure, supine and erect.
- Plasma electrolytes.
- Plasma renin activity*.

Salt-losing Disorders

Persistent hyponatraemia with hyperkalaemia may be discovered during the assessment of an infant who presents with failure to thrive.

Differential Diagnosis

Adrenal: disorders of aldosterone synthesis
- Associated ambiguous genitalia (pp. 41–42).
- Associated glucocorticoid deficiency (pp. 48–49).
- Primary hypoaldosteronism (corticosterone 18-methyl oxidase II deficiency, CMO II deficiency).

Renal
- Renal tubular insensitivity (pseudohypoaldosteronism).
- Obstructive uropathy.
- Prematurity.
- Post-transplantation.

Initial Investigations

Blood
- Electrolytes, urea, creatinine.
- Cortisol, ACTH*.
- 17-Hydroxyprogesterone.
- Renin activity, aldosterone*.

Urine
- Electrolytes.
- Adrenal steroids: corticosterone and aldosterone derivatives.

Imaging
- Renal ultrasound.
- Adrenal area ultrasound.

Optional investigations
- P-450c11 gene probe.
- Monocyte mineralocorticoid receptor studies.

Interpretation

CMO II deficiency is suggested by raised plasma renin activity with low aldosterone levels but elevated 18-hydroxycorticosterone. Urine steroid HPLC confirms elevated tetrahydro-18-hydroxy-11-dehydrocorticosterone and reduced tetrahydroaldosterone.

Pseudohypoaldosteronism is distinguished by renal salt-wasting and hyperreninaemia but with elevated plasma aldosterone and urinary tetrahydroaldosterone levels. Measured renal salt loss continues despite the administration of fludrocortisone.

Premature or Excessive Adrenal Activity: Androgen Excess

Clinical features of increased adrenal androgen activity include premature pubic hair growth, childhood acne and height acceleration. Inappropriate virilization is more ominous.

Differential Diagnosis

Isolated adrenarche (pubarche) (p. 45).

Late onset congenital adrenal hyperplasia:
- 21α-hydroxylase deficiency: non-classical
- 11β-hydroxylase deficiency
- 3β-hydroxysteroid dehydrogenase deficiency

Adrenal tumour.

Gonadal tumour.

Drugs.

Initial Investigations

Blood
- 17-Hydroxyprogesterone.
- Testosterone, androstenedione.
- LH, FSH.

Urine
- Adrenal steroid profile.

Imaging
- Bone age.
- Adrenal area USS.
- Ovarian and uterus USS.

Interpretation

Premature adrenarche implied when an otherwise normal 6–8 year old child shows early pubic hair growth accompanied by modest growth acceleration and bone age advance (< 2 years). Adrenal androgens, for example androstenedione, are elevated for age but compatible with early puberty.

Late-onset congenital adrenal hyperplasia is suggested by marked growth acceleration and bone age advance (> 2 years). Baseline 17-hydroxyprogesterone, testosterone, and androstenedione levels are usually abnormally elevated. It may be necessary to perform an ACTH stimulation test to differentiate homozygote from heterozygote levels. Basal or ACTH stimulated urinary steroid profiles are also helpful.

Optional Investigations

Blood
- P-450c21 gene probe.

Dynamic test
- ACTH stimulation.

Interpretation

Adrenal cortical adenoma/carcinoma is suggested by a rapid progression of sexual hair growth often accompanied by features of glucocorticoid excess. A clinical picture or preliminary biochemistry which does not exclude this diagnosis calls for detailed adrenal imaging.

Further Investigation

Imaging
- Adrenal area CT/MRI.

Premature or Excessive Adrenal Activity: Glucocorticoid Excess

Obesity with normal or modestly accelerated height growth is likely to be nutritional rather than endocrine mediated. Growth failure, facial plethora, striae, proximal muscle weakness and hypertension require full investigation.

Differential Diagnosis

Adrenal (ACTH independent)
- Adrenal adenoma/carcinoma
- Bilateral micronodular dysplasia:
  Isolated,
  Familial – associated with pigmented skin lesions.

Hypothalamic-pituitary (ACTH dependent).

Ectopic ACTH syndromes.

Drug
- ACTH.
- Glucocorticoids.

Initial Investigations

Blood
- Electrolytes, urea.
- Cortisol and ACTH* at 09.00 h and 24.00 h.
- Testosterone, androstenedione.

Dynamic tests
- Overnight low-dose dexamethasone suppression test.
- Two-day dexamethasone suppression test.

Urine
- Two overnight or 24-h free cortisol levels.
- Adrenal steroid profile.

Imaging
- Plain abdominal X-ray.
- Bone age.
- Adrenal area USS.

Interpretation

The key issues are the demonstration of an increased cortisol secretory rate with loss of diurnal rhythm, ACTH dependence, and whether the negative feedback loop is intact. Persistently elevated cortisol levels, suppressed ACTH, and absent dexamethasone induced suppression point to ACTH-independent adrenal pathology.

Adrenal adenoma/carcinoma is suggested by a mixed glucocorticoid and androgen pattern.

Further Investigations

Imaging
- Adrenal area CT/MRI: high resolution, thin-section scans usually define tumours but they cannot determine function, i.e. an adenoma may be non-functioning.
- ^{131}I-labelled cholesterol scans are unreliable.

Interpretation

Bilateral micronodular dyplasia presents as a rare ACTH-independent cause of Cushing's syndrome. The adrenal glands are normal or slightly enlarged on imaging, and the nodular pattern may not be evident.

ACTH-dependent Cushing's syndrome usually has a slowly progressive course in which there are few androgen mediated features. Early morning cortisol and ACTH levels are often normal but nocturnal levels are abnormally elevated. Urinary free cortisol is increased.

Further Investigations

Dynamic tests
- High-dose dexamethasone suppression test.
- CRF test.

These are specialist centre procedures.

Imaging
- Pituitary area CT/MRI to define microadenomata (< 10 mm).
- Adrenal area CT/MRI may show either bilateral diffuse hyperplasia or bilateral macronodular hyperplasia. The latter can be asymmetrical and lead to false interpretation as an adenoma.

Adrenal Reference Values

See Table 3.7.

Table 3.7 Adrenal reference values: blood and urine (age and pubertal stage related standards are available)

		Comments
Blood		
Cortisol (nmol/l)		Diurnal rhythms
Normal 08.00–09.00 h	150–700	are not established
Normal 18.00 h or later	< 250	until 6 months and are difficult to confirm in young children
Appropriate stress level	> 275	Higher values do
Adrenal failure	< 140	not exclude failure
ACTH (pmol/l)		
Normal 08.00–09.00 h	4–22	
Normal 18.00 h or later	< 2	
17-Hydroxyprogesterone (nmol/l)		Elevated in stress, notably in
Age 0–48 h	< 40	hyponatraemic
Age > 48 h	< 15	and LBW infants
11-Deoxycortisol (nmol/l)	< 60	
Androstenedione (nmol/l)		
Prepubertal	< 3.6	
Male adult	4–10	
Female adult	4–13	
Testosterone (nmol/l)		Infants under age 6
Prepubertal	< 0.7	months may have
Male adult	8–27	pubertal levels
Female adult	< 3.0	
Urine		
Free cortisol (nmol/day)	< 300	
Andrenal steroids		GC-MS urinary steroid analysis needs to be interpreted by a reference laboratory

Adrenal Dynamic Tests

- Short synacthen (tetracosactrin) test:

Purpose:	Screening test for adrenal failure.
Condition:	Non-fasting, no exogenous hydrocortisone.
Dose and route:	Single dose tetracosactrin 250 mcg or 35 mcg/kg BW IM or IV.
Samples:	Plasma at baseline, 30, 60 min.
Normal response:	Cortisol increase ≥ 200 nmol/l; cortisol peak ≥ 500 nmol/l.

- Long synacthen (tetracosactrin) test:

Purpose:	Differentiates primary from secondary adrenal failure.
Condition:	Careful observation in case of adrenal insufficiency.
Dose and route:	Six 12 hourly depot tetracosactrin 0.5 mcg/m^2 SA IM.
Samples:	Plasma at 08.00 h on days 1, 2, 3.
Normal response:	Cortisol peak ≥ 500 nmol/l. Depressed response with elevated endogenous ACTH levels confirm primary failure.

- Low-dose dexamethasone suppression test: overnight screening test:

Purpose:	Confirms normal suppression of adrenal cortex.
Condition:	Stress in normal patients may prevent suppression.
Dose and route:	22.00 h dexamethasone 10 mcg/kg BW single dose orally.
Sample:	Plasma at 08.00 h.
Normal response:	Cortisol < 100 nmol/l.

- Low-dose dexamethasone suppression test (48 h test):

Purpose:	Failure of suppression confirms Cushing's syndrome.
Condition:	Check for complicating drug therapy, e.g. carbamazepine.
Dose and route:	Dexamethasone 5 mcg/kg BW 6 hourly for 48 h orally.
Samples:	Baseline plasma cortisol and 24-h urine free cortisol. Plasma at 48 h for cortisol, ACTH. 24-h urine on day 3 for free cortisol.
Normal response:	48 h plasma cortisol < 140 nmol/l, ACTH < 5 pmol/l urine cortisol to less than half baseline.

- High-dose dexamethasone tests are used to differentiate adrenal from pituitary causes of Cushing's syndrome, but there are many potential pitfalls in interpretation.

THYROID DISORDERS

Infants Detected by Thyroid Screening Programmes

An elevated capillary blood TSH level collected at age 5 to 7 days provides the most sensitive screen for primary hypothyroidism. Screening based on umbilical cord or capillary thyroxine levels has the theoretical advantage of detecting hypopituitarism, but the disadvantage of being less sensitive. Of hypothyroid infants, 10–20% have thyroxine levels in the low normal range.

Screening programmes should be organized so that affected infants start treatment by age 20 days.

Initial Investigations

Blood
- TSH
- Free T4 (or derived free T4).

Imaging
- Knee X-ray for epiphyseal maturation.

Optional Investigations

Blood
- Thyroid binding globulin.

Imaging
- Thyroid isotopic scan.

Interpretation

The majority of infants detected by screening have unequivocal biochemistry, TSH above 50 mU/l and a low T4. Subnormal T4 and delayed skeletal maturation correlate with the severity of intrauterine hypothyroidism and a greater likelihood of neurodevelopmental handicap. Thyroid scans may clarify aetiology and need to be performed at the start of therapy while TSH levels are still high. Scans differentiate between hypoplastic and ectopic glands, infants with the former are reported to have a higher requirement for T4 replacement. Normal sized glands associated with elevated TSH levels suggest defects of thyroxine synthesis (10–15% of Caucasian infants detected by screening).

Infants with Borderline TSH Elevation (20–50 mU/l)

Differential Diagnosis

Transient TSH elevation due to hypothalamic immaturity (preterm infants).

Hypoplastic or ectopic thyroid.

Inherited defects of thyroid hormone synthesis (dyshormonogenesis).

Transient hypothyroidism:
- Maternal antithyroid or goitrogen exposure.

- Maternal iodine deficiency.
- Topical iodine exposure.

The introduction of thyroxine therapy must be guided by history and clinical features. Serial TSH and T4 measurements usually clarify the picture; age matched normal T4 levels and falling TSH support an expectant policy. Low T4 levels justify thyroxine replacement with the option of stopping therapy and reviewing thyroid status later in infancy.

Infants with Normal TSH and Low T4

Differential Diagnosis

Preterm.

Severe systemic illness.

Hypothalamic/hypopituitary hypothyroidism.

TBG deficiency.

T4 levels in preterm infants need to be judged against gestation matched reference ranges. Laboratories providing a service to neonatal departments need to define these ranges according to the assay used. It is uncertain whether low T4 levels in sick preterm infants are of functional significance. The fetal brain has a specific deiodinase which preferentially converts T4 to T3 so that cerebral tissue is relatively protected. Hypopituitarism is usually suggested by additional features such as micropenis, cryptorchidism, hypoglycaemia and persistent cholestasis.

Treatment Note: Monitoring Thyroxine Therapy in Primary Hypothyroidism

- Activity and development.
- Growth rate.
- Bone age.
- Thyroxine dose in expected range $100-110 \, mcg/m^2$ SA per day.
- T4 levels in the upper normal adult range.
- TSH in euthyroid range.

Juvenile Hypothyroidism

Hypothyroidism may present as growth failure with obesity, or because of a goitre, lethargy, or constipation.

Differential Diagnosis

Goitre present
- Autoimmune thyroiditis.

- Inherited defects of thyroid hormone synthesis (dyshormonogenesis).
- Goitrogen exposure.
- Endemic iodine deficiency.

Goitre absent
- Hypoplastic or ectopic thyroid.
- Hypothalamic/hypopituitary hypothyroidism.

Initial Investigations

Blood
- T4, TSH.
- Thyroid microsomal (peroxisomal) and thyroglobulin antibody titres.

Imaging
- Left-hand bone age

Interpretation

Autoimmune thyroiditis is the commonest cause of acquired hypothyroidism in regions without iodine deficiency. Autoimmune thyroiditis produces a firm bosselated goitre in 80–90%, and over 90% have antithyroid antibodies.

Optional Investigations

Blood
- Other organ specific autoantibodies
- LH, FSH, prolactin: elevated in precocious puberty (hormone overlap)
- CPK: elevated in muscular hypertrophy (Kocher–Debre–Semelaigne syndrome)

Dynamic tests
- TRH stimulation test: indicated if low free T4 and low or normal TSH. Autoimmune thyroiditis with compensated hypothyroidism produces an augmented TSH response to TRH.

Imaging
- Isotopic thyroid scan: spotty uptake pattern in autoimmune thyroiditis; defective organification secondary to thyroiditis results in abnormal perchlorate discharge.

Thyroxine-binding globulin deficiency, an X-linked condition, is suggested by a low total T4 but normal free T4 and TSH.

Inherited defects of thyroid hormone synthesis are suggested by positive family history, goitre and negative thyroid antibodies.

Hypothalamic/hypopituitary hypothyroidism is probable when a low T4 is accompanied by an inappropriately low TSH. There are usually other features of hypopituitarism.

Optional Investigations

Dynamic tests
- TRH stimulation as part of full pituitary assessment (p. 38).

Imaging
- Pituitary CT/MRI.

Hyperthyroidism

Hyperthyroidism is easily recognized when signs such as proptosis, tremor and a goitre are present. Other clues include growth acceleration, abnormal choreiform movements and altered behaviour.

Differential Diagnosis

Autoimmune thyroiditis (Graves' disease).

Drug induced:
- Thyroxine.
- Iodine.

Viral subacute thyroiditis

Initial Investigations

Blood
- T4.
- TSH: sensitive assay to confirm suppressed level.
- Thyroid microsomal (peroxisomal) and thyroglobulin antibody titres.

Imaging
- Left-hand bone age.

Interpretation

Autoimmune thyroiditis accounts for the large majority; a positive family history is common.

Viral subacute thyroiditis may be wrongly labelled as Graves' disease. Typically it presents with thyroid area pain and tenderness; thyroid antibodies are negative and the hyperthyroid phase is transient.

Optional Investigations

Blood
- T3 if T4 normal but TSH depressed.
- Other organ specific autoantibodies.

Dynamic tests
- TRH stimulation to confirm depressed TSH response. This test is largely redundant now that sensitive TSH assays are available.

Imaging
- Isotopic thyroid scan: uptake diffusely increased in Graves' disease.

Treatment Note: Monitoring Carbimazole Therapy in Childhood Hyperthyroidism

- Correction of symptoms and growth rate.
- T4 and TSH in euthyroid range.
- Carbimazole in dosage range 0.1–0.3 mg/kg BW per day.

Hyperthyroidism in Fetus and Neonate

The paediatrician will often be alerted by maternal thyroid disease or by the detection of fetal tachycardia or growth failure in an at-risk pregnancy. The newborn may present promptly or after a delay with tachycardia, irritability and poor feeding.

Initial Investigations

Blood
- Birth and serial T4 levels.

Interpretation

Birth T4 levels may be low, normal or elevated depending on the interplay of thyroid stimulating and suppressing antibodies as well as maternal carbimazole therapy.

Table 3.8   Thyroid reference values: blood*

Free T4 (pmol/l)	
FT cord	25–58
1–4 weeks	24–30
Childhood	Upper adult range
Adult	9–24
Total T4 (nmol/l)	
FT cord	105–205
1–4 weeks	85–280
Childhood	Upper adult range
Adult	55–150
Total T3 (nmol/l)	
Adult	0.8–2.4
TSH (mu/l)	
Adult	0.5–4.5

*Free thyroid hormones are more readily interpreted. Each laboratory has to establish an age related reference range.

Elevated T4 is usually evident by 5–7 days but has to be compared with age and gestation matched normal data.

Monitoring carbimazole therapy in infantile hyperthyroidism is largely based on clinical observation.

Thyroid Reference Values

See Table 3.8.

CALCIUM DISORDERS

Hypocalcaemia

A child with hypoparathyroidism may present acutely with convulsions, tetany and stridor or gradually with failure to thrive, developmental delay, signs of raised intracranial pressure, cataracts and poor dentition.

Differential Diagnosis of Hypoparathyroidism

Transient neonatal
- Prematurity, hypoxia.
- Maternal diabetes and hyperparathyroidism.

Permanent
- Congenital
  Isolated hypoplasia sporadic or familial,
  Complex Di George syndrome.
- Acquired
  Autoimmune,
  Transfusion haemosiderosis,
  Post-thyroidectomy.

Pseudohypoparathyroidism.

Functional hypoparathyroidism:
- Magnesium deficiency.

Initial Investigations

Blood
- Calcium, phosphate, alkaline phosphatase, magnesium.
- Creatinine, albumin.
- PTH (sensitive two-site immunoassay).

Urine
- Calcium: creatinine and phosphate (derived Tm_p/GFR).

Imaging
- Chest X-ray.
- Skeletal survey.

ECG
- QT prolongation.

Interpretation

Hypoparathyroidism is confirmed by hypocalcaemia, hyperphosphataemia, and normal renal function together with low PTH levels using a sensitive assay. Associated findings include an elevated urinary phosphate and low serum $1,25\text{-}(OH)_2D$ levels. Increased duration of disease results in basal ganglia calcification.

Optional Investigations

Blood
- Calcium ionic activity.
- $1,25\text{-}(OH)_2D$.
- T4, TSH.
- Autoantibody screen.
- Immune studies including T-cell profile.

Dynamic test
- PTH infusion.

Imaging
- Cardiac USS.
- Cranial CT/MRI.

Tissue
- G_s activity.

Interpretation

Idiopathic isolated hypoparathyroidism may be sporadic or familial. The increased availability of reliable PTH assays has reduced dependence on PTH infusion studies previously used to confirm the diagnosis and make the distinction from pseudohypoparathyroidism.

Di George syndrome varies in the severity and persistence of hypoparathyroidism. Identified by chromosome analysis for deletion within 22q11.

Autoimmune hypoparathyroidism may occur in isolation or in association with adrenal insufficiency, or more rarely hypothyroidism and insulin-dependent diabetes. Other associations include vitiligo, alopecia and chronic mucocutaneous candidiasis.

Pseudohypoparathyroidism refers to a heterogenous syndrome in which several mechanisms produce endorgan unresponsiveness to PTH and other peptide hormones. Patients with characteristic clinical and skeletal X-ray features have reduced tissue guanine nucleotide-binding protein (G_s).

Treatment Note: Monitoring Vitamin D Analogue Therapy in Hypoparathyroidism

- Relief of neuromuscular symptoms.
- Maintain plasma calcium in range 2.0–2.2 mmol/l.

- Alfacalcidol dose range 40–50 ng/kg BW per day.
- Urine calcium/creatinine ratio < 0.7 mmol/mmol.
- Renal USS to monitor nephrocalcinosis.

Hypercalcaemia

Hypercalcaemia presents with anorexia, failure to thrive, polydipsia, polyuria, weakness and renal calculi. A positive family history may be an important clue.

Differential Diagnosis

Hyperparathyroidism
- Primary:
  Sporadic – adenoma, hyperplasia.
  Familial – Multiple endocrine neoplasia (MEN 1, 2).
  Familial hypocalciuric hypercalcaemia (FHH).
  Neonatal primary hyperparathyroidism.
- Secondary – chronic renal failure.
- Ectopic.

Non-parathyroid
- Syndromic (Williams syndrome)
- Vitamin D (and A) excess
- Malignancy
- Sarcoidosis
- Other endocrine; thyrotoxicosis, adrenal insufficiency

Initial Investigations

Blood
- Serial calcium, phosphate, alkaline phosphatase.
- Electrolytes, creatinine.
- PTH (sensitive two-site immunoassay).

Urine
- Calcium: creatinine and phosphate (derived Tm_p/GFR).

Imaging
- Wrist and hand X-ray, skull X-ray.
- Renal tract X-ray and USS.
- Cardiac USS.

Optional Investigations

Blood
- Vitamin D metabolites.

Urine
- cAMP clearance.

Interpretation

Hyperparathyroidism is confirmed by finding persistent hypercalcaemia without suppression of PTH levels.

Other findings are hypophosphataemia, increased urinary calcium and cAMP, subperiosteal erosions and skull demineralization.

Multiple endocrine neoplasia, types 1 and 2, are inherited as autosomal dominant disorders but seldom manifest endocrine problems before age 18 years. Gene probes are available for family screening.

Familial hypocalciuric hypercalcaemia (FHH) is also an autosomal dominant in which hypercalcaemia occurs in the first decade, and is associated with inappropriately normal PTH secretion but low renal calcium clearance.

Neonatal primary hyperparathyroidism is partly accounted for by homozygous FHH leading to generalized parathyroid hyperplasia.

Calcium Reference Values

See Table 3.9.

Table 3.9 Calcium reference values: blood and urine

Blood		
Total calcium (mmol/l)	2.2–2.6	
Ionized calcium (mmol/l)	1.0–1.5	
Phosphate (mmol/l)		
Children	1.3–2.3	
Adults	0.6–1.5	
PTH (ng/l)	10–65	
1,25-(OH)$_2$D (pmol/l)	70–215	
Urine		
Calcium/creatinine ratio (mmol/mmol)	<0.7	In second void morning sample
Maximal rate of tubular phosphate reaborption, Tm_p/GFR (mmol/l)		
Children	1.3–2.6	
Adults	0.8–1.4	

Calcium Dynamic Test

- PTH infusion test

Purpose:	To differentiate PTH deficiency and unresponsiveness, and to classify pseudohypoparathyroidism types 1 and 2.
Condition:	Overnight fast followed by water hydration, empty bladder at start of test.
Dose and route:	Synthetic N-terminal PTH 5 U/kg BW (maximum 200 units) IV infusion in normal saline over 10 min (check manufacturer's instructions).

Samples: *Plasma and/or urine before PTH infusion*
Plasma at −30 and −5 min for cAMP, calcium, phosphate and PTH.
Two 30-min urine collections before PTH infusion for calcium, phosphate, creatinine and cAMP
Plasma and/or urine after PTH infusion
Plasma at +5 and +10 min for cAMP, calcium, phosphate.
Urine at 30 and 60 min for cAMP, phosphate and creatinine.

Interpretation: PTH increases plasma and urinary cAMP and urinary phosphate in both normals and hypoparathyroidism.
Pseudohypoparathyroidism type 1 blunted plasma and urine cAMP rise and phosphaturic response.
Pseudohypoparathyroidism type 2 normal cAMP rise, blunted phosphaturic response

GLUCOSE DISORDERS

Hyperglycaemia

Florid hyperglycaemia manifest by thirst and polyuria, and accompanied by ketonuria is indicative of insulin-dependent diabetes. It is unusual to have to consider alternative causes of hyperglycaemia in childhood.

Diabetes Classification

Insulin-dependent diabetes (IDDM).

Non-insulin-dependent diabetes of the young (NIDDMY) also known as maturity-onset diabetes in the young (MODY).

Secondary
- Pancreatic disease, e.g. cystic fibrosis, haemosiderosis.
- Endocrine, e.g. Cushing's syndrome.
- Syndromatic, e.g. DIDMOAD.
- Receptor abnormalities, e.g. associated virilization and acanthosis nigricans.
- Drug-induced, e.g. corticosteroids.

Other causes of hyperglycaemia:
- Stress-related, e.g. post-convulsive.
- Drug-induced, e.g. sympathomimetics, TPN-induced.

Initial Investigations

Initial investigation of suspected diabetes will be guided by clinical assessment of severity of dehydration and ketoacidosis.

Blood
- Glucose.
- Electrolytes, urea and osmolality.
- FBC.
- Blood gas analysis.

Urine
- Ketones.

Optional Investigations

Blood
- HbA1.
- Islet cell antibodies.
- Autoantibody screen including gliadin antibodies.
- Fasting insulin, C-peptide.

Interpretation

Diabetes in childhood seldom requires confirmation by glucose tolerance tests. Serial blood glucose levels usually resolve borderline cases. More formal tests may have a place in the monitoring of children with predisposing disease, for example cystic fibrosis.

Dynamic test

- Fasting, random and oral glucose loading tests. See Table 3.10.

Hypoglycaemia

In suspected hypoglycaemia it is essential to organize laboratory confirmation (blood glucose < 2.6 mmol/l), and to collect simultaneous blood and urine samples to enable a specific diagnosis.

Differential Diagnosis of Endocrine Mediated Hypoglycaemia

Deficiency
- GH – hypopituitarism (p. 37).
- ACTH/cortisol – hypopituitarism (p. 37).
- Cortisol – adrenal failure (p. 48–49).

Excess
- Insulin – endogenous; exogenous.

Table 3.10 Hyperglycaemia dynamic test: WHO criteria (glucose, mmol/l)

	Whole blood		Plasma	
	Venous	Capillary	Venous	Capillary
Diabetes				
Fasting	⩾ 6.7	⩾ 6.7	⩾ 7.8	⩾ 7.8
Random or 2-h after glucose load	⩾ 10.0	> 11.1	> 11.1	> 12.2
Impaired glucose tolerance				
Fasting	< 6.7	< 6.7	< 7.8	< 7.8
2-h after glucose load	6.7–10.0	7.8–11.1	7.8–11.1	8.9–12.2

Glucose load in oral GTT 1.75 g/kg body weight up to a maximum of 75 g over 5 min.

Initial Investigations

Blood
- Glucose.
- Intermediary metabolites (acetoacetate, 3-hydroxy-butyrate, FFA).
- Cortisol, GH, T4, TSH.
- Insulin, C-peptide.

Urine
- Ketones.
- Metabolic screen including reducing substances (freeze sample).

Interpretation

Hyperinsulinism in the newborn may be anticipated because of high birthweight or clinical features of Beckwith syndrome. It is also suggested by an intravenous glucose requirement exceeding 8 mg/kg BW per minute. In older children, the absence of ketonuria favours hyperinsulinism and this will be confirmed by finding low plasma free fatty acid and ketone body levels. The insulin assay must be of sufficient sensitivity to measure levels which may be low in absolute terms but inappropriate for hypoglycaemia.

Endogenous hyperinsulinism is confirmed by parallel elevation of both insulin and C-peptide levels. Covert insulin administration has been discovered by finding elevated insulin but low C-peptide levels.

Cortisol and GH deficiencies produces a ketotic hypoglycaemia with elevated ketone bodies and FFAs.

Optional Investigations

Blood
- Toxicology screen.
- Intermediary metabolites, free and acyl carnitines.

Dynamic test
- Monitored fast with serial glucose, metabolite and hormone levels.

Metabolic disorders.

Hypoglycaemia Reference Values

See Table 3.11.

Table 3.11 Hypoglycaemia reference values: blood

Insulin (mu/l)	
Fasting	5–20
Hypoglycaemia	< 5
C-peptide (nmol/l)	
Fasting	0.08–0.85

REFERENCES

Brook CGD (1989) *Clinical Paediatric Endocrinology*, 2nd edn. Blackwell Scientific Publications, Oxford.

Grossman A (1992) *Clinical Endocrinology*. Blackwell Scientific Publications, Oxford.

Ranke MB (1992) *Functional Endocrinologic Diagnostics in Children and Adolescents*. J&J Verlag, Mannheim.

Wilson JD, Foster DW (1992) *Williams Textbook of Endocrinology*, 8th edn. WB Saunders, Philadelphia.

4

Metabolic Disease

J E Wraith

INTRODUCTION

Inborn errors of metabolism are a family of genetic disorders characterized by an enzyme deficiency which leads to an accumulation of a "toxic" intermediary compound. In some conditions, e.g. the lipid storage disorders, the accumulation occurs within subcellular organelles. In addition, for certain disorders an essential end-product is not produced in adequate amounts.

Individually metabolic disorders are rare, but as a group they are sufficiently common to be considered in the differential diagnosis of many neonatal and childhood illnesses. The conditions are typically multisystem in effect, but the brain and nervous system seem particularly vulnerable to metabolic insult.

As individual disorders are rare their specific diagnosis often depends on enzyme assays available in only a few regional centres. However, as outcome, particularly in the newborn period, may depend on speed of diagnosis prompt clinical consultation between colleagues in district hospitals and the regional centres is essential if diagnosis is to proceed smoothly (Green 1989).

For the majority of conditions prenatal diagnosis is possible, emphasizing the importance of establishing an accurate diagnosis in affected infants (Cleary and Wraith 1991).

THE ACUTELY ILL NEONATE

Metabolic disease should always be considered in the differential diagnosis of any neonate with unexplained acute illness. Metabolic investigations should be undertaken at the same time as investigations aimed at the diagnosis of more common neonatal upsets, such as, sepsis, cerebral haemorrhage or necrotizing enterocolitis. A number of clues may be obtained from the history, clinical examination, "bedside" tests and simple laboratory investigations.

Clues from the History

The following questions should be asked when metabolic disease is suspected in the neonatal period:

1. Are the parents related?
2. Is there a previous family history of unexplained death in infancy?
3. Was the child well immediately after birth?
4. Has there been a change in feed?
5. Has the infant been subjected to a catabolic stress such as surgery or prolonged fasting?
6. Did the infant improve when feeds were discontinued?
7. Was there a relapse on restarting milk?

Most inherited disorders are inherited as an autosomal recessive and a history of consanguinity is important. The exception in the neonatal period is the urea cycle defect ornithine carbamoyl transferase deficiency which is X-linked. In the latter case there is often a family history of early death in male infants on the maternal side of the family.

Most infants with metabolic disease are born normally at term. Initially the infant appears in good condition and usually remains well for a number of days. This period of relative well-being is due to a number of factors. Firstly, there is placental protection from the metabolic lesion. The placenta effectively haemodialyses the fetus, preventing the build up of toxic intermediary products. Secondly, the fetus is in an anabolic state and this minimizes flux through amino acid degradative pathways. Finally, the fetus has not been in contact with protein-containing feeds, the digestion of which leads to an unmasking of the metabolic lesion in affected infants. This does not mean that investigation for metabolic disease is not indicated in infants presenting with illness on the first day of life. In some conditions placental protection does not occur. In particular those disorders that have a profound primary effect on the central nervous system, e.g. non-ketotic hyperglycinaemia can cause symptoms *in utero* and lead to severe illness from the moment of birth. Infants with lactic acidosis can cause particular problems with diagnosis in the newborn period and are considered separately (see later).

Clues from the Examination

Physical examination rarely leads to a specific diagnosis in the newborn period. The finding of cataracts should immediately suggest a diagnosis of galactosaemia. Occasionally the characteristic odours associated with maple syrup urine disease or isovaleric acidaemia will be detected, but most neonates who have an offensive odour do not have an underlying metabolic problem and physical examination is usually unhelpful in those disorders presenting acutely in the neonatal period. Usually the clinical picture is one of a rapidly progressing encephalopathy with no localizing features.

Simple "Bedside" Tests

The most useful bedside test is a urine examination for ketones (e.g. acetest or ketostix). The neonate does not produce ketones readily, and a strongly positive result should be followed up immediately by urgent organic acid analysis.

The finding of reducing substances within the urine can lead to a diagnosis of galactosaemia, but this should never be relied upon and if this disorder is suspected a specific screening test for the disorder must be performed as soon as possible. Untreated galactosaemia causes renal tubular disease which can limit the value of testing for reducing substances. Conversely, we have seen a number of severely ill galactosaemic infants who had no reducing substances detected in their urine.

Simple Laboratory Investigations

A whole range of biochemical investigations will be performed as a routine on sick neonates. The anion gap, $(Na + K) - (HCO_3 + Cl)$, can be useful. Usually this will be below 16 mmol/l and a value greatly in excess of 20 mmol/l is strongly suggestive of an organic acidaemia. A patient who is acidotic with a normal anion gap is likely to have renal tubular acidosis or intestinal bicarbonate loss. A full blood count and film can be helpful; infants with propionic acidaemia are often profoundly neutropenic and thrombocytopenic.

Other metabolic disorders can lead to hypocalcaemia or disturbance in liver function and these investigations along with regular acid–base estimations are essential in the investigation of infants suspected to be affected by metabolic disease.

It is good practice to collect and freeze all urine passed by the infant and also to collect a sample of blood for metabolic investigations in any infant about to undergo exchange transfusion for hyperbilirubinaemia.

The Metabolic Screen

Most laboratories will require a sample of urine (5–10 ml) and blood (1–2 ml in a lithium heparin tube) to perform a basic metabolic screen. This should be subsequently augmented by a 5 ml EDTA sample for DNA extraction and storage.

The metabolic laboratory will estimate amino acid concentrations in blood and urine (by various methods) as well as performing urinary organic acid analysis. Blood ammonia should be estimated and a portion of urine kept for orotic acid estimation if ammonia is found to be elevated.

Very occasionally more specialized investigations will be required, e.g. using CSF as the diagnostic fluid, and in this case it is best to discuss the clinical problem with the metabolic unit to ensure that the correct samples are collected.

What to do until the Results are Available

If the child presents with severe encephalopathic symptoms and the possibility of metabolic disease is high the infant should be transferred to a specialized metabolic unit.

In infants who have mild symptoms, protein containing feeds should be discontinued and a dextrose infusion started. Acidosis should be corrected by an infusion of sodium bicarbonate aiming to totally correct the base deficit over 12 h. Hypernatraemia is always a risk in infants with severe acidosis, but if the acidosis is so resistant to treatment dialysis should be considered early.

The most important aspect of management is to try to induce an anabolic state quickly. This can be achieved by high concentrations of dextrose (15–20%) combined with insulin (1 u per 3 g of dextrose, or approximately 0.05 u/kg body weight per hour). It is essential that a large central vein is cannulated as this regimen rapidly damages the vein and vascular access is essential at all times.

If the infant is hyperammonaemic sodium benzoate

250 mg/kg (as a bolus dose over 15 min) should be given IV and followed by an infusion of 250 mg/kg per 24 h. Ammonia nitrogen is diverted from the urea cycle by conjugation to glycine and excreted in the urine as hippurate. This can curb a rapidly rising blood ammonia in an infant with a urea cycle defect or hyperammonaemia from other causes. It is not effective in the anuric infant and other methods of toxin removal need to be employed. If more aggressive measures are indicated these should be performed at the specialist centre. Arteriovenous haemoperfusion is currently the method of choice for toxin removal with peritoneal dialysis reserved for infants in whom vascular access is impossible. Exchange transfusion is useless in the acute management of metabolic disease in the newborn period, producing at best only a very transient effect.

Although a number of disorders are known to have vitamin responsive forms it is no longer justifiable to give infants pharmacological dosages of such vitamins whilst awaiting results. The ready availability of metabolic investigations in most regions should allow for diagnosis to proceed rapidly and be followed by the use of the appropriate vitamin once diagnosis is confirmed.

What to do if the Child is Deteriorating Rapidly and Seems Likely to Die

If death seems inevitable it is vitally important to gather as much information about the child as possible. Autopsy is essential and should be discussed with the parents before the child dies. It is important to collect the appropriate samples to attempt a *post-mortem* diagnosis and this should be discussed with the metabolic unit, again before the actual death of the child. Any urine must be saved, even a few drops can be useful. If no urine is available CSF can be collected and frozen. Blood should be collected, separated and frozen. A skin biopsy should be performed, ideally this should be collected into tissue culture medium, but if none is available sterile saline can be used as long as the sample is transported rapidly to the metabolic laboratory. In only very rare circumstances is biopsy of other organs indicated and the need for muscle or liver biopsy should be discussed with the metabolic unit. If the child is dysmorphic photographs should be taken, including a close up of the facial appearance. Ideally the medical illustration department should be involved as the quality of print from a Polaroid "snap" is rarely good enough to allow a dysmorphic diagnosis to be made. A radiographic skeletal survey is also essential and can provide important clues to diagnosis.

Very occasionally disorders that usually present in a subacute way can cause profound neonatal illness. This is particularly true of lysosomal storage disorders which can present as hydrops fetalis. The investigation of infants with non-immune hydrops fetalis is not complete until these conditions have been considered in the differential diagnosis (Burton 1987).

THE INFANT OR CHILD WITH LACTIC ACIDOSIS

The lactic acidoses present a difficult problem as it is often impossible to distinguish a primary defect in pyruvate metabolism from lactic acidosis secondary to other hypoxic insults. In practice one has to treat the child aggressively for possible underlying causes whilst monitoring blood and urinary lactate levels. Patients with primary defects rarely show any improvement in their biochemistry with supportive therapy, whereas infants with a secondary lactic acidosis will improve as the underlying cause is treated. Often, however, one is faced with no clear distinction and then diagnosis relies on the assay of the enzymes associated with pyruvate metabolism. In many cases no specific diagnosis is made even though the history strongly suggests a primary defect.

Lactic acidosis is the hallmark of mitochondrial dysfunction and an increasing number of disorders have been described reflecting primary pathology in this organelle (Clarke 1992). A child of any age can be affected and disease of any organ produced, although a multisystem presentation is more common in childhood. The defect may involve one of the components of the respiratory transport chain coded for by nuclear DNA or may be due to a mutation within the mitochondrial genome itself. Investigation of patients with suspected mitochondrial disease is highly specialized and requires close cooperation between neurologist, metabolic specialist, pathologist, biochemist and molecular biologist (Tulinius et al 1991).

It is important to remember that blood lactate is extremely sensitive to the method of collection. Venous stasis due to tourniquet or restraint can cause a rapid elevation in blood lactate by 2–5 fold. Fasting, arterial samples are more reliable and children with a level > 2.0 mmol/l should be investigated further. In some disorders the CSF lactate may be considerably elevated when blood lactate is normal or only marginally increased. Such infants with "cerebral" lactic acidosis may have no disturbance of peripheral acid–base balance and it is assumed that their primary defect is limited to the brain. Pyruvate dehydrogenase deficiency, for instance, commonly presents in this way.

The Metabolic Causes of Cardiomyopathy

It is appropriate to consider cardiomyopathy within the group of disorders presenting with lactic acidosis (Table 4.1). It occurs in respiratory transport chain defects where it is associated with lactic acidosis as well as in some of the fatty acid oxidation defects and carnitine deficient states. In infants with *long chain fatty acyl-coA dehydrogenase deficiency (LCAD)*, the cardiac disease is also associated with recurrent episodes of hypoglycaemia, vomiting and encephalopathy. In addition there is usually significant skeletal muscle disease as well as a hypertrophic cardiomyopathy. The enzyme defect can be readily demonstrated in skin fibroblasts. *L-Carnitine* is a small water-soluble amine obtained from the diet and synthesized in the body from the amino acid lysine. It has a critical role in the transfer of fatty acids across the inner mitochondrial membrane. Primary carnitine deficiency is due to a defect in the transport or biosynthesis of the molecule. Because of carnitine's important role in metabolism, such disorders often lead to severe hepatic encephalopathy, cardiomyopathy and skeletal muscle disease (systemic carnitine deficiency). In some patients the defect appears to be limited to the heart or skeletal muscle alone (myopathic carnitine deficiency). Supplementation with L-carnitine can lead to a remarkable improvement in some patients. Secondary carnitine deficiency occurs in organic acid defects and other inborn errors of metabolism where increased acyl-carnitines are excreted in the urine. If defects of carnitine metabolism are suspected detailed metabolic investigation becomes essential and the metabolic laboratory should be contac-

Table 4.1 Some metabolic causes of cardiomyopathy

Fatty acid oxidation defects
  Especially long chain fatty acyl CoA dehydrogenase deficiency

Carnitine deficiency
  Primary
  Secondary

Some organic acid disorders
  e.g. propionic acidaemia

Glycogen storage disease
  Type II (Pompe's disease)
  Type III (Debrancher enzyme deficiency)

Mucopolysaccharidosis
  Type I
  Type VI

Acute hereditary tyrosinaemia

ted about the need for further investigation. Organic acid analysis can be perfectly normal even in children with severe symptoms of primary carnitine deficiency. In secondary carnitine deficiency organic acid analysis will usually reveal the underlying metabolic defect.

Glycogen storage disease type II (Pompe's disease) is a generalized defect resulting in the lysosomal storage of glycogen due to a deficiency of the lysosomal enzyme acid glucosidase. There is profound muscular hypotonia and macroglossia as well as progressive cardiac failure due to cardiac muscle involvement. Hypoglycaemia is not a feature of this type of glycogen storage disease. Affected infants usually die within the first 12 months of life from cardiac failure.

Very rarely some other lysosomal storage disorders result in severe, early onset cardiomyopathy. This has been reported in mucopolysaccharidosis types I (Hurler's syndrome) and VI (Maroteaux-Lamy syndrome). In these children the cardiomyopathy was symptomatic before the other characteristic features of the disorders.

The investigation of children with cardiomyopathy must include a detailed metabolic work-up which should include blood lactate, blood for acid glucosidase assay, total and free carnitine, urine organic acids and glycosaminoglycans. Further detailed enzyme assay may be indicated depending on the results of these preliminary investigations.

THE INFANT WITH AN ACUTE ENCEPHALOPATHY

Encephalopathy is a common presentation of metabolic disease (Table 4.2). In the newborn period it is most often associated with organic acid disorders or urea cycle defects and the investigation of these disorders has been discussed above. In older children encephalopathy can cause a diagnostic conundrum and metabolic conditions must not be forgotten as potential causes of this often devasting neurological disorder.

Children with fatty acid oxidation defects can present with recurrent episodes of encephalopathy or *Reye's syndrome* (see p. 83). The most common defect, medium chain fatty acyl coA dehydrogenase deficiency (MCAD),

Table 4.2 Some metabolic causes of acute encephalopathy

Amino acid disorders
Organic acid defects
Urea cycle defects
Fatty acid oxidation, including MCAD deficiency
Mitochondrial encephalomyopathies

usually presents between the ages of 6 and 24 months. There is often a prodromal illness, usually gastrointestinal, which precipitates metabolic imbalance. A quarter of affected infants will die in the first episode, often as a result of the profound hypoglycaemia associated with the disorder. The biochemical hallmarks of the disease are a poor ketotic response to hypoglycaemia and the excretion of characteristic dicarboxylic acids in the urine, detected on urine organic acid analysis. The pathological clue to diagnosis is the finding of a fatty liver and this condition has been linked to sudden infant death (SIDS) (see below), but the actual number of positive cases has been very small. Unlike many metabolic conditions there is a common genetic mutation responsible for 90% of the abnormal alleles in the Caucasian population. As a result the disorder lends itself to rapid diagnosis by direct DNA analysis and as a result a specimen of blood for DNA extraction (5 ml EDTA) should be collected from all infants suspected of having this disorder.

Late-onset variants of disorders more usually presenting in the newborn period must also be considered in the differential diagnosis of encephalopathy in infancy. In particular, hyperammonaemia due to ornithine carbamoyl transferase deficiency can occur for the first time in older children. This X-linked disorder can manifest in heterozygous females after protein loading or catabolic stress leading to acute encephalopathy and death if not considered as a diagnostic possibility.

What Metabolic Investigations Should be Done in SIDS Patients?

It is likely that metabolic disorders account for no more than 2–3% of all sudden infant deaths. Previous estimates with much higher suggested frequencies are not supported by recent large surveys (Bonham and Downing 1992). There is no doubt, however, that metabolic disorders can lead to an acute severe disturbance in metabolic homeostasis which, if it occurs during a period of additional catabolic stress such as infection, could be rapidly fatal.

Two groups of disorders are particularly prone to present in this way: fatty acid oxidation defects, and disorders of hepatic glycogen metabolism (glycogen storage disease types Ia, Ib and Ic).

Detailed metabolic investigation in all cases of SIDS cannot be justified and a selective approach to diagnosis is suggested (Table 4.3). It is important that all infants are examined post-mortem by an experienced paediatric pathologist. The significance of potentially informative findings, e.g. hepatic fatty change or excess glycogen deposition in liver or muscle, may not be appreciated by

Table 4.3 A protocol for investigation of sudden infant death syndrome

Propositus	
Blood	5–10 ml; separate plasma and freeze at −20°C
Urine or CSF	For amino and organic acid investigations; freeze at −20°C
Skin biopsy	
Needle liver biopsy	Liquid nitrogen, dry ice or freeze at −20°C
Subsequent siblings	
Urine	For organic acids
DNA analysis	For MCAD mutation (parents and siblings)

colleagues with little knowledge of the pathology of inborn errors of metabolism. Very detailed metabolic investigation is justified in infants with suggestive pathological findings, parental consanguinity, or previous unexplained death of a sibling, or who present outside the common age range for SIDS (i.e. < 1 or > 9 months of age).

Of course one cannot wait for the results of necropsy before collecting the appropriate samples for biochemical investigation and it is suggested that a routine is followed in all cases, but that not all of the samples are referred for further study. It is important to liaise closely with the metabolic laboratory if there is uncertainty about which samples to send. As a routine, blood (5–10 ml) should be collected and the plasma separated and frozen at −20°C. Any available urine should be frozen at the same temperature, if urine is not available CSF should be obtained by cisternal puncture and treated in the same way. A full thickness skin biopsy (1–2 mm × 1–2 mm) should be obtained after thorough cleaning of the skin with spirit. The chance of bacterial contamination increases rapidly after death and in infants who present > 12 h after death a small piece of fascia may grow more successfully. This can be taken at *post-mortem*. Finally, a needle liver biopsy specimen should be snap frozen in liquid nitrogen or dry ice. Usually the latter are not readily available and the only compromise in these circumstances is to place the biopsy specimen in the −20°C fridge immediately.

Subsequent siblings should be examined for evidence of metabolic disease in the newborn period. Urine should be sent for organic acid analysis, but a negative result does not exclude a disorder of fat oxidation. Most centres would also look for evidence of the common MCAD mutation in the parents and siblings, although the diagnostic yield is small.

THE CHILD WITH ISOLATED GLOBAL LEARNING DIFFICULTY

Metabolic disease very rarely leads to global learning difficulty alone. Screening laboratories receive many samples from patients with either "developmental delay" or "epilepsy" as the only clinical finding. The diagnostic pick-up rate in these particular groups is extremely small and either condition alone barely justifies metabolic screening.

Sometimes, however, the learning disorder may be apparent before other physical signs appear. For instance, *homocystinuria* due to cystathionine synthase deficiency can present with developmental problems alone, before the onset of lens dislocation and the marfanoid habitus make the diagnosis clinically obvious.

Depending on the country of birth, children may not have been screened for phenylketonuria in the newborn period and may present with developmental delay in infancy. *Maternal phenylketonuria* should always be considered in families where a number of siblings have global learning difficulty. A number of women with phenylketonuria avoid the devastating neurological damage associated with the untreated disorder and are diagnosed after having children affected by the teratogenic influence of phenylalanine in pregnancy. In some cases the women may have been on diet in childhood which has been relaxed in teenage years, but more commonly they have been born before the introduction of newborn screening programmes and have thus remained undetected within the community. A strict low phenylalanine diet from before conception is necessary to prevent fetal damage in this disorder.

Infants with *biotinidase deficiency* can present with a seizure disorder which is refractory to anticonvulsant treatment and in some patients mimics infantile spasms. The biochemical defect is due to a failure to release dietary protein-bound biotin as well as an inability to recycle endogenous biotin. Biotin is a water soluble B complex vitamin which has an essential co-factor role in the activities of four carboxylase enzymes necessary for gluconeogenesis, fatty acid metabolism and amino acid catabolism. Affected infants produce a characteristic organic aciduria and the enzyme defect can be readily demonstrated in serum. Untreated the disorder leads to severe learning difficulty, seizures, optic atrophy, sensorineural deafness, alopecia and conjunctivitis. Treatment with biotin 5–20 mg/day rapidly reverses most of the abnormalities, although in the late-diagnosed case recovery may not be complete. In-keeping with other vitamin-responsive disorders, the mother should be given the vitamin in subsequent pregnancies to treat the fetus prenatally.

Boys affected by *Lesch–Nyhan syndrome*, a disorder caused by a deficiency of hypoxanthine guanine phosphoribosyl transferase, usually present in the first 6 months of life with developmental delay. The choreiform movement disorder follows after a variable interval, but is usually present by the age of 2 years. The characteristic self-mutilation is usually present by the age of 4 years, but can occur considerably later. The combination of the dystonia, athetosis and self-injury make the diagnosis obvious but diagnosis can be delayed in those boys who present these characteristic features at a late age. This disorder is another of the few metabolic disorders inherited in an X-linked manner.

Mucopolysaccharidosis type III (Sanfilippo syndrome) presents with developmental delay. The mild somatic features associated with this variant result in diagnosis being considerably delayed when compared with other mucopolysaccharidoses. Often families have had two or more affected children before the diagnosis is established. Typically the developmental problems are associated with middle ear disease due to serous otitis media, sleep disturbance and often a tendency to diarrhoea. The disorder evolves into one of profound behavioural disturbance with neurodegeneration at which time the diagnosis is usually established. Very rarely, infants with disorders that usually present with encephalopathy in the newborn period avoid the acute neonatal presentation. This is most often seen in infants with *vitamin responsive organic acid defects*. Affected children fail to thrive and are often developmentally delayed. The diagnosis comes to light usually as a result of routine screening of such patients or because the infant suddenly becomes encephalopathic secondary to intercurrent infection.

As a routine, therefore, uric acid, urine amino and organic acids plus urine glycosaminoglycans are indicated in the investigation of children with global learning difficulty and in some children with epilepsy. It is difficult to justify detailed lysosomal enzyme studies in children with these features alone.

NEURODEGENERATIVE DISEASE

Many metabolic disorders present in a subacute way. After a period of normal development, progress slows, plateaus and then deteriorates. A history which includes loss of skills is always of ominous significance, and in these children detailed metabolic investigation is indicated. The majority of the metabolic neurodegenerative disorders are associated with abnormal lysosomal storage, but there are a few important exceptions that need to be remembered as the manner of investigation differs.

Canavan's disease is a progressive degenerative disease of cerebral white matter which presents in infancy with progressive enlargement of the head, spasticity, dementia and optic atrophy. The pathological hallmark of the disease is a spongiform leukodystrophy with grossly swollen astrocytes. Recently affected patients have been shown to excrete increased amounts of N-acetylaspartic acid in their urine and have a deficiency of the enzyme aspartylacylase in skin fibroblasts. The relationship between the biochemical abnormalities and the neuropathology is uncertain, but the former offer an opportunity for accurate pre- and post-natal diagnosis. In infants suspected of having this disorder, urinary organic acids should be requested with the additional information that Canavan's disease needs to be excluded.

A number of *other organic acid defects* can present with a neurodegenerative course. A variant of methylglutaconic aciduria produces basal ganglia disease, optic atrophy, sensorineural deafness and a progressive loss of skills leading to death in early childhood. Organic acid analysis should be part of the routine investigation of patients with neurodegeneration.

The *lysosomal storage disorders* are the commonest metabolic disorders to present in this way. In some disorders associated clinical features allow the clinician to predict the diagnosis, e.g. mucopolysaccharidoses or mucolipidoses. For other disorders the presentation is one of neurodegeneration alone and, although one can attempt to predict the diagnosis and test selectively, most metabolic laboratories perform a lysosomal enzyme screen (Table 4.4). In this way a large range of conditions can be excluded on a single sample of blood (5 ml EDTA tube). This should be supplemented by other tests as

appropriate, e.g. urinary oligosaccharides or glycosaminoglycans.

There are two other clinical situations which lead to frequent contact with the metabolic laboratory: "coarse" facial appearance and hepatosplenomegaly.

The Metabolic Investigation of the Child with a "Coarse" Facial Appearance

The mucopolysaccharidoses are associated with a characteristic facial appearance which is usually described as "coarse", although this is a term most parents find offensive. Typically there is a retroussé nose, large mouth and tongue and an increased head circumference with frontal bossing. A persistent nasal discharge is often an additional unattractive finding. The hair is thick in texture and patients are often hirsuite with a synophrys. When fully developed the appearance is so characteristic that it is immediately identified by the majority of clinicians. In younger children the signs can be subtle. It is important to remember that the facial phenotype evolves slowly with time. A "coarse" facial appearance at birth is not due to a mucopolysaccharidosis; it strongly suggests a diagnosis of either GM1-gangliosidosis or mucolipidosis II (I-cell disease). In addition there are a number of lysosomal storage disorders that produce a similar phenotype. The glycoproteinoses, mannosidosis and fucosidosis are associated with a mild "Hurler phenotype" with "coarse" facies, hepatosplenomegaly, bone dysplasia and variable mental retardation. Other less common disorders which are occasionally confused with mucopolysaccharidoses include aspartylglycosaminuria, sialic acid storage disease and mucolipidosis III. The first step in the differentiation of these conditions is urine analysis for oligosaccharide and glycosaminoglycan excretion. Abnormalities are then followed up with specific enzyme assay. A number of non-lysosomal conditions have caused difficulty in differential diagnosis. These include hypothyroidism, Soto's syndrome, William's syndrome, Coffin–Lowry syndrome and geleophysic dysplasia.

If initial investigations are normal, but a storage disorder is still strongly suspected a number of other procedures may help in diagnosis. Radiological investigations can be extremely helpful. The skeletal dysplasia associated with lysosomal storage disease, dysostosis multiplex, is very characteristic. The most useful X-rays are a lateral skull, lateral thoracolumbar spine, hips, pelvis and metacarpals (Figure 4.1). The characteristic abnormalities include expansion of the sella turcica (J-shaped sella), anterior beaking of the vertebral

Table 4.4 A lysosomal enzyme screen (assays performed on leukocytes unless otherwise stated)

Plasma β-hexosaminidase (Sandhoff's disease)
Plasma acid phosphatase (ACP deficiency)
Plasma β-mannosidase (β-mannosidosis)
Plasma MUGS (Tay–Sach's disease)
β-Glucuronidase (Sly's disease)
β-Galactosidase (GM1-gangliosidosis)
α-Mannosidase (α-mannosidosis)
α-Galactosidase (Fabry's disease)
α-Fucosidase (fucosidosis)
Acid esterase (Wolman's disease)
Aryl sulphatase A (metachromatic leucodystrophy)
β-Glucosidase (Gaucher's disease)
Sphingomyelinase (Niemann–Pick disease types A and B)
β-Galactocerebrosidase (Krabbe's leucodystrophy)
α-N-Acetylgalactosaminidase (Schindler's disease)

The 15 assays are performed on the material obtained from a single 5-ml sample of blood collected into an EDTA tube and transported by first-class post.

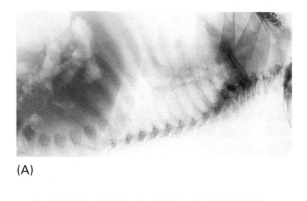

(A)

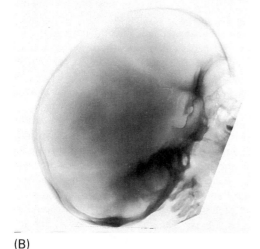

(B)

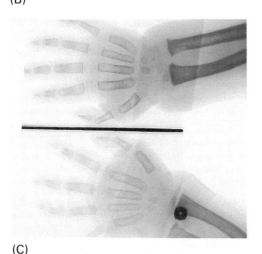

(C)

Figure 4.1   Dysostosis multiplex in a child of 18 months with Hurler's syndrome. (A) Lateral thoracolumbar spine showing characteristic hooked vertebrae. (B) Skull showing scaphiocephalic appearance with enlargement of the sella turcica. (C) Hands showing proximal pointing of the metacarpals.

bodies and pointing of the proximal end of the metacarpals. Dysostosis multiplex is often considered diagnostic of the mucopolysaccharidoses, but this is not so, the findings are non-specific and are found in a number of other lysosomal storage disorders. Occasionally a blood film can be helpful. Inclusions within the white blood cells are a feature of some of the mucopolysaccharidoses, whereas vacuolation of the lymphocytes is common in mucolipidoses and mannosidosis. Bone marrow examination may be even more productive in revealing storage phenomena. If all these investigations are normal and storage is still considered to be a possible diagnosis, biopsy is indicated. A skin biopsy, taken under local anaesthetic, should be divided and one part set up in culture (for subsequent enzyme studies). The remaining portion should be examined under the electron microscope where characteristic lysosomal distension is usually obvious and diagnostic of lysosomal storage disease.

The Child with a Large Liver and Spleen

The majority of children with hepatosplenomegaly do not have a metabolic disorder (see Chapters 1 and 8). Hepatosplenomegaly is a feature of a number of lysosomal storage disorders, it is *not* a feature of glycogen storage disease. In many cases the organomegaly is only one part of a characteristic phenotype, e.g. in the mucopolysaccharidoses and diagnosis is usually not in doubt. Occasionally enlargement of the liver and spleen may be the presenting feature of the metabolic disturbance and this is seen most commonly in non-neuronopathic Niemann–Pick and Gaucher's disease. Typically in storage disorders the liver and spleen are firm with easily defined edges. In some cases the enlargement may be massive and fill the whole abdomen. Vacuolated lymphocytes in the peripheral blood and foam cells in the bone marrow are characteristic of Niemann–Pick disease. In Gaucher's disease there is often associated hypersplenism and the characteristic Gaucher cell is seen in bone marrow aspirates. Lysosomal enzyme studies are indicated in these patients to confirm diagnosis.

Patients with the hepatic forms of glycogen storage disease (types I, III, VI and IX) present with hepatomegaly alone. The liver may be massively enlarged, but is very soft in consistency, often making it difficult to define the edge clearly. It may extend right across the abdomen, particularly in types I and III and is often confused for hepatosplenomegaly rather than gross hepatomegaly alone. If there is doubt an ultrasound examination usually quickly resolves any dilemma. Patients with glycogen storage disease types I and III usually have associated hypoglycaemia and other metabolic disturbance, whereas in types VI and IX isolated hepatomegaly in an otherwise well child is the usual mode of presentation. The biochemical confirmation of a suspected case of glycogen storage disease should be discussed with the metabolic laboratory, although there are a number of screening tests (e.g. glucose tolerance test, and glucagon stimulation test) helpful in diagnosis.

THE DYSMORPHIC CHILD

Many inborn errors of metabolism are associated with dysmorphic manifestations and a metabolic work-up should be considered in any undiagnosed infant with multiple congenital anomalies or dysmorphic appearance (Clayton and Thompson 1988). Dysfunction in a wide range of metabolic pathways can interfere with embryogenesis. The basic mechanism in some cases appears to be a direct teratogenic effect of toxic intermediary compounds, whilst in others interference with fetal energy metabolism is responsible. For many, however, the relationship between the biochemical defect and the anomalies associated with it remains obscure.

In one variant of glutaric aciduria type II (multiple acyl-CoA dehydrogenase deficiency) congenital anomalies have included a "Potter's-like" facial appearance, polycystic kidneys, cerebral dysplasia and abnormalities of the genitalia and anterior abdominal wall. In addition severe hypoglycaemia and acidosis lead to death in the first week of life in affected infants.

3-Hydroxyisobutyryl CoA deacylase deficiency and 3-hydroxyisobutyric aciduria are disorders of valine metabolism in which it is thought that the accumulation of a teratogenic intermediary compound leads to congenital malformation. The reported defects include cerebral dysgenesis due to defects in neuronal migration.

Agenesis of the corpus callosum is found frequently in infants with non-ketotic hyperglycinaemia. The underlying mechanism behind the association is obscure, but the biochemical defect is known to be based in the CNS. Infants with this particular neurological finding must be screened closely for non-ketotic hyperglycinaemia. Glycine is considerably elevated in body fluids, particularly in cerebrospinal fluid and the ratio of plasma to CSF glycine is usually diagnostic (between 5 : 1 and 10 : 1, as opposed to the normal 35 : 1).

Disorders of peroxisomal metabolism can also produce characteristic dysmorphic features which are present at birth (unlike the majority of lysosomal storage defects), indicating a prenatal onset of insult (Theil et al 1992). Peroxisomes are small ovoid or round organelles found in most mammalian cells. They are slightly smaller than mitochondria and have a single limiting membrane. Biochemical function includes plasmalogen biosynthesis, β-oxidation of very long chain fatty acids (VLCFAs), and glyoxylate catabolism. A number of well-recognized syndromes are associated with defects in this organelle. In some instances the biochemical defect is due to a failure to manufacture peroxisomes (biogenesis), and in others individual enzymes are defective. In Zellweger's syndrome the organelle is virtually absent and the clinical picture is dominated by severe neurological dysfunction characterized by profound hypotonia. In addition, the facial appearance is characteristic with large open fontanelles, flat occiput, epicanthic folds and a high forehead. The liver is enlarged and macrogyria and polymicrogyria are common CNS findings. X-ray examination of the knee reveals stippled epiphyses.

In rhizomelic chondrodysplasia punctata the punctate epiphyseal changes are associated with severe proximal shortening of the limbs. In addition, the forehead is prominent, the nasal bridge is flat and there is often malar hypoplasia and cataracts. The biochemical defect includes a deficiency in plasmalogen biosynthesis and a defect in phytanic acid oxidation. Many other peroxisomal disorders have been described, some of which have similar dysmorphology to that outlined above. These conditions must be considered in the differential diagnosis of the dysmorphic infant. To screen for peroxisomal disorders a combination of tests aimed at assessing the function of two peroxisomal pathways is usually performed. Plasma levels of VLCFAs give a crude indication of fatty acid oxidation and assay of the enzyme dihydroxyacetonephosphate acyl transferase (DHAP-AT) assesses plasmalogen synthesis. Both these investigations can be performed on a single 5-ml sample of blood (EDTA tube). More detailed investigation of peroxisomal function may be necessary in certain cases, and this should be discussed with the metabolic laboratory.

REFERENCES

Bonham JR, Downing M (1992) Metabolic deficiencies and SIDS. *J Clin Pathol* 45 (Suppl): 33–38.

Burton BK (1987) Inborn errors of metabolism: the clinical diagnosis in early infancy. *Pediatrics* 79: 359–369.

Clarke LA (1992) Mitochondrial disorders in pediatrics. *Pediatr Clin N Am* 39: 319–334.

Clayton PT, Thompson E (1988) Dysmorphic syndromes with demonstrable biochemical abnormalities. *J Med Genet* 25: 463–472.

Cleary MA, Wraith JE (1991) Antenatal diagnosis of inborn errors of metabolism. *Arch Dis Child* 66: 816–822.

Green A (1989) Guide to diagnosis of inborn errors of metabolism in district general hospitals. *J Clin Pathol* 42: 84–91.

Theil AC, Schutgens RBH, Wanders RJA et al (1992) Clinical recognition of patients affected by a peroxisomal disorder: a retrospective study in 40 patients. *Eur J Paediatr* **151**: 117–120.

Tulinius MH, Holme M, Kristiansson B et al (1991) Mitochondrial encephalomyopathies in childhood. I. Biochemical and morphological investigations. *J Paediatr* **119**: 242–250.

5
Clinical Chemistry

A Green

INTRODUCTION

With the exception of specialist metabolic, endocrine, toxicological and immunological investigations (see Chapters 3, 4 and 12), the clinical chemistry investigations undertaken in infants and children at most acute district hospitals are usually carried out by a non-specialist general clinical chemistry department which serves the whole unit. Such departments may ideally have a biochemist with a special interest in paediatric clinical chemistry and, hopefully, be a point of contact for the paediatricians. Paediatrics has different requirements for clinical chemistry compared with adult medicine and the laboratory needs to be aware of these needs and provide accordingly. Frequent dialogue between laboratory and paediatricians is important if the best possible service is to be obtained.

Test Repertoire and Service Provision

With modern instrumentation most laboratories are now able to carry out a range of the most commonly requested biochemical tests on very small specimen volumes, i.e. 500 μl whole blood. However, special care needs to be taken when processing small volume specimens to minimize risk of evaporation, and methodologies provided should be those which are least likely to be interfered with by bilirubin, haemoglobin and lipids. The concentration of an analyte in a 100 μl plasma specimen left uncovered for 1 h may change by as much as 10%. For certain assays, methodologies must be chosen carefully to provide the required level of sensitivity (e.g. plasma creatinine at the lower end of the normal range for infants or young children) and linearity at high concentrations (e.g. bilirubin). Blood for bilirubin measurement should be protected from light.

Although capillary specimens can be used for several analytes it is important to remember the limitations of such specimens. Large volumes (i.e. in excess of 2 ml whole blood) are best taken as a venous specimen and for some analytes venous blood is preferred as there are significant differences from the concentration in capillary blood, e.g. potassium concentration in capillary blood is on average 1.0–1.5 mmol/l higher than that in venous blood, although greater discrepancies can occur even without visible haemolysis. Results from badly collected specimens will reflect release of electrolytes from red cells, especially potassium and magnesium, and dilution with tissue fluid, e.g. low albumin or sodium. Sweat contamination may produce "abnormal" ammonia and amino acid results.

It is important to remember that older children may actually prefer venepuncture, especially if a large number of investigations are required on a single blood specimen. Capillary collections should certainly not be undertaken in patients who are known to be, or are at high risk of being, hepatitis B or HIV positive.

Analytes which are possible on capillary blood and which should be available in most laboratories are listed in Table 5.1.

Table 5.1 Clinical chemistry analytes usually available on blood obtained by capillary puncture

Alanine aminotransferase	γ-Glutamyl transpeptidase
Albumin	Glucose
Alkaline phosphatase	Hydrogen ion (pH)*
Aspartate aminotransferase	Osmolality
Bicarbonate	$p\text{CO}_2$*
Bilirubin (total and direct/ conjugated)	Phosphate
Calcium	Potassium
Chloride	Sodium
Cholesterol	Total protein
Creatinine	Urea

*Special collection tube required.

All specimens must be accompanied by full patient information data; age or date of birth is particularly important as reference ranges may be very different. Provision of clinical information and the particular reason for a request will enable the clinical biochemist to interpret results correctly and the clinician will get the best out of the service.

Extra-Laboratory Equipment

Units with a special care baby unit or high dependency unit will require on-site monitoring of acid–base/blood gases, and require rapid turnaround for sodium, potassium, glucose, calcium and bilirubin.

Provision of equipment within such units or in a nearby side room should be the responsibility of the laboratory. Quality assurance, training of designated staff, maintenance and troubleshooting are vital functions best performed by the laboratory to ensure reliable and safe working practices.

Reference Ranges

Reference range data are difficult to obtain for neonates, infants and children. The variables which affect reference ranges include the population (e.g. genetic background), well/sick, diet, the conditions of the subjects at the time of sampling (e.g. fasting), the type and handling of specimen collected, and the analytical method used. It is likely that your local laboratory has not been able to obtain its own reference data and will rely on data produced by others.

If a series of results for a particular patient has been obtained from more than one laboratory it is important to check for comparability of reference ranges. The "apparent" change in concentration of an analyte can be misleading if this is not appreciated. Particular examples of this problem are for enzymes, e.g. alkaline phosphatase and creatine kinase. The data given in the Appendix to this chapter have been found by the author to be relevant for methods commonly in current usage. However, they will *not* be valid for some laboratories, so care must be exercised in their use.

NEONATAL SCREENING

All babies in the UK are offered screening for phenylketonuria (PKU) and congenital hypothyroidism at around 6–10 days of age. The tests (phenylalanine and TSH) are performed on blood obtained by capillary puncture of the heel. Most babies are tested in the home by the midwife/health visitor. Those babies in hospital, particularly those on special care units need to be tested and mechanisms should be set up to ensure that they are not missed. If the baby is not on full milk, testing should not be deferred although it will be important to re-test for PKU when feeding has been fully established.

In some parts of the UK testing for sickle cell disorders and cystic fibrosis is also undertaken using the same specimen.

Phenylketonuria

Cases of PKU should be referred to a paediatrician/metabolic team with particular expertise in management. Dietary treatment requires frequent monitoring of plasma phenylalanine and strict control to maintain plasma concentrations in the recommended range report of the MRC Working Party (1993).

Approximately 1–3% of hyperphenylalaninaemia is caused by defects in the synthesis or metabolism of tetrahydrobiopterin, a cofactor for phenylalanine hydroxylase. The diagnosis requires measurement of blood dehydropteridine reductase and blood/plasma pterins.

Congenital Hypothyroidism

See Chapter 3.

SODIUM, POTASSIUM AND OSMOLALITY

Sodium and potassium are commonly measured by specific ion-selective electrodes (ISE). The "older" method of flame photometry is less likely to be available. Although most methods compare well and give similar results, significant differences can occur between direct and indirect reading ISE systems for sodium measurement. This is particularly likely if ward-based instruments are used. Such instruments should never be introduced into extra-laboratory areas without laboratory involvement as comparisons with the main laboratory analyser will be required.

If your patient has an unexpected sodium result – contact your laboratory to discuss.

Sodium

A normal plasma sodium concentration is compatible with either salt depletion or overload if there are associated changes in body water.

Postoperative *hyponatraemia* (Table 5.2) is frequently dilutional secondary to excess water retention. Young infants with renal immaturity are at particular risk of hyponatraemia as they are unable to retain sodium as efficiently as older children and may require sodium administration.

An artefactually low plasma sodium may result from the hyperlipidaemia associated with intravenous lipid administration or endogenous primary or secondary hyperlipidaemia. This "pseudohyponatraemia" can be confirmed by measurement of sodium using a direct ion selective electrode analyser.

Hypernatraemia (Table 5.3) nearly always occurs with associated fluid loss. It rarely occurs due to high solute load.

Iatrogenic hypo- or hyper-natraemia, i.e. inappropriate intravenous replacement, should always be considered in the differential diagnosis.

Potassium

Plasma should always be separated from red cells as promptly as possible as delays can cause leakage of potassium from the red cells and an artificially elevated plasma level. Analysis of haemolysed specimens should be avoided and a repeat specimen requested. Capillary blood even without visual haemylosis may have an artificially elevated potassium concentration and true deficiency may be masked.

Hypokalaemia is usually the result of potassium depletion. It can occur without depletion if there is shift into the cells as happens in alkalotic states (Table 5.4).

Hyperkalaemia occurs mainly as a result of renal failure or after severe trauma (Table 5.5).

Urine Sodium and Potassium

There is no "normal" range for sodium and potassium excretion – output depends on state of hydration, dietary

Table 5.2 Causes of hyponatraemia

Sodium depletion	Gastrointestinal tract loss
	Renal loss:
	    Renal tubular dysfunction
	    Diuretics
	Adrenal cortical insufficiency:
	    Inappropriate ADH
	    Cystic fibrosis

Water excess	Excess hypotonic intravenous fluids
Pseudohyponatraemia (artefact)	Contamination (intravenous fluids) Hyperlipidaemia Hyperproteinaemia Hyperglycaemia

Table 5.3 Causes of hypernatraemia

Water deficit	Diarrhoea (low sodium) Diabetes insipidus Insensible water loss, e.g. overhead heater Fluid deprivation/starvation
Sodium excess	High solute diet Sodium bicarbonate administration Use of saline as emetic Child abuse – salt administration

Table 5.4 Causes of hypokalaemia

Excess loss	Gastrointestinal losses Renal tubular defect/diuretics Adrenocortical excess
Inadequate intake	
Redistribution	Glucose/insulin Alkalosis
Iatrogenic	Glucose/insulin

Table 5.5 Causes of hyperkalaemia

Failure of renal secretion	Renal failure Adrenal insufficiency
Excess intake	Excess therapy
Redistribution	Acidosis Diabetes
Tissue injury/cell death	Hypoxia Catabolism Tumour lysis Dehydration Trauma/bruising Haemorrhage
Iatrogenic	Exchange transfusion
Pseudohyperkalaemia	Delay in plasma separation Haemolysis Capillary blood specimen

intake and gastrointestinal tract losses. There is excessive sodium excretion in preterm neonates, particularly in the first 2 weeks of life. Highest levels are seen in the most immature infants in the first week. Isolated values as concentrations in a random urine are of little use except when extremely high or low values are obtained. The urinary sodium/potassium ratio is about 1.0 in full-term neonates. In the face of an abnormally low plasma concentration a urinary potassium greater than 20 mmol/l suggests a renal cause. In hyponatraemic states the expected response is a urine sodium < 10 mmol/l.

Concentrations are more usually expressed as a ratio to potassium or for sodium (Na) as a per cent fractional excretion (FE-Na). For measurement of FE-Na collect a random urine as close as possible to a blood specimen and measure both sodium and creatinine in both plasma and urine.

$$\text{FE-Na}\ (\%) = \frac{\text{Urinary Na}}{\text{Plasma Na}} \times \frac{\text{Plasma creatinine} \times 100}{\text{Urine creatinine}}$$

Note: all concentrations must be in mmol/l.

Osmolality

Measurement of urine and plasma osmolality is performed manually and is not part of the repertoire of automated clinical chemistry analysers. Measurement of plasma osmolality should be restricted to those situations where its value adds to measurement of individual plasma electrolytes. The major contributor to plasma osmolality is sodium and its associated anions (Table 5.6).

Table 5.6   Contribution to plasma osmolality

	Analyte concentration (mmol/l)	Osmolality (mmol/l)
Sodium	135	135
Potassium	4	4
Calcium (ionized)	2.5 (1.25)	1.25
Magnesium	0.75	0.75
Urea	5	5
Glucose	4	4
Chloride, bicarbonate and other associated anions of		141
Protein	65 g/l	≃ 1
Total		292

An approximate rule-of-thumb is that plasma osmolality mmol/l = plasma concentration (sodium and potassium) × 2 plus 10 mmol/l, assuming glucose and urea concentrations are normal. A major discrepancy between this calculated value and measured osmolality suggests the presence of exogenous molecules such as prescribed drugs (e.g. mannitol), poisoning, or contrast media.

Urine Osmolality

Infants above 1 month of age should be able to concentrate urine above 800 mosmol/kg provided they are on a normal solute intake.

Collection of an early morning urine after a dry supper and no fluids overnight enables assessment of the urinary concentrating ability. A result > 870 mosmol/kg confirms that the pituitary secretion of ADH and response by the kidney are normal. Inability to concentrate to this degree after overnight fluid restriction suggests the need for a more formal water deprivation test. This test is potentially dangerous and must be performed under close medical supervision (see p. 40).

ACID–BASE STATUS AND BLOOD GASES

Causes of Acid–Base Disturbances

Acid–base disturbances may arise from respiratory or non-respiratory causes, or a combination of both. The neonate is particularly vulnerable to acidosis because of the relative immaturity of the organ systems. Respiratory inadequacy is exacerbated if there is superimposed organ failure, e.g. congenital renal disease, or if accompanied by poor perfusion.

Acidosis due to respiratory and non-respiratory causes are shown in Tables 5.7 and 5.8.

Table 5.7   Some causes of respiratory acidosis

Neonate	Intrapartum asphyxia
	Prematurity
	Drugs (maternal analgesics, sedatives, anaesthetics)
	Trauma to CNS
	Congenital abnormalities
	Anaemia
	Primary muscle disease
Infant	Upper airway disease
	Bronchitis
	Asthma
	Pneumonia

Table 5.8 Metabolic causes of acidosis

Hypoxia	
Hypoperfusion	Hypothermia Poor cardiac output Infection
Renal dysfunction	↓ GFR (e.g. prematurity) Tubular defect
Over-production/ administration of acid	Inherited metabolic disorder Diabetes mellitus Poisoning, e.g. salicylate
Bicarbonate loss – G.I. tract	Gastroenteritis

Alkalosis is most likely to be iatrogenic caused by over-ventilation or bicarbonate therapy; other causes are included in Table 5.9.

Acid–Base Blood Gas Measurement

For intensive care, particularly of the preterm neonate, it is essential to have rapidly available pH and blood gas analyses. The quality of specimens for these analyses is paramount. The best specimen is arterial, collected through an indwelling catheter. Capillary blood, if collected properly from a well perfused limb, can be useful for pH and pCO_2 measurement; but is *not* suitable for pO_2. Capillary blood must be collected into special heparinized tubes, taking great care not to trap air bubbles. If the blood-gas analyser is on a remote site, the blood should be transported on ice (see p. 91).

pO_2

The best way to ensure that excessive oxygen tensions are avoided is to provide continuous pO_2 measurement. This can be done by providing a continuous recording pO_2 electrode attached to an indwelling catheter or by transcutaneous measurement.

Transcutaneous pO_2 ($TcpO_2$) electrodes are useful particularly in neonates because the skin is thin and permeable. They must, however, be checked regularly for accuracy by comparing with arterial specimens collected from an indwelling catheter.

If the baby is shocked or poorly perfused, reliable $TcpO_2$ will be impossible. Measurement is also not reliable in infants with thicker skin and subcutaneous tissue. The electrode is heated to 43°C and great care must be taken, particularly in the preterm baby, to avoid burns.

Monitoring of Oxygen Saturation (Oximetry)

98% of oxygen is carried by haemoglobin as oxygenated haemoglobin with the remaining 2% transported physically dissolved in the blood. The release of oxygen to tissues is determined by the oxygen tension (pO_2) and the ability of oxygen to be released from oxyhaemoglobin.

Direct measurement of the percentage of haemoglobin able to transport oxygen (sO_2) provides an indication of the adequacy of oxygen being carried. sO_2 is normally approximately 96–98%. Measurement of oxygen saturation can be useful as an additional parameter to pO_2.

Factors influencing sO_2 are the oxygen tension (pO_2), pH, pCO_2, temperature and haemoglobin concentration and composition (i.e. fetal, carboxy, Met etc.). Tissue oxygen supply will be compromised if sO_2 is < 80%; sO_2 measurements are useful to decrease risk of hypoxia and optimise treatment, i.e. transfusion needs, cardiac output, ventilation needs.

Measurements of sO_2 is undertaken either by "Pulse" oximetry at the bedside (uses a light emitting probe attached to a hand or foot) or by direct measurement in a blood sample (co-oximetry).

Table 5.9 Acid base disturbances

	pH	[H+]	pCO_2	HCO_3^-	
Respiratory acidosis	↓	↑	↑	N/↑	Hypoventilation
Metabolic acidosis	↓	↑	N/↓	↓	Hypoperfusion Renal impairment GI tract loss bicarb Inh.Metab.Disease
Respiratory alkalosis	↑	↓	↓	N/↓	Over-ventilation Hyperammonaemia
Metabolic alkalosis	↑	↓	N/↑	↑	Bicarb.admin Pyloric stenosis Hypokalaemia

Table 5.10   Differential diagnosis of metabolic acidosis.

Cause	Supporting biochemical evidence
Hypoxia/poor tissue perfusion	↑ Anion gap, ↑ Blood lactate
Renal – Glomerular failure	n/↑ plasma creatinine ↑ plasma chloride
– Tubular dysfunction	Anion gap normal N/↑ Urine pH
Gastrointestinal	Normal anion gap
Excessive acid production/administration	↑ Anion gap* ketonuria
Inherited metabolic disorder	Hypoglycaemia, hyperammonaemia
Diabetes mellitus	Hyperglycaemia
Salicylate poisoning	Initially a respiratory alkalosis

↑, increased
*The anion gap is calculated as shown below and is normally < 20 mmol/l
$([Na^+] + [K^+]) - ([Cl^-] + HCO_3^-])$

sO_2 can be approximated by a blood gas analyser if the haemoglobin concentration is known and assuming *normal* proportions of Hb derivatives. This can be misleading however if these assumptions are not true. Co-oximetry will measure Hb and derivatives and calculate sO_2, and provide a more accurate assessment of the oxygen content of blood.

Intravascular pO_2 Electrodes

Umbilical artery catheters which have an "inbuilt" pO_2 electrode in their tip can be useful to provide continuous pO_2 whilst the catheter remains in situ. It is necessary to calibrate against directly measured pO_2.

pCO_2

Normal pCO_2 is 4.5–6.0 kPa. A low level, due to over-ventilation, may be an important clue to a primary metabolic acidosis (see below). Increased pCO_2 is usually due to hypoventilation.

Metabolic Acidosis

Metabolic acidosis (Table 5.10) is evident from a low plasma bicarbonate, a low pCO_2 and a low pH (↑ [H$^+$]). Metabolic acidosis is most often secondary to disorders producing hypoxia or poor tissue perfusion with lactic acid accumulation. Differential diagnosis of lactic acidosis is considered in Chapter 4 (see p. 63). Renal tubular acidosis (proximal or distal) may be suspected from an associated hyperchloraemia and alkaline urine (i.e. pH > 6.5) (see Chapter 6).

It is important to consider inborn errors of metabolism if there is unexplained or particularly severe metabolic acidosis and investigate accordingly (see Chapter 3).

PARENTERAL NUTRITION

Intravenous feeding is now widely used in the extremely preterm or low-birth-weight infant. The term neonate/infant may be fed parenterally if there is compromised gastrointestinal function. In older children, parenteral nutrition may be used if enteral feeding alone cannot maintain adequate nutrition.

Many metabolic complications have been associated with parenteral nutrition (Table 5.11) and as a result regimes have been developed to take account of the differing needs for the preterm and term baby. Neonates, particularly if preterm, are at risk of developing biochemical abnormalities and monitoring should be geared to identifying these problems.

Table 5.11   Metabolic complications of parenteral nutrition in neonates/infants

Common findings
Sodium depletion*
Potassium depletion*
Hyperglycaemia*
Glycosuria*
Jaundice*
Hypophosphataemia*
Metabolic acidosis
Calcium depletion

Less common problems
Hyperphenylalaninaemia (± tyrosine)*
Hyperlipidaemia (cholesterol ↑, triglycerides ↑)*
Zinc deficiency
Copper deficiency
Selenium deficiency
Hyperammonaemia

*Particularly important in extremely preterm infants.
↑, increased.

Glucose

Very low-birth-weight babies are at particular risk of hyperglycaemia and glycosuria. Regular blood and urine glucose monitoring (6 hourly) will be required. Although most of this monitoring will be with stix tests on the ward, it is important that any apparently abnormal (low or high) results are confirmed by sending a specimen to the laboratory for quantative glucose.

Lipids

The most widely used source of lipid in the UK is Intralipid (Kabi Vitrum). Parenteral lipid should be introduced gradually in babies who are preterm or small for gestation, and in those with jaundice or liver dysfunction. When lipid is infused faster than the lipoprotein lipase can metabolise, then clearance is reduced. Both hypertriglyceridaemia and hypercholesterolaemia have been reported.

A visual inspection of plasma collected during the infusion will reveal if there is a major problem with triglyceride tolerance, although it does not correlate well with a quantitative level. If there is evidence from this visual inspection of poor tolerance to lipids, plasma triglycerides should be measured.

Jaundice

Unconjugated hyperbilirubinaemia occurs in neonates, particularly if on parenteral nutrition for more than a few days. The risks of bilirubin deposition in the CNS will be influenced by many factors including free fatty acids. For this reason lipid infusion should be stopped if the bilirubin exceeds 170 μmol/l and reduced if 100–170 μmol/l.

Conjugated hyperbilirubinaemia may be a problem in some infants on long-term parenteral nutrition. Absence of enteral feeding may enhance this risk.

Amino Acids/Ammonia

Abnormalities of plasma amino acids have been reported primarily when using products not particularly formulated for the neonate especially if preterm. A particular problem reported is increased plasma phenylalanine in some babies on Vamin 9 glucose. The newer products (e.g. Vaminolact) are formulated to resemble the natural protein source for premature infants and have a reduced phenylalanine and taurine supplements compared with formulae for the older infant.

It is advisable to monitor plasma amino acids (qualitative) when the parenteral nutrition regime has been established for 3 days to check for excessively high levels particularly phenylalanine. Any apparent increase should be confirmed quantitively.

Hyperammonaemia is a rare complication with modern formulae and if liver function is normal. If the baby has compromised liver function or develops symptoms suggestive of hyperammonaemia, then the plasma concentration should be measured. At-risk infants should be monitored if the amino acid intake is being increased.

Trace Metals

Selenium, copper and zinc deficiency may occur as a result of long-term parenteral nutrition. Plasma concentrations should be measured if parenteral nutrition continues beyond 3 weeks.

Electrolytes

Hyponatraemia, hypokalaemia and hypocalcaemia frequently occur and regular monitoring should be done. Hypophosphataemia is also a common abnormality. Biochemical monitoring in the assessment of parenteral nutrition should be complementary to the daily evaluation of intake and output. The extent of monitoring will depend on the particular clinical circumstances and must be minimized in patients on long-term parenteral feeding in order to minimize blood loss.

In infants who are clinically stable a conservative approach to investigation can be taken (Table 5.12). For those who are very low birth weight, unstable, have major organ failure or abnormal losses then more frequent and extensive monitoring may be indicated.

LIPIDS

The commonly requested lipid investigations are plasma total cholesterol, high-density lipoprotein (HDL) cholesterol and triglycerides. Low-density lipoprotein (LDL) cholesterol is sometimes "calculated". Specific apolipoprotein quantitation and lipoprotein electrophoresis is only necessary for the accurate "typing" of primary lipid disorders and hence rarely required in the general setting. Increased lipid levels occur secondarily to many disorders (Table 5.13). Visual hyperlipidaemia should always be noted as it may be a clue to disease and may produce artefactually low plasma sodium concentrations (see p. 73).

Table 5.12   Protocol for routine biochemical monitoring of term neonates/infants on parenteral nutrition (PN)

Before PN
Blood – sodium, potassium, bilirubin, phosphate
Urine – sodium, potassium

After 3 days or more full PN
Plasma amino acids (qualitative)

Each week of PN
Blood – sodium, potassium (twice weekly)
              phosphate, bilirubin (once weekly)
              glucose (BM stix) (daily first week or more
              frequently if unstable or pre-term)

Additional tests after 2 weeks PN
Blood – calcium, alkaline phosphatase, then weekly

Additional tests after 3 weeks PN
Blood – selenium, zinc, copper; then every 3 weeks

Notes:
1. Preterm infants will require additional monitoring, particularly plasma phosphate and glucose and urine glucose (clinistix).
2. More frequent phosphate monitoring will be required if phosphate is low.
3. Apparently low glucose results by BM stix (i.e. < 2 mmol/l) *must* be confirmed with a quantitative laboratory result.
4. Frequency of glucose monitoring can be reduced after first week unless glucose intake is being increased or baby is preterm.

Table 5.13   Secondary causes of hyperlipidaemia in children

Glycogen storage disorders
Hypothyroidism
Nephrotic syndrome
Diabetes mellitus
Cholestatic disease

Cholesterol

Plasma cholesterol is low in neonates and young infants. It increases rapidly in the first month of life, and then gradually over the first few years. Concentrations vary little throughout the day or in response to meals and random non-fasting specimens can be used. Capillary blood can be used as an alternative to venous.

Increased levels due to familial hypercholesterolaemia will usually be observed after the age of one year. The diagnosis of familial hypercholesterolaemia (FH) can only be made after the secondary causes have been excluded (see secondary hyperlipidaemia Table 5.13).

Diagnosis of FH cannot be made from an isolated total cholesterol concentration in an individual child even after other causes have been excluded. It can be inferred if there is a family history of increased LDL cholesterol. Dietary

and possibly drug treatment should be considered for children over 2 years if plasma cholesterol concentrations are persistently above 6.0 mmol/l especially if there is a family history of atherosclerosis.

Low cholesterol may be suggestive of certain inherited disorders of cholesterol absorption/metabolism, e.g. Wolman's disease (a beta lipoproteinaemia), and peroxisomal disorders Mevalonic aciduria and Smith–Lemli–Opitz syndrome.

HDL Cholesterol

The value of HDL-cholesterol measurement is solely for the management of hypercholesterolaemia.

Triglycerides

A fasting specimen (at least 8 h) is essential for meaningful interpretation. Total parenteral nutrition may produce hypertriglyceridaemia (see p. 77). More rarely, increased levels are due to a primary disorder of lipid metabolism, which requires further investigation and treatment.

Type I hyperlipidaemia (lipoprotein lipase deficiency) is characterized by milky plasma and may be a fortuitous finding in a young infant. Clinical presentation is usually in the older infant/child with eruptive xanthoma, lipaemia retinalis and abdominal pain. Acute pancreatitis can occur and may be the presenting feature. Hyperlipidaemia in such a situation is a significant finding and a primary lipid disorder should be considered.

TRACE METALS

Measurements of plasma and urine trace metals can be useful in certain situations to detect deficiency or toxicity states and help diagnosis of certain metabolic disorders. Special collection containers are usually required to avoid exogenous contamination.

Copper

Plasma copper is low at birth and increases rapidly within the first week and then more slowly to reach adult levels by 3 months. Concentrations then increase with the highest levels found at 1–5 years. Levels then decline throughout childhood to reach adult levels by puberty.

Copper Deficiency

Clinical copper deficiency is characterized by hypochromic anaemia, hypotonia, neutropenia and bone disease. It is rare in term infants but is sometimes seen in preterm neonates and those on parenteral nutrition. It should be considered in the differential diagnosis of bone fractures in young infants, but the suspicion rarely negates a diagnosis of non-accidental injury.

Other causes of low plasma copper concentrations include Menke's kinky-hair syndrome, Wilsons' disease, tyrosinaemia type I, and zinc supplementation.

Zinc

At birth plasma zinc is in the normal range of adults but it decreases within the first week and continues to decline for the first 3 months. By late infancy levels have increased to those of adults. During puberty boys have lower levels than girls.

Zinc Deficiency

Clinical deficiency is characterized by dermatitis, poor growth, poor wound healing, alopecia and immune defects. Causes include malnutrition, malabsorption and inadequately supplemented parenteral nutrition.

Low alkaline phosphatase activity may be a clue to zinc deficiency.

Acrodermatitis enteropathica is a rare inherited disorder of zinc absorption which manifests as a zinc deficiency state.

Selenium

Plasma selenium measurement should rarely be required. Deficiency states can occur after prolonged parenteral nutrition (> 3 weeks) and prolonged severe deficiencies can result in cardiomyopathy and death. Earlier signs may be thinning of hair, muscle pain and tenderness.

SPECIFIC PROTEINS

Non-specific increases of many plasma specific proteins occur as an acute phase response and may "mask" a low level.

C-Reactive Protein (CRP)

CRP is a non-specific marker of an acute phase response and concentrations increase rapidly in response to inflammation. Increases in plasma CRP occur in many situations. Measurement of plasma CRP can be used to:

● Confirm the presence of a systemic bacterial infection

as the major disease process or co-existing with another condition.
● Differential diagnosis of meningitis.
● Diagnosis and monitoring of rheumatoid disorders (see Chapter 18).

Serial measurement to look at trends are the most useful way to use this test as individual results may be difficult to interpret. In certain situations a rapid result can be extremely useful for patient management, e.g. to assess response to treatment, or to provide early evidence of infection in high risk groups.

Caeruloplasmin

Plasma concentrations are normally low in early infancy. When interpreting levels it is important to use age-specific ranges. Pathological low levels are seen in most cases of Wilson's disease, although a normal result should never be used to exclude the disease. Investigation should always include measurement of plasma and urine copper.

Ferritin

Ferritin is a sensitive indicator of body iron stores. It is decreased in the very early stages of iron deficiency and increases during overload. Ferritin is produced by tumour cells and in patients with neuroblastoma the serum concentration at diagnosis is used as an index of prognosis. Serum ferritin can also be used as a measure of tumour mass and hence to monitor response to treatment. Single estimations may be difficult to interpret and it is best used as serial measurements to monitor trends.

α_1-Antitrypsin

Diagnosis of α_1-antitrypsin deficiency is important in the investigation of persistent neonatal jaundice (see p. 128). Plasma α_1-antitrypsin phenotyping should be carried out when the concentration is < 1.0 g/l. The identification of an α_1-antitrypsin deficient child should be followed up by typing of parents and siblings.

α-Fetoprotein

Levels are high at birth and normally fall rapidly over the first 3 months to reach adult levels by about 8 months of age. Very high levels occur in infants with hepatocellular carcinoma or yolk sac tumours. Serum levels fall dramatically following resection and serial measurements can be useful to check for evidence of recurrence. High levels also occur in ataxia telangiectasia and tyrosinaemia type I.

ENZYMES

Alkaline Phosphatase

Activity changes markedly throughout childhood and reference ranges are highly method dependent. Preterm infants may have very high peak levels, up to five times the upper limit for adults. Activity is increased in intra- and extra-hepatic biliary obstruction, hepatocellular damage or increased osteoblastic activity. Isoenzymes can be measured by a variety of techniques but are rarely required in routine practice. The liver origin of an increased activity can usually be inferred by measurement of serum γ-glutamyltranspeptidase. Low levels may occur in zinc deficiency and are characteristic of the inherited defect hypophosphatasia.

Transient Hyperphosphatasia

Marked isolated increases in alkaline phosphatase in the absence of associated pathology have been described. The activity is often dramatically increased, exceeding 10-fold the upper limit of normal and usually returns to normal usually within 4 months. The absence of clinical and biochemical liver and bone disease allows this diagnosis to be made by exclusion provided that the levels return to normal. In contrast, a persistently elevated level (> 6 months) with no liver or bone disease is possibly persistent hyperphosphatasia. This is an inherited condition probably with dominant inheritance; alkaline phosphatase should be measured in parents and siblings.

Amylase

Virtually no amylase is produced in the neonate and plasma concentrations are low during the first year of life. Grossly increased levels usually occur in acute pancreatitis, although beware of false-negative results as levels may be only transiently increased and the peak sampling may have been missed. Urine amylase/creatinine ratio may be useful in this situation.

Persistently increased levels are suggestive of pseudocyst or chronic pancreatitis. Low concentrations may indicate pancreatic insufficiency. Raised levels in the absence of pancreatic disease occur in mumps, macro-amylasaemia or inflammatory bowel disease.

Aminotransferases

Aspartate aminotransferase (AST) and alanine aminotransferase (ALT) are both produced by the liver. AST is also found in other tissues, notably muscle. AST is a more sensitive indicator of liver injury than ALT, but ALT is more specific. Falling levels usually indicate that the pathology is improving.

In chronic disease, e.g. glycogen storage disease, amino transferase levels may only be slightly/moderately increased.

γ-Glutamyltranspeptidase (γ-GT)

This enzyme is a sensitive indicator of biliary tract injury and can be useful in interpreting increases in alkaline phosphatase. Values in the normal neonate are much greater than those in the older child.

Drugs which induce hepatic microsomal systems increase γ-GT concentrations, e.g. phenytoin.

VITAMINS

Vitamin-deficiency states rarely require measurement of the vitamin for diagnosis. Groups at risk of nutritional deficiency, e.g. those receiving parenteral nutrition, on special diets, on a poor diet, or due to malabsorption, are usually treated with supplements to minimize risk of clinical deficiencies. The possibility of vitamin toxicity is becoming of more concern with the widespread use of vitamin supplements and the potential for overtreatment.

Vitamin A (Retinol)

Retinol circulates as a complex with retinol binding protein (RBP). The main storage site is the liver and serum concentrations provide only an approximate assessment of body stores. In deficiency states serum levels of both retinol and RBP are low. Serum retinol values < 0.7 μmol/l are considered low.

Excess vitamin A is toxic and can occur acutely or chronically. Toxicity is thought to occur when the binding capacity of RBP has been exceeded and the free retinol damages cell membranes. Plasma retinol levels tend to plateau with toxicity, RBP levels are not altered.

Serum carotene concentration usually mirrors vitamin A level. However, excess carotene in the presence of low serum vitamin A suggests the inherited defect of carotenaemia where there is an endogenous inability to convert carotene to retinol.

Vitamin E

Vitamin E activity is associated with the tocopherols and tocotrienols. Normally α-tocopherol accounts for the majority of vitamin E activity (90%), although this may differ in patients on Intralipid as a significant percentage of total tocopherol is as other isomers. Methods for measuring plasma vitamin E may measure total or α-tocopherol.

Interpretation of plasma concentrations is complicated by the association of tocopherol with lipoproteins. Absorbed tocopherol is taken up by the liver and re-secreted within lipoprotein moieties (very low density lipoproteins (VLDL), LDL and HDL). It remains with the lipoprotein and in plasma is mainly associated with LDL and HDL. When lipoprotein levels are low little tocopherol can be carried and hence plasma concentrations will underestimate body stores. In hyperlipidaemic states, e.g. cholestasis, higher plasma levels occur and may mark a true deficiency. This relationship between vitamin E and lipoprotein can be corrected for by determining the ratio of vitamin E to total lipids.

Vitamin E deficiency most commonly occurs in association with fat malabsorption e.g. cholestatic liver disease, cystic fibrosis, coeliac disease. Deficiency is important to detect because neurological deterioration due to deficiency is treatable.

Isolated vitamin E deficiency should be considered in children with unexplained progressive ataxia.

In extreme deficiency states of lipoproteins, e.g. a β-lipoproteinaemia, a measure of the red cell membrane resistance to oxidation can be used (e.g. hydrogen peroxide haemolysis test).

Vitamin D

Indirect tests, i.e. urine and plasma calcium and phosphate, should be the initial approach to assessing vitamin D status. Measurement of vitamin D metabolites should rarely be required to demonstrate deficiency or toxicity.

In the absence of liver damage serum total 25-hydroxy vitamin D is the best assessment of vitamin D status. The method used must measure the 25-hydroxylated forms of both D_2 and D_3.

1,25-Dihydroxy vitamin D is a poor indicator of vitamin D status. Measurement should be restricted to those situations where abnormal metabolism (i.e. defective 1-hydroxylase) is suspected.

B Vitamins (Niacin, Pyridoxine, Riboflavin, Thiamin, Vitamin B₁₂)

Direct measurement of the water soluble B vitamins in plasma is generally unhelpful in assessing deficiency or toxicity states. The best test of clinical deficiency is to see if clinical symptoms improve after supplementation. Measurement of vitamin-dependent enzymes, e.g. red cell transketolase, glutathione reductase, and alanine aminotransferase, are sometimes used as an indirect measure of vitamin levels.

Thiamine deficiency as a result of inadequate intake from parenteral nutrition may result in an acute neurological deterioration.

Vitamin B_{12} deficiency is characterized by an increase in urinary methylmalonic acid and clinical and biochemical deficiencies may occur in children who are strict vegetarians and infants who are breast-fed by vegan mothers.

Vitamin C

There is no good test of vitamin C deficiency. Plasma concentrations reflect recent intake rather than body stores and leucocyte assays require large blood volumes.

Suspected vitamin C deficiency should initially be treated. Vitamin C supplements are rarely contraindicated except in oxalate stone formers and patients with renal failure where high intake may be a risk.

DRUGS AND TOXICOLOGY

Measurement of plasma drug concentrations should be restricted to situations where it is essential for management or toxicity is suspected.

Toxicology

Emergency assays for salicylate, paracetamol and iron should be available. Screening for overdose of some other drugs will be available, but not necessarily on site and you will need to discuss carefully with your local clinical chemist or clinical toxicology centre. If your immediate management will not be altered by confirmation of a drug level then the assay can wait until the next working day. Often the most important action is to take blood (heparin) and urine specimens and store safely.

Salicylate

Acute ingestion of less than 150 mg/kg is unlikely to result in toxic symptoms; 150–300 mg/kg will cause mild to moderate symptoms. Stimulation of the respiratory centre occurs resulting in hyperventilation and respiratory alkalosis. This is transient and is followed by metabolic acidosis. The possibility of chronic over ingestion should be checked for in children on salicylate therapy or where symptoms suggest this.

Diagnosis is confirmed by measurement of serum salicylate concentration (this will be available from the laboratory on an emergency basis). Salicylate is rapidly absorbed and hydrolysed and has a half-life of 15–20 min. The plasma level should be measured as soon as possible. Peak levels are delayed by up to 2 h following ingestion of enteric-coated capsules and, therefore, if this is suspected the patient should be observed and plasma concentrations should be re-tested 1–2 h later. Urine will give a positive reaction in the ferric chloride test ($FeCl_3$) (purple colour) and this may be useful for very rapid confirmation. However, caution is needed as the $FeCl_3$ screening test is not specific for salicylate. Treatment with alkaline diuresis to produce an alkaline urine (pH > 7) should be considered if plasma levels exceed 2.5 mmol/l (35 mg/100 ml).

Levels of > 7.2 mmol/l (100 mg/100 ml) may require more aggressive treatment such as dialysis.

Treatment should be monitored with blood-gas, sodium, potassium, calcium, glucose and prothrombin-time measurements.

Paracetamol

Children of < 12 years of age are generally less susceptible to the hepatotoxic effects of paracetamol than adults. Blood paracetamol should be measured 4 h after ingestion (specimens taken before 4 h may not represent peak concentrations). The antidote, N-acetylcysteine (NAC), should be given if the paracetamol level falls in the potentially toxic range between 4 and 15 h post injection (see Figure 5.1). After 15 h, liver status is best assessed by measurement of prothrombin time. Early treatment (within 8 h) is crucial for a good outcome. If doubt persists, a Poisons Centre should be consulted.

Iron

Serum iron > 60 μmol/l is associated with toxicity. The specific antidote, desferrioxamine, is given if there are symptoms and the level is > 60 μmol/l. Patients with levels of > 90 μmol/l should always be treated. Subsequent serum iron measurements are required to monitor the effectiveness of treatment.

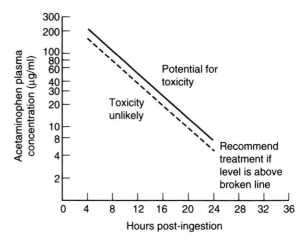

Figure 5.1 Nomogram relating plasma or serum acetaminophen (paracetamol) concentration and time since ingestion. Reproduced from Rumack and Matthew (1975), by permission.

Lead

Lead poisoning in childhood results from exposure to lead containing dust, paint or soil. It is more likely to occur in children residing in inner-city areas particularly in poor housing where there is a possibility of aging paint work. The possibility of poisoning is important to consider in children with unexplained acute onset of convulsions or coma, and in those presenting with gradual drowsiness or irritability of unknown cause.

Supporting radiological findings are increased density at the metaphyses of the long bones; and radio-opaque material in the gut. Haematology may show basophilic stipling of the red cells and/or iron deficiency anaemia; the latter may also be a primary event due to associated nutritional iron deficiency.

Secondary biochemical findings are glycosuria and amino aciduria due to renal tubular damage. Although lead exposure is associated with an increase in urinary δ-ALA and erythrocyte protophorphyrin, these should not be used as alternatives to requesting a blood lead.

The reference or *normal* range for blood lead in children in the UK has been steadily falling over the years, with 95% currently having a concentration < 10 μg/100 ml (< 0.5 μmol/l). Although the current UK action limit is 25 μg/100 ml (1.2 μmol/l) it is probably abnormal for children to have a level above 10 μg/100 ml and evidence for increased lead exposure should be sought.

At blood lead concentrations greater than 60 μg/100 ml (3 μmol/l), clinical symptoms may be apparent and encephalopathy can occur if greater than 100 μg/100 ml (5 μmol/l).

In acute poisoning, rapid treatment with chelation therapy is essential and advice should be sought from a specialist centre. It is also important to test siblings.

In chronic poisoning it is important to test other family members in the same house and to find the source of the lead and remove it.

BIOCHEMICAL INVESTIGATION OF SUDDEN INFANT DEATH SYNDROME (SIDS) (Green 1993)

Many inherited metabolic disorders are associated with acute life-threatening events (see Chapter 4). The group that has been documented as a possible cause of SIDS are the fatty acid oxidation defects. The pathologist should consider metabolic disorders in all cases, but particularly where there is a previous clinical history, or more than one unexplained death in a family.

Investigation for metabolic disorders should be considered in the following groups of newborn siblings (Green, 1993):

- Symptomatic siblings, e.g. unexplained hypoglycaemia, acidosis failure to thrive, illness precipitated by infection/stress, drowsiness.
- Asymptomatic siblings with one/more of the following:
  (a) sudden expected sibling death with history suggestive of metabolic disorder,
  (b) SIDS in a sibling with *post-mortem* findings suggestive of IMD,
  (c) more than one case of SIDS in family,
  (d) previous sibling with Reye-like illness or unexplained cardiorespiratory arrest, and
  (e) family history, i.e. close family member has an inherited metabolic disorder.

The investigations should be discussed with a specialist laboratory (see Chapter 4).

BIOCHEMICAL INVESTIGATION OF REYE'S OR REYE-LIKE SYNDROMES

It has become increasingly apparent that a significant number of patients who present with a Reye-like illness have an underlying metabolic disorder. Data from the British Paediatric Surveillance Unit has shown that 10% of patients initially reported with Reye's syndrome between 1981 and 1991 were subsequently found to have a metabolic disorder (Green and Hall 1992). These dis-

orders include organic acid metabolism, including fatty acid oxidation, and those of urea cycle, amino acid and carbohydrate metabolism.

The *possibility* of an inherited metabolic disorder should therefore be considered in *all* patients who present with Reye-like illness. The presence of certain features are particularly suggestive (Table 5.14).

First-line biochemical tests should include:

- Plasma aspartate (or alanine) aminotransferase.
- Plasma alkaline phosphatase.
- Plasma γ-Glutamyltranspeptidase.
- Blood glucose.
- Plasma ammonia.
- Acid–base status.
- Blood lactate.
- Urinary ketones.

The presence of severe and/or unresolving metabolic acidosis, hypoglycaemia, hyperammonaemia and lactic acidosis are clues to possible IMD, although not specific, abnormalities. At this stage, the clinical chemistry laboratory should be asked to store, deep frozen, any spare urine and plasma specimens that have been collected.

Further investigations should include:

- Urine – amino acids (qualitative) and organic acids by gas chromatography/mass spectrometry (essential to refer to a specialist centre).
- Plasma – amino acids (initially qualitative with quantitation if indicated).

In addition, if there is hypoglycaemia a plasma sample (collected in fluoride) should be taken for quantitative 3-hydroxybutyrate, free fatty acids and lactate. If there is a metabolic acidosis, a plasma sample (collected in fluoride) should be taken for lactate.

Table 5.14 Features suggestive of inherited metabolic disorders in patients presenting with a Reye-like illness

Young age (< 3 years) at onset of Reye-like illness

Past history of: encephalopathic episodes; vomiting in association with viral infections; unexplained failure to thrive; neurodevelopmental disorder; "near-miss" SIDS

Family (both immediate and extended) history of: Reye's syndrome; unexplained encephalopathy; SIDS

Absence of a history of a viral prodrome clearly separated from the onset of encephalopathy

SIDS, sudden infant death syndrome. With permission.

SPECIMEN COLLECTION AND REQUIREMENTS

Blood Collection (Alstrom et al. 1987; Blumenfeld et al. 1979; Meites et al. 1979)

Most clinical chemistry analyses are performed on plasma rather than whole blood. Limited availability of specimen, particularly in neonates, means that consideration needs to be given when making repeated requests, e.g. monitoring of total parenteral nutrition. The risk of infection from repeated heel stabs should be remembered. An additional problem which affects specimen volumes required is the haematocrit which may be as high as 75% in the newborn. Anticoagulated blood is preferred to clotted for the majority of analyses as it will yield a larger plasma sample. Most biochemical tests require heparinised blood, the notable exceptions being glucose (fluoride oxalate) and lead (EDTA). Do *not* transfer blood from one type of tube to another. Discussion with the clinical chemist will allow the best use of a particularly precious specimen. For the more specialized assays it is necessary to find out the local arrangements *before* any specimen is collected.

Capillary blood should only be taken by trained personnel who are performing skin punctures on a regular basis. It is best provided as a joint collection for clinical chemistry and haematology in order to minimize punctures for an individual patient. Provision of the service by the laboratory has the advantage of optimizing the organization of specimen collection; allowing best use of medical staff time and enabling laboratory staff to have an appreciation of the difficulties of specimen collection. The importance of a good collection from a well perfused limb cannot be overstated. A badly collected specimen from excessive squeezing or scraping of the tube across the skin is likely to be haemolysed and contaminated with tissue fluid and sweat. Blood should not be collected from the same limb as is receiving intravenous solution. When collecting blood via an in-dwelling catheter, to avoid dilution it is essential to flush with a small volume of blood before collecting the specimen.

Blood Collection by Capillary Puncture (Green and Morgan, 1993; Clayton and Pound, 1994)

General

If specimens for both clinical chemistry and haematology are to be collected, then the blood for haematology collection must be collected *first*. (*Beware* possible contami-

nation from potassium EDTA.) This arrangement should minimize the extent to which the platelet count falls in shed blood after skin injury and provide results similar to those from a venous specimen (see also blood gas analysis, p. 75).

For a neonate the puncture depth *must not exceed* 2.4 mm, and preferably be not greater than 1.6 mm, in order to avoid penetration of bone and hence the potential complication of osteomyelitis.

Several puncture devices are available, e.g. Medipoint, Vacutainer safety flow or Microlance lancets. The disposable lancets and platform must be discarded after each puncture and on no account should they be re-used.

Every attempt should be made to collect clinical chemistry specimens without haemolysis. This is possible even when great pressure is needed to obtain blood.

If a baby has skin problems consider whether capillary collection is reasonable.

Selection and Preparation of Site for Skin Puncture

Capillary Heel Stab Neonate/Infant

Make sure that the baby is lying in a secure and comfortable position so that the heel is easily accessible. An area of heel, free from previous puncture sites, should be selected. Check if the ankle has been used for venous access, as there is a danger of re-opening wounds. Punctures should not be performed on the posterior curvature of the heel where the bone is closest to the skin.

Capillary Finger Puncture (Infant)

Above the age of 1 year the thumb or finger can be used provided there is sufficient flesh.

Before attempting any blood collection, the site should be warm and well perfused – this may be achieved by rubbing, immersion in warm (< 40°C) water or wrapping in a warm (< 40°C) nappy or towel. A dirty heel or finger should be prewashed with soapy water, rinsed with clean water and thoroughly dried.

The site must be cleaned with an antiseptic solution (isopropyl alcohol – Sterets) and wiped completely dry with clean cotton wool to prevent haemolysis. Sterets can be used in an incubator; give the heel a quick wipe and then immediately remove the Steret from the incubator.

Skin Puncture

Before performing the puncture, check that all the necessary items are ready and in close proximity:

- Steret.
- Lancet.

- Cotton wool.
- Specimen tube, e.g. Sarstedt lithium, heparin CB 300.

Check the name and registration number of the baby or child before starting the puncture.

Heel

Stand facing slighly away from the baby's head and hold the heel with the nearest hand. Grip the baby's heel firmly by holding around the ankle with the index and middle fingers so that the sole of the foot is against the palm of the hand and the heel exposed. The thumb is placed around the heel and pressure is controlled with the thumb and index finger. Whilst maintaining tension on the heel make the puncture as one continuous deliberate motion in a direction slightly off perpendicular to the puncture site. Release pressure and wipe off the first drop of blood as it appears.

Finger

Hold the infant's fingers flat, with the thumb or chosen finger slightly separated from the rest. The phlebotomist's thumb and fingers should be placed so that pressure compresses the flesh of the infant's finger. Maintain the tension and prick the side of the finger just where it begins to curve and about ⅛ in. from the nail bed, this is less painful for the patient and gives a better flow. Release pressure and wipe away the first drop of blood as it appears.

Blood Collection

Hold the collection tube between thumb and forefinger. Obtain a hanging drop of blood and touch the *side* of this drop which faces away from the patient against the inside of the tube which is furthest from the patient. "Pluck" off the drop of blood and knock it down to the bottom of the tube by giving the tube a sharp tap on a hard surface. Using a minimum of pressure, obtain further drops of blood and touch them against the same site inside the neck of the tube. They will follow the track of the initial drop. Pressure around the heel or finger should be eased and then slowly and gently reapplied to allow more drops of blood to flow. Excessive "milking" or "massaging" is not recommended as this causes haemolysis. Should blood become smeared over the heel/finger *during* collection do not be tempted to scrape it off – wipe with clean dry cotton wool (*not* a Steret!) and start again. Periodically flick the blood gently in the tube using the little or other free finger of the hand holding the tube. This is to ensure mixing of the blood with anticoagulant. Blood

will flow more easily if the heel is held low. The blood volume required is obviously dependent on which specific tests are required. When the collection is finished, push the cap into the tube and invert gently several times to ensure mixing. Press a wad of dry clean cotton wool firmly against the puncture site and hold the baby's heel/finger above the body for a few minutes to stop the flow of blood. A plaster may be applied to the puncture site but this is best avoided if possible; neonates have sensitive skin and a plaster, if it becomes detached, is a potential item for ingestion.

Make sure that the tube is labelled either with a felt-tipped pen or by writing on a narrow adhesive label as a "flag" (i.e. wrap the label around the tube close to the top so that a portion overhangs at the side).

Urine

Useful results can often be obtained from random or overnight urine specimens by relating analytes to the creatinine concentration.

The need for a 24-h, or shorter, timed collection should be restricted to those situations which demand it. An *accurately* timed collection over a shorter time period is far better than an "incomplete" 24-h collection.

An infant below 6 months of age will have a total daily urine output of less than 500 ml and hence apparent "small" losses from timed collections in newborns or young infants may be significant.

In neonates several millilitres can be collected by cotton wool balls. In older infants urine bags can be used. In certain circumstances, e.g. fasting for metabolic studies or protein load, where the urine collection is an *essential* part of the test, it may be important to catheterize the child.

Some analytes, e.g. catecholamines and trace metals, require special bottles with particular preservatives. It is important to check with the laboratory *before* collecting the specimen. *Do not* transfer urine from one bottle to another type in the hope of overcoming the "wrong" collection bottle!

Other Specimens

Cerebrospinal Fluid (CSF)

Protein analysis should not be undertaken on a bloody specimen as the protein from lysed blood and plasma will give falsely high results. Corresponding blood specimens are often required, e.g. glucose, lactate, glycine, in order to interpret CSF concentrations. For these analytes if the test is not undertaken immediately cloudy specimens should be centrifuged and the supernatant stored deep frozen.

Faeces

Collection of timed faecal specimens should rarely be necessary. Random collections, e.g. for reducing substances or steatocrit, are best collected on to a polythene sheet to ensure that the liquid portion of the specimen is not lost.

Sweat

Measurement of sweat sodium *and* chloride is an essential test for diagnosis of cystic fibrosis. Measurement of sodium alone can give misleading results. Sweat collection should be performed by skilled, trained staff, preferably laboratory staff who undertake such collections regularly. Sweat should be collected for 15–20 min after stimulation by pilocarpine iontophoresis (Gibson–Cooke procedure).

At least 100 mg of sweat should be collected to ensure there has been an adequate sweat rate. Weights less than this may give misleading results. Normal children aged between 4 weeks and 13 years have sodium concentrations of < 60 mmol/l and chloride concentrations of < 50 mmol/l.

The results are consistent with cystic fibrosis if sodium is greater than 60 mmol/l and chloride is greater than 70 mmol/l. In cystic fibrosis the chloride concentration is usually greater than the sodium, whereas in normal subjects the reverse usually applies.

ACKNOWLEDGEMENTS

Much of the information in this chapter reflects "departmental practice" and I would like to thank numerous staff (past and present) in the Department of Clinical Chemistry at the Children's Hospital, Birmingham, who have contributed to the collection and analysis of data over many years and have helped develop and establish procedures and protocols for children.

I am grateful to many colleagues who have contributed to the data in the following appendix, in particular to Sue Keffler (Clinical Biochemist) at Birmingham Children's Hospital.

REFERENCES

Alstrom T, Dahl M, Grasbeck R et al (1987) Recommendation for collection of skin puncture blood from children, with special reference to production of reference values. *Scand J Clin Lab Invest* 47: 199–205.

Blumenfeld TA, Turi GK, Blanc WA (1979) Recommended site and depth of newborn heel skin punctures based on anatomical measurements and histopathology. *Lancet* i: 230–233.

Bonham JR (1993) The investigation of hypoglycaemia during childhood. *Ann Clin Biochem* 30: 238–247.

Clayton BE, Pound JM (1994) *Clinical Biochemistry and the Sick Child* Blackwell Scientific, Oxford.

Dodd KL (1993) Neonatal jaundice – a lighter touch. *Arch Dis Child* 68: 529–533.

Green A, Dodds P, Pernock C (1985) A study of sweat sodium and chloride: criteria for the diagnosis of cystic fibrosis. *Ann Clin Biochem* 22: 171–176.

Green A, Hall SM (1992) Investigation of metabolic disorders resembling Reye's syndrome. *Arch Dis Child* 67: 1313–1317.

Green A (1993) Biochemical screening in newborn siblings of cases of SIDS. *Arch Dis Child* 68: 793–796.

Green A, Morgan I (1993) *The Neonate and Clinical Chemistry*. Venture Publications, Association of Clinical Biochemists.

Henderson MJ, Dear PRF (1993) Role of the clinical biochemistry laboratory in the management of very low birthweight infants. *Ann Clin Biochem* 30: 341–354.

Medical Research Council Working Party on Phenylketonuria (1993) Recommendations on the dietary management of phenylketonuria. *Arch Dis Child* 68: 426–427.

Meites S, Levitt MJ, Blumenfeld TA et al (1979) Skin puncture and blood collecting techniques for infants. *Clin Chem* 25: 183–189.

Meites, S (ed) (1989) *Paediatric Clinical Chemistry Reference (Normal) Values*, 3rd edn. Washington DC., American Association for Clinical Chemistry.

Puntis JWL, Hall SK, Green A et al (1993) Biochemical stability during parenteral nutrition in children. *Clin Nutrit* 12: 153–159.

Rumack BH, Matthew H (1975) Acetaminophen poisoning and toxicity. *Pediatrics* 55: 871–876.

Scott PJH, Wharton BA (1992) Biochemical values in the newborn. In: Roberton N (ed) *Textbook of Neonatology*, 2nd edn, pp. 1213–1227. Churchill Livingstone, Edinburgh.

Walter JH (1992) Metabolic acidosis in newborn infants. *Arch Dis Child* 67: 767–769.

Appendix: Biochemical Reference Ranges

The values quoted below are a guide to interpreting data for neonates, infants and children and apply to laboratory methods currently in use at Birmingham Children's Hospital; they will not necessarily apply to methods in use at other Hospitals. Ranges will differ *significantly* for some analytes for different methods – **you must consult your local laboratory**.

Table A5.1

	Units	Reference Range	Comments
Blood			
Hydrogen ion (pH)	nmol/l	35–44	Arterial (see Table A5.2)
pCO_2	kPa	0–3 yr 3.7–5.3 >3 yr 4.3–5.5	Arterial
Bicarbonate	mmol/l	1–4 yr 17–25 4–8 yr 19–27 >8 yr 21–29	
Base excess	mmol/l	− 3 to + 3	
PO_2	kPa	11–14.0	Arterial Generally lower in neonates.
Alanine aminotransferase (ALT)	U/l	≤ 40	Range will vary with method
Albumin	g/l	Neonate 25–45 Child 35–55	Neonate: depends on gestational age
Alkaline phosphatase (ALP)	U/l	Neonate 150–700 1 m–1 yr 250–1000 2–9 yr 250–850	High levels in first week due to placental ALP. Range can vary widely with method. Preterm levels higher
17-α-Hydroxyprogesterone (17-OHP)	nmol/l	Neonate 0.7–12.4 Child 0.4–4.2	*Note:* There is a rapid fall from the very high concentrations (maternally derived) in the first 24–48 h of life. This is therefore an inappropriate time to measure 17-OHP for diagnostic purposes. Premature infants also have 2–3 fold higher levels of 17-OHP compared with values for full term infants.
α-1-Antitrypsin	g/l	Neonate/infant 0.9–2.2 Child 1.1–2.2	Phenotype should be assessed if < 1.0 g/l
α-Fetoprotein	ug/l (1 ng = 1.09/U)	Term neonate: 500–55 000 1 month 70–12 000	Higher if premature. Depends on gestational age. Normal "adult" levels are reached by 8 months.

Within the Alkaline phosphatase row:

Year	Females	Males
10–11	250–950	250–730
12–13	200–730	275–875
14–15	170–460	170–970
16–18	75–270	125–720
>18	60–250	50–200

Table A5.1   continued

	Units	Reference Range	Comments
Blood – *contd*			
Ammonia	μmol/l	Neonate ≤ 100 Infant/Child ≤ 40	May be higher if preterm and/or sick
Amylase	I.U/l (Phadebas)	Neonate ≤ 50 1–3 m < 100 > 1 yr 100–400	Method dependent.
Anion gap, i.e. (sodium + potassium) (bicarbonate + chloride)	mmol/l	< 20	
Aspartate aminotransferase (AST)	U/l	≤ 50	In neonates and early infancy values may be up to 2-fold higher.
Bilirubin (total)	μmol/l	0–14 days ≤ 200 Infant/child ≤ 20	
Bilirubin (conjugated)	μmol/l	0–14 days < 40 Infant/child < 2	Conjugated hyper-bilirubinaemia should always be investigated.
Caeruloplasmin	g/l	Neonate 0.08–0.23 Infant/child 0.15–0.40	
Calcium (total)	mmol/l	After 1 week 2.15– 2.60	There is often a marked fall after birth with lowest conc. (1.8) at around 24–48 h of age.
Calcium (oinized)	mmol/l	1.18–1.32	
Chloride	mmol/l	96–110	
Cholesterol (total)	mmol/l	Neonate 1.5–4.0 1–6 yr 2.0–4.8 > 6 yr 2.8–6.4	Gradual increase from birth.
Copper	μmol/l	Neonate 3–11 Infant 7–25 Child 12–26	
Cortisol	nmol/l	a.m. 200–700 Midnight < 140	Diurnal variation, important in assessing adrenal cortical function.
Creatine kinase	U/l	Infant/child 60–300	Range dependent on methodology. High levels in neonates up to 10 × those in infancy/childhood. Marked fall during first week of life following peak at 24–48 h. From puberty levels tend to be higher in boys than girls.
Creatinine	μmol/l	Infant 20–55 Child 20–80	Neonate – depends on gestational age. Method dependent.
C-reactive protein (CRP)	mg/l	≤ 10	Values in 1st two weeks may be 2–3 fold higher.
Ferritin	ug/l	Neonate 90–640 Child ≤ 150	Values fall throughout infancy.
Glucose	mmol/l	Neonate 2.5–5.5 Child 3.0–6.0	
Gamma glutamyl transpeptidase (γGT)	U/l	6–14 days ≤ 250 2 wk–2 m ≤ 150 2–12 m < 80 > 1 yr ≤ 30	

Table A5.1   continued

	Units	Reference Range	Comments
Blood – *contd*			
Immunoglobulins			
(IgG)	g/l	Neonate 5.0–17.0 ≤3 m 2.7–7.7 3 m–6 m 2.4–8.8 6 m–1 yr 3.0–9.0 1 yr–3 yr 3.1–13.8 3 yr–6 yr 4.9–16.0 >6 yr 5.4–16.0	
(IgA)	g/l	Neonate up to 0.08 ≤3 m 0.05–0.40 3 m–6 m 0.10–0.60 6 m–2 yr 0.3–1.2 2 yr–3 yr 0.3–1.3 3 yr–6 yr 0.4–2.0 6 yr–12 yr 0.5–2.5 >12 yr 0.7–4.0	
(IgM)	g/l	Neonate 0.05–0.2 ≤3 m 0.15–0.7 3 m–6 m 0.2–1.0 6 m–1 yr 0.6–2.1 1 yr–3 yr 0.5–2.2 3 yr–6 yr 0.5–2.0 6 yr–12 yr 0.5–1.8 >12 yr 0.5–2.2	
(IgE)	KU/L	Neonate ≤5 ≤3 m ≤15 3 m–6 m ≤25 6 m–1 yr ≤35 1 yr–3 yr ≤125 3 yr–7 yr ≤175 >7 yr ≤200	
Iron	μmol/l	Neonate 10–30 Infant 5–25 Child 10–30	
Lactate (fasting)	mmol/l	0.5–2.0	
LDH	U/l	Infant ≤900 Child ≤700	Method dependent. High levels in neonate. Gradual fall throughout infancy.
Magnesium	mmol/l	0.6–1.0	
Osmolality	mosmol/kg	275–295	
Phosphate	mmol/l	Neonate 1.4–2.6 Infant 1.3–2.1 Child 1.0–1.8	
Potassium	mmol/l	Neonate/infant 3.5–6.5 Child 3.3–4.7	Capillary blood Venous or arterial blood and not haemolysed.

Table A5.1   continued

	Units	Reference Range	Comments
Blood – *contd*			
Protein (total)	g/l	Neonate 54–70 Infant 59–70 Child 60–80	Depends on gestational age.
Sodium	mmol/l	133–145	
Thyroid stimulating hormone (TSH)	mU/l	0.3–4.5	Higher levels occur in first week of life.
Thyroxine (total) tT4	nmol/l	1–3 days 142–296 1–4 wks 116–203	
Thyroxine (free) fT4	pmol/l	11–24	Higher at 1–3 days
Triglycerides (fasting)	mmol/l	0.3–1.5	
Tri-iodothyronine fT3	pmol/l	3–9	
Immunoreactive Trypsin	ng/ml	upper limit 70 (dried blood spot). upper limit 130 (plasma)	
Urea	mmol/l	Neonate 1.0–5.0 Infant 2.5–8.0 Child 2.5–6.5	Infants fed on cows milk formula may have higher levels.
Urate	μmol/l	Infant/child 120–350	Values are higher at birth. Levels are higher in boys after puberty.
Zinc	μmol/l	11–24	
Urine			
Calcium	mmol/kg/24 h	< 0.1	24 h urine
Calcium : creatinine ratio	mmol/mmol	≤ 0.7	Second urine after overnight fast
Copper	μmol/24 h	≤ 1.0	
Osmolality	mosmol/kg	> 870	Following overnight water deprivation.
Phosphate tubular reabsorption	%	> 80	
Potassium	mmol/kg/24 h	Neonate: ≤ 5 Child: ≤ 2	Depends on potassium intake and gestational age.
Protein/creatinine	mg/mmol	≤ 20	
Sodium	mmol/kg/24 h	Neonate < 1 ≤ (full term) < 3 ≤ (preterm)	Depends on sodium intake and gestational age.
Fractional sodium excretion	%	Neonate ≤ 1 Child < 0.1	Higher if pre-term
Urate : creatinine ratio	mmol/mmol	Neonate up to 2.0 Infant 0.5–1.5 Child 0.3–0.8	
CSF			
Protein	g/l	2–4 m < 0.6 5 m–10 yr < 0.25 11 yr–18 yr < 0.3	

Table A5.1 continued.

	Units	Reference Range	Comments
Blood – *contd*			
Glucose	mmol/l	2.5–4.5	Normally ~ 75% of blood glucose.
Sweat			
Sodium	mmol/l	1 m–5 yr < 50	Older children may have sodium concentrations up to 60 mmol/l.
Chloride	mmol/l	1 m–5 yr < 50	Sodium and chloride concentrations increase with age.

Values are for children unless specified.
Neonate up to 4 weeks.
Infant 1 month – 2 years.
Child 2 years and above.

Table A5.2 Relationship of pH to hydrogen ion $[H^+]$ concentration

Approximate reference values 38–44 mmol/l.

pH	H^+ nmol/l
6.85	140
6.87	135
6.89	130
6.90	125
6.92	120
6.94	115
6.96	110
6.98	105
7.00	100
7.03	95
7.05	90
7.07	85
7.10	80
7.13	75
7.15	70
7.19	65
7.22	60
7.26	55
7.30	50
7.35	45
7.40	40
7.45	35
7.52	30

1. Ideally, arterial blood taken anaerobically in a heparinized syringe is required. *Free flowing* capillary blood, collected carefully in special tubes, may also be used.
2. Blood *must* be taken to the laboratory promptly.

6
Nephrology

J T Brocklebank

RENAL FAILURE

Acute renal failure is rare in childhood. In the newborn period sepsis and surgery, particularly cardiac surgery, are the commonest causes. Haemolytic uraemic syndrome occurs frequently in the toddler age group. Nephrotoxic drug treatments should be considered at all ages. The investigation of acute renal failure may be considered in three categories:

1. Establish the presence of acute renal failure by urine examination. The urine flow rate is generally reduced, less than 0.5 ml/kg per hour, but a higher urine flow rate does not exclude acute renal failure.
2. Urine testing will identify blood and protein and microscopy will show many granular casts and red blood cells (see below).
3. Chemical analysis of the urine may help to define whether the oliguria is due to the pre-renal or parenchymatous renal failure (Table 6.1). The results give a useful guide but should be interpreted with caution.

Glomerular filtration rate (GFR) can be estimated from the plasma creatinine concentration. In parenchymatous renal failure the creatinine concentration increases steadily by more than $30\,\mu mol/l$ per day. The blood urea concentration has little value in assessing GFR but, when it is greater in comparison to the plasma creatinine,

dehydration and pre-renal failure or increased protein catabolism are suggested.

To Establish the Cause of Acute Renal failure

The cause of renal failure is generally apparent from the history of a precipitating event or exposure to nephrotoxic drugs. Investigations will include:

Blood Film

In the diagnosis of haemolytic uraemic syndrome, typically fragmentation of the red blood cells is seen together with a low platelet count. A high white cell count (greater than $20 \times 10^9/l$) may indicate the severity of the disease. Examination of the blood film may also give information about other haematological disorders including sickle cell disease.

Infection

This is both an important cause and a complication of acute renal failure. Blood culture and urine cultures should always be obtained and, where appropriate, stool culture. The verotoxin producing *Escherichia coli* 0157 has been shown to be present in the faeces of up to 60% of children with haemolytic uraemic syndrome.

Renal Ultrasound

This should be done to exclude obstructive uropathy which may require urgent drainage procedures. Bilaterally small kidneys suggest chronic renal failure.

Renal Biopsy

This may be indicated when the cause of the renal failure is not apparent, or a drug-induced interstitial nephritis or rapidly progressive glomerulonephritis is suspected.

Table 6.1 Reference ranges for serum creatinine ($\mu mol/l$)

	Urine sodium concentration (mmol/l)	FENa (%)	U/P creatinine
Renal	> 60	> 3	< 20
Pre-renal	< 20	< 1	> 20

U/P = Urine concentration/Plasma concentration.

Investigations to Plan Management

Plasma creatinine and electrolytes provide an indication of the severity of renal failure. When the plasma creatinine concentration is greater than three times normal for the patient's age or is rapidly rising, then dialysis treatment may be required and the patient should be referred to an appropriate centre. Similarly a plasma potassium greater than 6.5 mmol/l or severe acidosis requires urgent treatment. Hypocalcaemia and a high plasma phosphate would suggest chronic renal failure.

CHRONIC RENAL INSUFFICIENCY

Glomerular Clearance

If a solute is cleared from the plasma only by the glomerulus, then its rate of appearance in the urine is equal to the product of the urine concentration (U) and the urine flow rate (V). It follows that the rate of its appearance in the urine must equal its rate of disappearance from the plasma which is the product of the plasma concentration (P) and the unit volume of plasma (C)

$$CP = UV$$
$$C = U(V/P)$$

The clearance of a solute will only measure true glomerular filtration rate (GFR) when it is totally filtered by the glomerulus, not bound to plasma proteins and neither reabsorbed nor excreted by the renal tubules. Inulin meets these requirements but, because its chemical analysis is difficult, its use is generally reserved for research purposes and other solutes are used for routine clinical practice.

Glomerular Filtration Rate

The GFR is the most widely used test of glomerular function. Its value gives useful information about the number of functioning nephrons. Under normal physiological conditions it varies with diet and posture, tending to be higher during the day than at night. It alters significantly with age. For these reasons it is important that it is measured under carefully standardized conditions to enable reproducible results to be obtained. It can be measured using a variety of different techniques.

Measurement of GFR

Standard Method

This requires the collection of a timed urine sample to obtain the numerator (UV) of the clearance formula. The plasma concentration of the solute should be measured at the midpoint of urine collection to give the denominator (P). This technique of measuring GFR is difficult in small children because accurate timed urine collections cannot be obtained easily, and alternative techniques have been devised.

Slope Disappearance Technique

This requires the intravenous injection of a solute. Three blood samples are then taken usually 2, 3 and 4 h afterwards. GFR is calculated from the terminal slope of the plasma disappearance curve or from the area under the curve. [^{125}I]othalomate [^{51}Cr]ethylenediamine tetraacetic acid ([^{51}Cr]EDTA) and [$^{99}_m$Tc]diethylenetriamine pentaacetic acid (DTPA) are most frequently used.

Constant Infusion Technique

This requires a solute to be infused at a constant rate which has been calculated to maintain a steady plasma concentration. GFR can then be calculated from the rate of infusion and the plasma concentration of the solute after a period of equilibration. It is a laborious method and not widely used. This technique is employed principally when measuring inulin clearances.

Creatinine Clearance

The estimation of GFR from creatinine clearance is widely used in clinical practice. Creatinine is a naturally occurring substance, formed in the muscles by conversion from creatine and creatine phosphate. Its rate of production has a direct relationship to the patient's muscle mass and body weight, and is constant for the same individual, assuming no change in muscle mass. As both weight and muscle mass increase with growth, the plasma creatinine will be expected to increase with age. It is freely filtered at the glomerulus but a significant amount is secreted by the proximal tubules. As a result the true creatinine clearance may be 30% greater than the inulin clearance. However, when creatinine is measured by methods that measure total creatinine chromogens, the plasma concentration is higher and, therefore, the P value is artificially high, making the calculated clearance value lower. It is fortuitous that the creatinine clearance then approximates more closely to the inulin clearance.

The chemical estimation of creatinine is interfered with by ketones and cephalosporin antibiotics which cause an inappropriately high creatinine. Conversely, bilirubin reduces the measured creatinine.

Plasma Creatinine Concentration

Although creatinine clearance can be measured by standard clearance methods, GFR can also be calculated from the plasma creatinine concentration. It has been shown that the ratio of patient's height (centimetres) and the plasma creatinine (micromoles per litre) has a constant relationship to GFR when it is corrected to 1.73 m^2 body surface area. Furthermore, when this ratio is multiplied by 40, the results approximate to the GFR. Thus:

$$\text{GFR (ml/min per 1.73 m}^2) = (\text{Height/Creatinine}) \times 40.$$

This formula has proved to be a clinically useful way of following the progression of renal disease in children (Parkin et al 1989). It cannot, however, be applied to infants and the newborn.

Urea

Urea is a major metabolite of protein catabolism. It is formed by the liver and both excreted and reabsorbed by the renal tubules. Its concentration in the plasma is influenced by the dietary protein intake, catabolism and the state of hydration as well as GFR. The urea level is not a reliable marker of GFR, but can provide useful information about the nutritional state of children with renal disease where it will be inappropriately high when compared with the plasma creatinine concentration.

B$_2$ Microglobulin

This has been proposed as an alternative to plasma creatinine to calculate GFR, but its value is limited because its rate of production and plasma concentrations are increased by other factors including inflammatory diseases and neoplasia.

Effects of Maturation on GFR

GFR is low at birth, averaging 3 ml/min in the term infant. It then rapidly increases during the first 6 months of life and thereafter there is a steady increment reaching normal adult values by the age of 14 years. So that some valid comparison of GFR can be made between different children of different ages, it is generally necessary to make a correction for body size. It is conventional to use the body surface area (SA) and to standardize GFR to 1.73 m^2 body surface area. Surface area can be computed from the height (centimetres) and weight (kilograms) and referring to a standard nomogram. During the neonatal period, however, there are strong arguments for standardizing GFR for body weight, rather than surface area, because this correction produces less variability. Normal values for plasma creatinine for children of different ages are shown in Table 6.2 and those for the GFR in Table 6.3.

Chronic renal insufficiency may be said to have occurred when the GFR has fallen below 25% of normal. This usually occurs when the plasma creatinine is three times the normal for age. Investigations may be categorized into those designed to establish the cause and those examining the consequence of renal insufficiency.

Table 6.2 Reference ranges for serum creatinine (μmol/l)

Age	Males Mean	Males Range	Females Mean	Females Range
1–3 months	43	19–67	44	29–59
3–6 months	45	28–62	43	29–57
6–12 months	44	23–65	43	20–66
1 year	48	22–74	45	24–66
2 years	46	26–66	46	21–71
3 years	49	32–66	49	26–72
4 years	51	28–74	51	35–67
5 years	53	34–72	50	32–68
6 years	55	34–76	51	36–66
7 years	56	39–73	54	36–72
8 years	57	38–76	58	43–73
9 years	60	38–82	57	45–69
10 years	64	40–88	60	47–73
11 years	63	47–79	63	44–82
12 years	66	46–86	60	51–69
13 years	69	44–94	66	53–79
14 years	70	52–88	69	48–90
15 years	77	53–101	69	54–84
16 years	80	52–108	72	51–93
17 years	81	62–100	76	59–93
18 years	86	64–108	76	59–95
19 years	89	68–110	77	59–95
20 years	85	63–107	75	53–97

Data from Savory (1990).

Table 6.3 Normal creatinine clearance (ml/min per 1.73 m^2)

Age	Mean	Range
1–3 months	51	27–69
3–6 months	73	61–84
6–12 months	93	77–126
>2 years	150	110–200

Investigations to Establish the Cause of Renal Failure

A detailed history is invaluable. Previous evidence of urinary tract infection would suggest chronic pyelonephritis. A family history of renal disease may give a clue to the nature of the underlying renal defect. Small stature, particularly dating from birth, may suggest renal dysplasia.

Urine Examination

This may show evidence of infection suggesting reflux nephropathy. Significant proteinuria, haematuria and red cell casts would point to glomerulonephritis. Normal urine can be found in the nephropathy associated with familial nephronophthysis and nephrocalcinosis.

Renal Ultrasound

This examination is done to show the kidney size. Small kidneys being the end-point of any renal pathology and merely indicating the irreversibility of the renal disease. Large hydronephrotic kidneys may require surgical drainage.

Micturating Cystourethrogram

This will show evidence of reflux nephropathy. Surgical correction of reflux does not delay the progression of the renal failure, but a cystogram is important to show the anatomy of the bladder if renal transplantation is considered in the future.

Renal Biopsy

This is rarely indicated in chronic renal insufficiency unless the onset has been relatively recent and drug toxicity or rapidly progressive glomerulonephritis is suspected.

Investigations to Examine the Consequences of Renal Insufficiency

Renal insufficiency is a debilitating illness with important effects on growth, nutrition and most organs in the body.

Anaemia

Serum ferritin concentration is regarded as the best indication of iron stores in renal failure. Higher levels than normal are found in renal failure when concentrations less than 100 μg/l suggest iron deficiency. Folate deficiency should also be excluded by measuring the red cell folate concentration. The assay of erythropoetin has very little value in the management of anaemia in renal failure.

Bone Disease

Renal bone disease develops when the GFR falls below 25 ml/min per 1.73 m^2. It is suggested when the plasma calcium is low or normal, the plasma phosphate and bone alkaline phosphatase concentrations are high. Plasma 1,25-dihydroxy vitamin D concentrations will be low and parathyroid hormone concentrations high. The N-terminal parathyroid hormone concentration should be measured regularly and its concentration controlled by reducing dietary phosphorus intake and using phosphate binders such as calcium carbonate. X-ray of the bone including chest, spine, pelvis and long bones will show evidence of rickets and/or hyperparathyroidism. Rickets is best seen in the X-rays of the wrists. The hyperparathyroid changes are manifested by subperiostial erosions in the phalanges of the fingers.

Cardiovascular Disease

Many children with renal insufficiency are hypertensive. Cardiac hypertrophy is common and uraemic cardiomyopathy may also occur. Regular chest X-rays are important to document cardiac size and pulmonary vasculature. Echocardiography provides information about cardiac function and should be done regularly, particularly in patients with hypertension treated by beta-blocker drugs.

Nutrition

Regular measurements of growth velocity and skin-fold thickness give information about the nutritional status and response to dietary manoeuvres. Although the blood urea concentration is a poor marker of GFR, it is valuable in the assessment of the nutritional status of patients with renal insufficiency. If the concentration is inappropriately high, compared with the plasma creatinine, then increased protein catabolism is implied. The protein catabolic rate can be calculated from the rate of rise of plasma urea and the urine excretion rates.

Neurological Disorders

These include uraemic myopathy, peripheral neuropathy and generalized seizures. The myopathy affects particularly the proximal muscle groups and is usually associated with advanced renal bone disease. Peripheral neuropathy is mixed motor and sensory, particularly affecting the lower limbs. It is important to exclude other causes for neuropathy, such as vitamin B deficiency and drug toxicity. Electrophysiological studies will identify these neurological abnormalities.

RENAL TUBULAR DISORDERS

Tubular Excretion and Reabsorption

If the glomerular clearance of a solute is greater than inulin then it follows that renal tubular secretion has occurred. Conversely, if a solute clearance is less than inulin clearance then tubular reabsorption has occurred. From these observations the concept of fractional clearance of a solute is derived. Thus the clearance of a solute (S) can be expressed as a fraction of inulin clearance:

$$FE^s = \frac{U^s V^s / P^s}{U^i V^i / P^i}$$

If the urine volume is the same for each measurement then V will cancel and the equation becomes:

$$FE^s = \frac{U^s / P^i}{P^s / U^i}$$

It can be expressed as a percentage by multiplying by 100. Conversely, the tubular reabsorption (TRP) of a solute is

$$TRP\% = 100 - FE^s$$
$$= 100 \left(1 - \frac{U^s / P^i}{P^s / U^i} \right)$$

Because of the difficulties of measuring inulin in clinical practice, creatinine is generally substituted.

Clinical Investigation

Disturbance of renal tubular function may be suspected when there is depletion of one or more plasma electrolytes which cannot be explained by gastrointestinal losses. There is frequently failure to thrive and polyuria. Renal tubular dysfunction can conveniently be categorized depending upon the site of tubular injury. Investigation requires, first, the characterization of the site of the tubular damage and, secondly, the identification of the pathological process which has caused it.

Proximal Tubular Disorders

The proximal tubule reabsorbs at least 85% of the glomerular filtrate. Sodium, bicarbonate, phosphate,

glucose, amino acid and water are all actively reabsorbed at this site. Proximal tubular damage may be associated with increased urinary loss of one or all of these solutes.

Tubular Proteinuria

See p. 101.

Proximal Renal Tubular Acidosis (Type-II RTA)

Under normal circumstances the plasma bicarbonate concentration is kept at a constant level. The threshold at which bicarbonate is no longer completely absorbed by the renal tubule alters with maturity. In adults the plasma bicarbonate does not exceed 25–26 mmol/l, in the newborn the threshold is 22 mmol/l, and children have a value somewhere in between. When the renal threshold is exceeded, urinary excretion of bicarbonate occurs. The fractional excretion of bicarbonate is then greater than normal.

The characteristic features of proximal RTA are:

- The threshold for bicarbonate is low. This can be investigated by bicarbonate infusion and determining the plasma concentration at which bicarbonate appears in the urine. This is a laborious technique and not used in routine clinical practice. A simpler way is to calculate the fractional excretion of bicarbonate which should not exceed the normal (10%).
- The urine is alkaline (pH > 5.5) in the presence of systemic acidosis, but in contrast to distal RTA, the urine can become acid (pH < 5.5) when the plasma bicarbonate falls below the renal threshold for bicarbonate and its tubular reabsorption is complete. Usually this occurs when the blood pH is less than 7.2.
- Treatment requires relatively large doses of bicarbonate compared with distal RTA, often in the region of 20 mmol/kg per 24 h. It is not generally possible fully to correct the plasma bicarbonate level by bicarbonate supplements.
- Hypokalaemia is a common association. Probably due to secondary hyperaldosteronism.

Hypophosphataemic Rickets (Vitamin-D-Resistant Rickets)

This is a familial disorder. It may be inherited as a dominant characteristic. Analysis of kindreds has shown that females are affected more than males indicating an X-linked dominant form of inheritance. Sporadic cases have also been described. Although the defect is present at birth, it does not usually present clinically until the second year of life when typical features of rickets become manifest. Muscle weakness may also be a feature, causing delayed motor development.

The characteristic features of hypophosphataemic rickets include:

- Radiological and biological evidence of rickets. The plasma calcium may be normal or low. The plasma phosphate is usually less than 0.7 mmol/l and the bone alkaline phosphatase is high.
- Increased urinary phosphate loss is indicated by a low tubular reabsorption of phosphorus (TRP). It is usually less than 60% (normal >75%). Alternatively, the tubular maximum of phosphate (TMP) corrected for GFR (TMP GFR) can be calculated and is similarly low (Shaw et al 1992).
- The plasma parathyroid hormone concentration is increased. This secondary hyperparathyroidism contributes to the increased urinary phosphate leak and generalized aminoaciduria which may also be found.
- Treatment with pharmacological doses of vitamin D, or its metabolites, is necessary to heal the rickets. Phosphate supplements are also necessary to maintain normal plasma phosphate concentrations.
- Growth is stunted but height velocity increases following successful treatment.

Aminoaciduria

Aminoaciduria may occur as result of two basic defects. Firstly, in inborn errors of metabolism which cause an increase in the plasma concentrations of specific amino acids and their consequent urinary excretion. The overflow aminoaciduria occurs in conditions such as phenylketonuria, tyrosinaemia, liver failure and during parenteral nutrition. Secondly, aminoaciduria occurs when there is a defect in renal tubular reabsorption of amino acids. This second group may be further classified according to the type of amino acids involved.

Generalized Aminoaciduria

In this group of disorders no one amino acid predominates. It usually indicates complex proximal renal tubular damage as occurs in the Fanconi syndrome and may be due to a variety of nephrotoxic insults. Renal tubular immaturity in the premature and newborn infant is associated with general amino aciduria.

Specific Aminoaciduria

Excess urinary excretion of specific amino acids is rare. Glycinuria and histidinuria have been described and are usually asymptomatic. More frequently there is excess excretion of groups of amino acids which share the same transport mechanisms. These include:

- *Cystinuria*. There is excess excretion of the dibasic amino acids cystine, lysine, arginine and ornithine. The sulphur containing amino acid cystine is insoluble in acid urine (pH < 7) and precipitates forming stones. Cystine stones are radio-opaque. The urinary excretion of cystine exceeds the normal of 300 mg/ 24 h. The diagnosis should be suspected when hexagonal crystals are seen on urine microscopy.
- *Hartnup disease*. The neutral amino acids alanine, threonine, valine, leucine, isoleucine, phenylalanine, glutamine, histidine, asparagine, tyrosine, tryptophane and citrulline are all present in the urine. The clinical features of cerebellar ataxia and a scaly photosensitive skin rash suggest the diagnosis.

Renal Glycosuria

This may occur in two situations. In the first the renal threshold of glucose is normal but, because of nephron heterogeneity, some individual nephrons leak glucose at lower plasma concentrations than others. This phenomenon causes an increased splay of the glucose titration curve. It is a phenomenon found in renal insufficiency and during infancy and has no clinical significance. In the second type of renal glycosuria (true renal glycosuria), the renal threshold for glucose is low. It is extremely rare except when it occurs as part of the Fanconi syndrome.

The Fanconi Syndrome

In this syndrome there is excess urinary loss of sodium, potassium, bicarbonate, phosphorus, glucose and water with generalized aminoaciduria. The primary clinical features are failure to thrive, rickets and polyuria. It is suspected when there is glycosuria in the presence of a normal plasma glucose, hypokalaemia, hypophosphataemia, aminoaciduria and acidosis. The urinary losses of these specific solutes may be investigated as outlined above. Tubular proteinuria will also be present.

The nature of the renal tubular injury causing Fanconi syndrome should be examined further. Many are idiopathic, but cystinosis is the commonest cause. This can be diagnosed by measuring the white blood cell cystine concentration and suspected when slit-lamp examination of the eye shows crystals in the cornea. Nephrotoxic drugs and heavy metals, such as lead and gold, should be considered. In tyrosinaemia there is an increased urinary excretion of succinylacetate and the renal Fanconi syndrome is a late feature in the course of the disease.

Distal Renal Tubular Abnormalities

The Syndrome of Nephrogenic Diabetes Insipidus

This is distinguished from pituitary diabetes insipidus by the inability of the kidney to produce a concentrated urine in the presence of high plasma levels of antidiuretic hormone (ADH). The diagnosis should be suspected when the urine flow rate is high or when episodes of hypernatraemic dehydration occur. It is confirmed by a water deprivation test and examining the renal response to antidiuretic hormone.

The water deprivation test should be carried out in the early morning. The patient is weighed and plasma and urine osmolalities measured. If the plasma osmolality is 290 mosm/kg of water or higher and the urine is dilute, then the diagnosis is confirmed and no further testing should be carried out. If the plasma osmolality is normal (< 285 mosm/kg of water) then the fluid deprivation test should proceed. The patient is weighed each hour and the urine and plasma osmolality measured. The test is positive and should be discontinued if the plasma osmolality reaches 295 mosm/kg of water or a weight loss greater than 4% occurs. Otherwise, after 7–8 h desamino 8 D-arginine vasopressin (DDAVP) is given by nasal inhalation in a dose of 5 μg to a neonate, 10 μg to an infant and 20 μg to older children. Normally this is followed by a further increase in urine osmolality to concentrations greater than 800 mosm/kg of water. A failure to respond suggests nephrogenic diabetes insipidus.

The measurement of plasma concentrations of ADH is not essential for the diagnosis. In patients with nephrogenic diabetes insipidus the plasma ADH levels are higher than normal for given urine and plasma osmolalities.

Nephrogenic diabetes insipidus may occur due to failure of the distal tubule to respond to ADH as a primary abnormality. This is inherited as a sex-linked disorder occurring predominantly in males, it rarely occurs in females. More frequently it occurs secondary to other kidney disorders, such as medullary cystic kidney disease, polycystic kidney disease, pyelonephritis and Fanconi syndrome.

The kidneys of infants during the first year of life are unable to concentrate urine to more than 300 mosm/kg of water. Adult levels are usually achieved by the age of 2–3 years.

Distal Renal Tubular Acidosis (Type-I RTA)

The distal renal tubule reabsorbs the 10–15% of bicarbonate which is not absorbed by the proximal tubule and secretes hydrogen ion which is titrated by the urinary buffers $NaHPO_4$ and NH_3 to NaH_2PO_4 and NH_4^+. Titratable acid refers to the hydrogen ion excreted as NaH_2PO_4. Ammonium is measured directly. Net acid excretion is the sum of the excretion of ammonium and NaH_2PO_4 minus the excretion of bicarbonate. The distal tubule excretes a relatively small amount of hydrogen ion (1–2 mmol/kg per 24 h) and this can easily be overwhelmed if relatively small amounts of bicarbonate are rejected by the proximal tubule. Because the distal tubule makes a small contribution to acid excretion, the acidosis of distal RTA can be corrected with relatively small amounts of bicarbonate (2–3 mmol/kg per 24 h). In some children with distal RTA large amounts of bicarbonate are required to correct the acidosis, this suggests there is a degree of proximal tubular rejection of bicarbonate as well. This mixed proximal and distal RTA is referred to as type-III RTA. It is a disorder frequently found in the neonatal period and is usually transient. Plasma potassium is low in RTA.

Distal RTA presents as failure to thrive and rarely as an acute emergency with severe acidosis, shock and hypokalaemia. It should be suspected when:

- There is severe systemic acidosis (blood pH < 7.2) in the presence of an alkaline urine (pH > 5.5).
- There is systemic acidosis with a high plasma chloride greater than 110 mmol/l and a normal anion gap of 7–15 mmol/l.

If both of these conditions apply, then the diagnosis of RTA is confirmed and no further investigations should be carried out. In the absence of systemic acidosis then an acid loading test should be performed. It should never be done if the patient is already acidotic.

Acid Loading Test

One of two blood and urine samples are obtained in the first hour for control levels before the administration of the acid load. The acidifying agent may be ammonium chloride 100 mEq/m² body surface area given orally or argenine hydrochloride 100–150 mEq/m² body surface area given intravenously. Blood and urine pH, urine ammonia, titratable acidity and bicarbonate are measured at hourly intervals. An adequate urine flow rate is ensured by providing water freely throughout the test. Normally the blood pH should be less than 7.2 3–4 h after the acid load when a urine pH less than 5.5 should be achieved. The titratable acidity is normally between 33–71 mEq/min per 1.73 m² and ammonium excretion between 46 and 100 mEq/min per 1.73 m². Patients with distal RTA will fail to acidify the urine and have reduced titratable acid and ammonium excretion rates.

Examination of the urinary anion gap (sodium plus potassium minus chloride) has been found to be a useful method of assessing ammonium excretion. As ammonium is excreted in association with chloride then the anion gap will become progressively more negative as ammonium excretion increases. The normal urinary anion gap after a three day ammonium chloride load (100 mg/kg body weight per day) is negative (−27 mmol/l) but in RTA it is positive because of the reduced ammonium excretion (Battle et al 1988).

Distal RTA is often secondary to other renal diseases including medullary cystic disease, pyelonephritis, and obstructive nephropathy. These should be excluded by renal ultrasound and DTPA scan. It is rare as a primary disorder when it is usually inherited as an autosomal dominant characteristic.

Type-IV RTA is now recognized as the commonest type in children. In contrast to the other types it is charcterized by hyperkalaemia rather than hypokalaemia. The defect in urinary acidification, acidosis and potassium retention have been attributed either to lack of or defective tubular response to aldosterone. It is commonly found in renal insufficiency. The kidneys of newborn infants have a reduced ability to excrete an acid load. This is due to a reduced net acid excretion rate, which rapidly matures and reaches adult values within the first month of life.

Miscellaneous Renal Tubular Disorders

Bartters Syndrome

This usually presents with a failure to thrive with weakness, polyuria and salt craving. It occurs in infancy and rarely in childhood. It is a syndrome characterized by hypokalaemic alkalosis with hypochloraemia and a tendency to hyponatraemia. The presence of hypertension excludes it as a diagnostic possibility. Glomerular filtration rate is normal, but there is an inappropriately high urinary excretion of potassium and an inability to concentrate the urine maximally. There is a high urinary excretion of prostaglandin E_2, and elevated plasma aldosterone and renin but these are secondary phenomena. The renal histology is characterized by hyperplasia of the juxtaglomerular apparatus and, in some cases, interstitial nephritis.

Proteinuria

Proteinuria is an important sign of renal disease. It is helpful both in the diagnosis of renal disease and in assessing its progress and response to treatment. Proteinuria can be evaluated both quantitatively and qualitatively.

Quantitative Evaluation

- *Dipstix*. This is a specific test for protein but correlates with quantitative measurements of proteinuria in only about two-thirds of cases. It measures the urinary protein concentration and is insensitive to levels less than 30 mg/dl.
- *Precipitation methods*. These techniques depend upon the characteristics of most proteins to precipitate when heated or in the presence of strong acids. They are generally performed by heating the urine and adding glacial acetic acid or 5% sulphosalicylic acid. The amount of flocculation is graded on a 0–4 scale. Protein concentrations as low as 10 mg/dl can be detected by these techniques. Radiocontrast materials and drugs, including penicillin, may give false-positive results. These methods are cheaper to perform than the dipstix, but are less convenient.
- *24-h Urine protein*. This is the standard way of quantifying proteinuria. The protein concentration is measured using standard flocculation techniques. Protein excretion is not constant during the day, it varies with posture and diet and, for these reasons, short urine collection periods may not be reliable. Proteinuria may be graded:

  Normal < 4 mg/m^2 per hour
  Significant proteinuria 4–40 mg/m^2 per hour
  Nephrotic proteinuria > 40 mg/m^2 per hour

- *Protein/creatinine ratio (PCR)*. This is a rapid and simple way of quantifying proteinuria in children. It has the advantage that it can be performed on a random urine sample, the first morning specimen is the best. In addition there is a good correlation between the PCR and the 24-h urine protein excretion. The normal protein (mg/l)/creatinine (mmol/l) ratio is less than 0.2. Some laboratories multiply the ratio by 1000. The result is then expressed as a protein creatinine index (PCI) which, when normal, is less than 200.

Qualitative Evaluation

Knowledge about the characteristics of proteinuria is helpful in determining the nature of the renal injury. Glomerular injury is characterized by high-molecular-weight proteins in the urine. Tubular proteinuria occurs when low-molecular-weight proteins are filtered at the glomerulus, not reabsorbed because of damage to the proximal renal tubule and appear in the urine. Mixed glomerular and tubular proteinuria indicates severe renal injury. The different types of protein may be characterized using polyacrylamide gel electrophoresis (PAGE) or by the measurement of specific proteins using radioimmunoassay (RIA) (Brocklebank et al 1991).

Glomerular Proteinuria

Of proteinuria in glomerular disease, 60% is albumin (molecular weight (MW) 60 kDa). The remainder is made up of variable amounts of haptoglobin, transferrin and immunoglobulins. Glomerular proteinuria can be further subdivided into selective or non-selective proteinuria depending upon the ratio of the glomerular clearances of a high-molecular-weight and low-molecular-weight protein. Albumin or transferrin are generally measured as being representative of low-molecular-weight proteins and Immunoglobulin G (IgG) as representative of high-molecular-weight proteins. The clearance of albumin is given by:

$$C_a = \frac{U_a V_a}{P_a}$$

and the clearance of IgG as

$$C_g = \frac{U_g V_g}{P_g}$$

If the same urine is used for each measurement, then the V term will cancel. Thus the selectivity ratio is:

$$S = \frac{U_g P_a}{P_g U_a}$$

A urine selectivity ratio less than 0.1 generally suggests steroid responsive nephrotic syndrome and greater than 0.3 steroid resistance. There is, however, considerable variability in the selectivity ratio in steroid responsive nephrotic syndrome, and for this reason the test has limited clinical usefulness.

Tubular Proteinuria

A pattern of proteinuria in which proteins of lower molecular weight than albumin occur is found when there is damage to the proximal renal tubule. These proteins are filtered at the glomerulus and appear in the urine because of failure of reabsorption. Many tubular proteins have been identified as useful markers of proximal tubular disease. β_2 microglobulin (MW 11.3 kDa), retinol binding protein (MW 21 kDa) and α_1 micro-

globulin (MW 31 kDa) can readily be measured by RIA. The presence of these low-molecular-weight proteins in the urine suggests renal tubular damage. Overflow proteinuria may occur when there is excess production of α_2 microglobulins due to sepsis or to immunological disorders.

Urinary Enzymes

Several urinary enzymes have been examined as markers of renal damage. N-Acetylglucosaminidase (NAG) has been widely investigated. It is an intracellular enzyme released from the lysozomes of the proximal tubular cell following injury. Although present in most cells, its molecular size excludes it from the normal glomerular filtrate. Increased excretion has been found in renal transplant rejection, drug toxicity and interstitial nephritis. It is a highly sensitive marker of early renal tubular damage and can be detected in the urine long before there is significant evidence of reduction in the GFR. Other enzymes including the brush border enzyme alanine aminopeptidase and intestinal-type alkaline phosphatase may prove to be helpful in determining the site of renal injury.

Clinical Types of Proteinuria

Intermittent proteinuria is a transient increase in urinary protein excretion, usually following strenuous exercise or fever. It occurs in the absence of significant renal disease.

Postural proteinuria is a type of intermittent proteinuria which is present only when the individual is in the upright posture. The amount of proteinuria seldom exceeds 20 mg/m^2 per 24 h. It can be detected by measuring the protein concentration in an early morning urine, after the patient has been recumbent all night, and comparing it with the concentration in the sample obtained at the end of the day. The early morning urine protein concentration should be normal (PCR < 0.2). Postural proteinuria is a phenomenon found frequently in adolescent boys and in the healing phase of acute glomerulonephritis.

In *persistent* proteinuria, protein excretion is between 4–40 mg/m^2 per 24 h. It can best be detected by asking the patient to record the urinary albustix measurement in an early morning urine sample for at least a week. The majority of patients do not have significant renal pathology on renal biopsy, unless there is also haematuria. A minority have been shown to have focal segmental glomerular sclerosis.

Nephrotic Syndrome

When the urinary protein excretion rate is 40 mg/m^2 per 24 h or greater, and there is associated hypoalbuminaemia and oedema, then the clinical picture of nephrotic syndrome is present. About 80% of childhood nephrotics have steroid responsive nephrotic syndrome. This group, in general, has minimal changes on renal histology (MCNS), the remaining 20% comprise a variety of other glomerular pathologies and this group, in general, have a much poorer prognosis. It includes focal segmental glomerular sclerosis, mesangiocapillary glomerular nephritis and other primary and secondary glomerular diseases. It is therefore important to determine into which of these two groups an individual patient fits. There are a number of clinical features that are helpful.

Age

The peak age of onset of MCNS is between 1 and 4 years of age. By the age of 8 years, about 50% of children with nephrotic syndrome have MCNS, the remaining 50% at this age fall into the poor prognosis group. Under the age of 1 year, congenital nephrotic syndrome is the most frequent cause.

Sex

MCNS is much more common in boys than girls with a male/female sex ratio of $3.5 : 1$.

Hypertension

This is rare in MCNS, but when present implies a poor prognosis.

Urinalysis

The presence of haematuria, granular or red cell casts, implies a disease in the poor prognosis group, but up to 10% of children with MCNS may have microscopic haematuria.

Heavy proteinuria is characteristic of all types of nephrotic syndrome. An albumin/IgG clearance ratio (urinary protein selectivity) of less than 0.1 suggests steroid responsive nephrotic syndrome and a ratio greater than 0.2 suggests a poorer prognosis. Although there are some exceptions to this guideline, it remains a useful test to apply to all new nephrotic patients.

Impaired glomerular filtration rate

This occurs rarely in MCNS, and an elevated plasma creatinine suggests a disease in the poor-prognosis group.

C_3 Complement

The C_3 complement is normal in minimal change nephrotic syndrome. When low it suggests mesangiocapillary glomerular nephritis and this can be confirmed by measurement of the C_3 nephritic factor. However, rarer causes of nephrotic syndrome, such as lupus nephritis and shunt nephritis, may also be associated with a low C_3 complement level.

Trial of Steroids

Of children with nephrotic syndrome, 80% will respond to steroids and it is always worth a trial of this drug in the absence of any adverse features. The majority of children will respond to a dose of prednisolone of 60 mg/m^2 within 4 weeks. Failure to do so suggests a disease in the poor-prognosis group.

Renal Biopsy

A renal biopsy should be undertaken early in those children with adverse clinical features and in those who fail to respond to prednisolone after 4 weeks of treatment.

Haematuria

Gross haematuria can easily be recognized by the typical coloration of the urine, but it is important to remember that vegetable dyes and some drugs may also stain the urine red. The dipstix test uses an orthotoluene impregnated paper strip and the peroxidase activity of haemoglobin facilitates the oxidation of the dye to a blue colour. Myoglobin produces a similar colour. The dipstix test is sensitive and will detect at least five red cells per high-powered field. If haematuria is suspected, then the presence of red blood cells should be confirmed by microscopy. Cells which have passed through the glomerulus tend to be damaged whereas those arising from the lower urinary tract appear intact. Red blood cells lyse quickly in an acid urine (pH < 6) and when the urine specific gravity is less than 1005. More than three red blood cells per high-powered field is considered to be abnormal. White blood cells are recognized as nucleated cells which are larger than red blood cells. Tubular cells are columnar in shape with the nucleus situated at the base. Epithelial cells are much larger with a centrally placed nucleus.

Haematuria is a common presenting feature of many renal diseases. It is convenient to consider the causes in four major categories: structural abnormalities of the urinary tract including renal calculi, urinary tract infection, nephritis including both glomerulonephritis and interstitial nephritis and finally haematological disorders. It is usually possible to distinguish between all of these by careful history and physical examination.

History

A full history of the onset is necessary. An infection occurring 2 or 3 weeks previously would suggest a post-infectious glomerulonephritis. If the infection coincides with the onset of haematuria, then an IgA nephropathy is likely, particularly if the haematuria is recurrent. Acute pyelonephritis is suggested when there is a history of high fever and dysuria. A family history of haematuria is found in autosomal dominant polycystic kidney disease and metabolic stone disease. When associated with deafness and a family history of renal failure, Alport's disease is likely. A family history of haematuria is also present in benign recurrent familial haematuria. When there is a history of drug ingestion it is important to consider the possibility of a drug-induced interstitial nephritis. The pattern of haematuria is also important. It may be gross or microscopic, intermittent or persistent. Persistent haematuria, whether gross or microscopic, usually represents a serious underlying pathology.

Urine Examination

When the haematuria is intermittent it can be confirmed by dipstix testing of urine at home. It is important to establish the presence of red blood cells by urine microscopy. Red blood cell casts indicate glomerular nephritis and pyelonephritis is suggested by the presence of bacteriuria. Significant proteinuria suggests glomerular nephritis and the protein to creatinine ratio should be measured. A third of children with isolated haematuria without proteinuria have hypercalciuria which is detected by a urine calcium to creatinine ratio greater than 0.7 mmol/mmol.

Haematological Disorders

Disorders of coagulation may be detected by clotting studies and a blood film should also be examined. Where appropriate the sickledex test is also indicated.

Renal Ultrasound

This should be done on all children to demonstrate structural abnormalities of the urinary tract or renal calculi. Renal scarring, due to chronic pyelonephritis, may also be demonstrated. Minor degrees of scarring can be confirmed by dimercaptosuccinic acid (DMSA) scan.

Immunological Investigations

Evidence of recent streptococcal infection suggesting poststreptococcal glomerulonephritis is indicated by a rise in antistreptolysin O titre. Raised levels of anti-hyalurolidase and antideoxyribonuclease B are more sensitive indicators of recent streptococcal infection. Postinfectious glomerular nephritis activates the alternative pathway of the complement cascade, depressing the serum C3 levels below 80 mg/dl for up to 3 months after the initial illness. If the level remains low for more than 3 months then either mesangiocapillary nephritis or lupus nephritis may be preseent. These can be confirmed by examination of the serum C3 nephritic factor and DNA binding, respectively.

When structural abnormalities have been excluded and both urinary calcium and clotting studies are normal, then the haematuria is most likely due to some form of glomerular nephritis. A renal biopsy is indicated only when the haematuria is persistent and associated with significant proteinuria when important types of glomerulonephritis are suspected. Isolated intermittent haematuria is generally present in benign forms of glomerular nephritis and do not always require a renal biopsy for confirmation.

Renal Stone Disease

Renal stone disease affects between 1 and 2 children per million population. Stones develop when the solubility coefficient of the solute is exceeded either due to excess concentration or change in the acidity of the urine. Precipitation is encouraged by the presence of cellular debris and other particles. Citrate, pyrophosphate and mucopolysaccharides are important inhibitors of urinary crystal growth and stone formation.

Infective Stones

Over 80% of renal stones are associated with urinary infection or stasis. It is important to exclude anatomical abnormalities of the urinary tract by ultrasound and diethylenetriamine pentaacetic acid (DTPA) scan will identify obstruction. The stones comprise either ammonium magnesium phosphate (struvite) or calcium hydrogen phosphate (apatite) and are radio opaque.

Hypercalciuria

This is the next commonest cause of renal calculi. It is defined as a urinary calcium excretion in excess of 0.1 mmol/kg per 24 h or a calcium/creatinine ratio greater than 0.7 mmol/mmol. The calcium excretion can also be corrected for changes in creatinine clearance rate and this is known as the calcium excretion index.

$$\text{Ca excretion index} = (U_{Ca}V)(P_{Cr}/U_{Cr}V)$$
$$= U_{Ca}P_{Cr}/U_{Cr}$$

where U_{Ca} and U_{Cr} are the urinary concentrations of calcium and creatinine, respectively, V is the urine volume, and P_{Cr} the plasma creatinine concentration. The upper limit of normal for the calcium excretion index is 35 mol/l (Shaw et al 1992).

Idiopathic hypercalciuria may result from increased gut absorption or an increased renal tubular secretion of calcium. They can be distinguished from each other by an oral calcium loading test but, in clinical practice, there is no advantage in distinguishing the two as treatment of both is identical.

Cystine Stones

This is a cause of radio-opaque renal calculi and has been discussed under the heading "Renal Tubular Disorders".

Hyperoxaluria

This may be due to one of two inborn errors of metabolism. In type-I hyperoxaluria there is a defect of the enzyme allanine glycolate aminotransferase which is located in the peroxisomes of the liver. In type-II disease there is excess urine excretion of glyceric acid as well as oxalate. A third type of hyperoxaluria occurs secondary to some types of malabsorption and inflammatory bowel disease. Oxalate renal calculi are radio-opaque and there is usually nephrocalcinosis. The normal urinary excretion of oxalate is between 0.2 and 0.5 mmol/1.73 m² per 24 h (Henderson 1993). Type-I hyperoxaluria has a much worse prognosis and often progresses to renal failure. The diagnosis can be confirmed by analysis of the enzyme content of a liver biopsy.

Purine Stones

These occur as a result of rare inborn errors of metabolism. Nevertheless they are important because of the availability of specific treatments. In a third of cases acute renal failure may be the presenting feature. All purine stones are radiolucent. Defects of the purine salvage enzymes hypoxanthine guanine phosphoribosyl transferase (HGPRT) (Lesch–Nyhan syndrome), adeninephosphoribosyl transferase (APRT) and xanthine oxidase deficiency (XO) are associated with increased urinary excretion rates of uric acid, dihydroxyadenine and xanthine respectively. The diagnoses are made by measurements of these specific metabolites in the urine (Henderson 1993).

Hypertension

Measurement of Blood Pressure

- *Mercury sphygmomamometer*. The systolic pressure is the appearance of the sounds. The diastolic pressure is

taken as the point of muffling of the sound (4th Korotkoff sound). The normal blood pressures of children of different ages are shown in Table 6.4. Until the age of 13 years, sex has no effect on blood pressure but after this age it is slightly higher in boys than girls.
- *Automatic*. Automatic machines use either a microphone to pick up the sounds or oscillometry to detect movements of the arterial wall. Both of these automatic methods tend to overestimate systolic and underestimate diastolic pressure.

It is important to use an appropriately sized blood pressure cuff. The recommendations of the American Heart Association are generally adopted. These state that the inflatable part of the cuff should cover at least three-quarters of the humerus length and should be approximately 40% of the arm circumference. The blood pressure should be recorded in the leg using a similar sized cuff. Interpretation of a blood pressure recording should be made in relation to the growth percentile of a child. A tall child with blood pressure on the 90th percentile would be considered to be normal, whereas a similar blood pressure in a small child is abnormal. There is great variability in blood pressure measurement during the day, and higher recordings are obtained in the recumbant posture. It is wise to obtain several recordings under standardized conditions before making a diagnosis of hypertension.

Cause of Hypertension

Over 80% of children with hypertension have a primary renal cause, in the remainder hypertension is largely due to coarctation of the aorta. Endocrine causes are rare. Essential hypertension is uncommon before adolescence.

Table 6.4   Normal blood pressure in children (mean ± SD)

Age	Systolic (mmHg)	Diastolic (mmHg)
Birth	73 ± 10	51 ± 9
6 months	93 ± 13	48 ± 11
1 year	94 ± 12	53 ± 9
5 years	94 ± 11	57 ± 10
8 years	99 ± 10	62 ± 10
10 years	102 ± 11	64 ± 10
13 years	108 ± 13	66 ± 11
16 years	115 ± 12	67 ± 11

Data from Task Force on Blood Pressure Control in Children (1987).

Investigation of Hypertension

The renal investigation of hypertension in childhood is conveniently divided into three stages.

Stage-one investigations establish a renal cause for the hypertension.

- Urine examination – significant proteinuria suggests a renal cause and the presence of granular or red cell casts indicate glomerular nephritis. Bacteriuria and white cells indicate pyelonephritis.
- The assessment of overall renal function by the measurement of plasma creatinine or a clearance technique.

Stage-two investigations are designed to identify the anatomical nature of the renal disease.

- An intravenous urogram, using a low osmolar contrast medium, is a good investigation for hypertensive patients. It provides information about the renal anatomy and, when early and late films are taken, delayed excretion, unequal kidney size and increased concentration of dye by one kidney are suggestive of renovascular disease. It is positive in about a third of cases and a normal intravenous urogram does not exclude a renovascular cause of the hypertension.
- Renal ultrasound provides information about anatomical abnormalities of the kidney and inequalities in their size.
- A DMSA scan shows the renal scarring of pyelonephritis. The percentage contibution each kidney provides to the overall renal function can also be calculated. This is important information when decisions are made about surgical treatment.
- A DTPA scan provides information about renal perfusion. Furthermore, the changes in renal perfusion before and after captopril treatment have been proposed as a helpful guide to identify the presence of renal vascular disease.

Stage-three investigations give more detailed information about the renal pathology and help with decisions about treatment. They are generally more invasive procedures and should be carried out in specialized centres. These investigations include:

- Renal biopsy if glomerular nephritis is suspected on urine examination.
- Renal arteriogram when the intravenous urogram and DTPA suggest renal vascular disease then this diagnosis should be confirmed by renal arteriography.
- Renal venous plasma renin activity (PRA). Renal venous blood is sampled at the time of the arteriogram. In typical renal hypertension the renin secretion of the healthy kidney is suppressed by the excess production of the diseased kidney. If the ratio of renin activity in the diseased/healthy kidney is greater than 1.5, then surgical intervention is likely to be helpful. Peripheral venous renin activity seldom provides useful additional information. Normal peripheral venous renin activity varies with age. It is much higher in the newborn and infants than in older children and adults.

Acute Urinary-Tract Infections

A urinary-tract infection is defined as "a pure growth of bacteria greater than 10^5 per microlitre". Counts less than this may occur during diuresis and occasionally in boys. When this occurs it is an indication for repeating the urine examination. The techniques of collecting urine and its examination are discussed below (see p. 106). There are two fundamental principles that underline the further investigations of a child with a proven urinary-tract infection. The first is to identify an anatomical abnormality which predisposes to infection, and the second to prevent renal scarring and its progression, which causes hypertension and renal insufficiency in adult life. Most renal scars are present when the children first present with urinary infection and it is most unusual for them to develop during the follow-up period. This has been interpreted as suggesting that damaging infections occur principally in young children at a time when the kidneys are maturing, i.e. during the first 2 years of life. It is also of note that this young age is a time when the clinical diagnosis of urinary-tract infections is difficult and can only be made by careful examination of the urine. For these reasons the plan of investigation of urinary tract infections is influenced by the patient's age (Royal College of Physicians 1991).

Renal Ultrasound

All children with a urinary-tract infection should have an ultrasound examination of the kidneys and bladder. This is done to demonstrate anatomical abnormalities of the urinary tract. Gross renal scarring may also be apparent but small scars will be missed. Renal calculi may be demonstrated and ultrasound examination is particularly useful in the demonstration of radiolucent metabolic stones.

X-ray of Abdomen

This will demonstrate radio opaque renal calculi. More importantly skeletal abnormalities of the spine, such as spina bifida, will also be detected. An abdominal X-ray should be done in all children with UTI.

DMSA Scan

This requires the injection of an isotope with a radiation dose of 1 mSv. It is taken up by the renal tubules and retained; less than 5% is excreted in the final urine. It is the preferred method of demonstrating renal parenchymal damage, but is not a good technique to show the renal anatomy. Renal scars will not take it up and will appear as cold areas on the scan. All children with urinary-tract infection under the age of two years should have a DMSA scan performed as the presence of scars will determine the future management. In older children it should be done if the ultrasound suggests scarring or when there have been repeated infections.

DTPA Scan

This solute is cleared by glomerular filtration, there is no tubular secretion or renal tissue retention. There are three phases of renal activity identified. The initial shows transit through the kidney and represents renal perfusion. The second phase occurs 1–3 min later and is a measure of renal function. The third phase represents the excretion of the solute through the urinary tract. The high concentration of the isotope in the urine provides good visualization of the anatomy of the urinary tract. When a diuretic such as frusemide is given, obstruction can be distinguished from non-obstructive dilatation of the urinary tract by failure of the diuretic to wash out the isotope from the obstructed kidney. A DTPA scan should be done when the renal ultrasound shows dilatation of the urinary tract and obstructive uropathy is suspected.

MAG₃ Scan

Technetium-99 mercaptoacetyl triglycine (MAG_3) is an analogue of hippuran. Unlike the other renal pharmaceuticals it is both filtered and secreted by the renal tubule. Thus effective renal plasma flow can be measured from blood samples taken after its injection. A correction factor is necessary to obtain results comparable with those obtained using hippuran. Because it is both filtered by the glomerulus and secreted it provides superior γ-camera images of the kidney at low levels of renal function than DTPA. However, it is a more expensive isotope and in practice it has no major advantages over DTPA.

Micturating Cystourethrogram

There are three techniques available. The direct contrast technique is the only one which demonstrates the anatomy of the lower ureter, bladder and urethra. A urethral catheter is inserted and the contrast injected into the bladder. The catheter is removed and the child encouraged to void urine under screening. The anatomy of the urethra can be visualized and vesicoureteric reflux demonstrated. The second technique uses a radioactive tracer instead of the contrast medium. It will demonstrate reflux but not the anatomy of the bladder or the urethra. In the third technique, the indirect radionucleotide cystogram, the tracer is injected intravenously and its appearance in the bladder and ureter detected during micturition. This method may prove to be useful to follow the progression and resolution of vesicoureteric reflux after it has been identified by contrast cystography.

Micturating cystourethrograms should be performed on all children under 2 years with urinary-tract infections. It will demonstrate important anatomical abnormalities of the bladder, such as urethrocoeles in girls and urethral valves in boys, both of which will require surgical treatment. It also demonstrates vesicoureteric reflux which, when present in children under 2 years of age, requires long-term prophylactic treatment.

Over 2 years, a micturating urethrogram is not recommended in all children. It should be done in those where anatomical abnormalities of the urinary tract have been demonstrated by renal ultrasound or in those who have had repeated infections where reflux is suspected and surgical treatment considered.

NOTES ON EXAMINATION OF THE URINE

Microbiology

It is essential to obtain the correct urine sample suitable for the type of investigation which is planned. If bacteriological examination is required then a clean sample should be collected after the perineum has been cleaned with soap and water. Antiseptic washes are avoided because the chemical contamination of the urine sample interferes with bacteriological growth. In cooperative children a midstream urine can easily be obtained, but in infants and small children a bag collection may be necessary. The bag should be checked regularly, at least every 15 min, and removed immediately to ensure an uncontaminated sample. Suprapubic urine samples may be obtained when alternative methods prove unsatisfactory. This procedure should be performed midway between feeds when the bladder might be expected to be full. A fine needle is introduced into the bladder, 1 cm above the pubic symphysis. Only one pass should be attempted to avoid unnecessary trauma and haematuria. Bladder catheterization is rarely necessary except when urethral obstruction is suspected or an accurately timed urine collection is considered essential and patient co-operation is not possible. A fine bore catheter is used. If it is left in place for any length of time, the bladder should be washed with chlorhexidine prior to catheter removal. Samples for bacteriological examination should be collected either into a sterile container or in 1.8% boric acid. Both samples may be kept refrigerated (4°C) for up to 24 h prior to examination if the samples are obtained at a time when the laboratory is closed.

Microscopic examination of the urine sediment provides useful information. When infection is suspected, microscopy of an uncentrifuged sample is adequate but a centrifuged sample is necessary to examine other urinary deposits. Bacteria are easily identified on microscopy of an uncentrifuged sample of urine. The presence of one organism in a high-powered field has been shown to correlate well with significant bacteruria. The dipstix chemical test for micro-organisms is based upon the presence of nitrites formed by the bateriological reduction of nitrates which are normally present in the urine. The urine must be incubated with the bacteria for at least 4 h so that the nitrite can be formed. This means that the test is best done on an early morning urine sample when the urine has been present in the bladder overnight. The sensitivity of the urinary nitrite test is about 90%. A positive test indicating significant bacteruria, but a negative test does not exclude a urinary tract infection.

Chemistry

For routine chemical urinalysis, the first morning urine sample is the best. When timed urine collections are necessary to quantify the urine excretion of some solutes, accurate timing of the collection period and complete bladder emptying are essential, but often difficult to achieve without resorting to bladder catheterization. The difficulties of obtaining a timed sample can be avoided by measuring the urine creatinine concentration as well as the solute under investigation and the result expressed as a ratio to creatinine. This creatinine correction assumes that the urine creatinine excretion rate is constant throughout the 24-h period. It is also important to ensure there is no ketonuria as ketones cross-react with the creatinine measurement, making it inappropriately high and the creatinine ratio will therefore be lower than expected. Specimens for protein examination are best collected with a preservative such as sodium azide or

toluene. It is important to check with the biochemistry laboratory before collections are obtained so that the appropriate preservatives are used.

Casts

Tubular casts are easily recognized but tend to migrate to the edge of the microscope coverslip. Hyaline tubular casts are found in normal urine and appear in increased amounts in diuretic states. Occasional granular casts may also be seen in normal urine but, when frequent or abnormally broad, suggest glomerulonephritis. Red blood cell casts are always abnormal indicating glomerular bleeding due to glomerulonephritis. White blood cell casts are seen in pyelonephritis.

Crystals

The identification of crystals in the urine is aided by the knowledge of the urine pH. Amorphous crystals in an alkaline urine are likely to be phosphates, but in acid will probably be urates. Square crystals with diagonal crosses imply calcium oxalate and hexagonal crystals are cystine.

ACKNOWLEDGEMENTS

The author would like to thank Miss Mandy Jones for her help and forebearance through a very difficult time during the preparation of this manuscript.

REFERENCES

Battle DC, Hizon M, Cohen E, Gutterman BS, Gupta R (1988) The use of the urinary anion gap in diagnosis of hyperchloraemic metabolic acidosis. N Engl J Med 1: 594–598.

Brocklebank JT, Cooper EH, Richmond K (1991) Sodium dodecyl sulphate polyacrylamide gel electrophoresis patterns of proteinuria in various renal diseases of childhood. Pediatr Nephrol 5: 371–375.

Henderson M (1993) Renal stone disease – investigation aspect. Arch Dis Child 68: 160–162.

Parkin A, Smith HC, Brocklebank JT (1989) Which routine test for kidney function? Arch Dis Child 64: 1261–1263.

Royal College of Physicians (1991) Guidelines for the management of acute urinary tract infection in childhood. Report of a working group of the Research Unit. J Royal Coll Physicians 25: 36–41.

Savory DJ (1990) Reference ranges for serum creatinine in infants, children and adolescents. Ann Clin Biochem 27: 99–101.

Shaw NJ, Wheeldon J, Brocklebank JT (1992) The tubular maximum for calcium reabsorption: A normal range in children. Clin Endocrinol 36: 193–195.

Task Force on Blood Pressure Control in Children (1987) Report from the Second Task Force on Blood Pressure Control in Children. Paediatrics 79: 1–25.

7

Gastroenterology

J W L Puntis and I W Booth

INVESTIGATION OF GASTROINTESTINAL SYMPTOMS

Abdominal pain, chronic diarrhoea, constipation, vomiting and gastrointestinal bleeding are the most common gastrointestinal symptoms leading to hospital referral. A meticulous history will often point to the most likely diagnoses and indicate a plan of investigation. If a differential diagnosis has not formed in the mind of the investigating doctor after the history has been taken, it is very unlikely to appear at the end of the examination. Although the following account cannot be comprehensive, we have suggested how to begin investigating these problems and which more detailed or specialized techniques are needed to pursue less common diagnoses. However, the distinction between first line and referral centre investigations is not meant to be too rigid, since available expertise and experience (in endoscopy for example) will often determine whether or not local investigation is appropriate. Referral to a paediatric gastroenterology unit may be necessary for some specialist investigations and in planning clinical management.

RECURRENT ABDOMINAL PAIN

Some organic causes of recurrent abdominal pain in childhood are shown in Table 7.1. Some are very esoteric and the list is lengthy. Clearly it is inappropriate to exclude each cause on the basis of investigation. Rather, a decision about who to investigate, and how, can only be made after a careful history and examination. Points for particular consideration are summarized in Table 7.2 and the probability of any one diagnosis must be weighed up on the basis of history and examination (Figure 7.1). Around 10% of schoolchildren suffer repeated episodes of self-limiting abdominal pain for longer than 3 months, which interferes with their activities and yet for which no

Table 7.1   Recurrent abdominal pain

Non-organic
Functional
Abdominal migraine
Constipation
Irritable bowel syndrome

Oesophagus and stomach
Oesophagitis
Oesophageal spasm
Gastritis
Duodenitis
Peptic ulceration

Small bowel
Intussusception
Malrotation
Duplication
Volvulus
Internal hernia
Stenotic bowel

Gall bladder
Cholecystitis
Cholelithiasis

Renal tract
Urinary tract infection
Pelvi-ureteric junctional obstruction
Urinary tract stones
Nephrotic syndrome

Gynaecological
Ovarian tumours/cysts
Salpingitis
Haematocolpos

Miscellaneous
Crohn's disease
Tuberculosis
Chronic pancreatitis
Lead poisoning
Porphyria
C1 esterase inhibitor deficiency
Myelitis
Sickle cell anaemia

Table 7.2   The child with recurrent abdominal pain: who to investigate

History

Pain with vomiting (with or without bile staining) and distension (barium meal, ? malrotation)

Nocturnal pain or a history of peptic ulcer in a first degree relative (? peptic ulcer or *Helicobacter pylori*)

Diarrhoea (? inflammatory bowel disease)

Blood in the stools (? inflammatory bowel disease)

Urinary symptoms

Growth failure or weight loss

Examination

Jaundice

Anus (? Crohn's)

Abdominal mass

Testes

Nutritional status

Fundoscopy (? space occupying lesion)

cause can be found (Apley 1959). The pain is non-specific, classically periumbilical and colicky, and does not wake the child from sleep. Psychogenic factors play a role in only a small proportion of patients; in most no obvious stress factors or emotional disturbance can be identified. As adults they are more likely than controls to suffer recurrent pain of one sort or another, frequently irritable bowel syndrome.

Helicobacter pylori

Recently it has become clear that infection with *Helicobacter pylori* is responsible for some cases of recurrent abdominal pain (Drumm 1990, Farrell 1993) and this organism may be found in around 10% of children undergoing endoscopy for upper gastrointestinal symptoms. Infection is, however, rare before 8 years of age except in developing countries where it may be associated with chronic diarrhoea. Prevalence is inversely related to socio-economic class. Serological testing may be helpful in diagnosis (see p. 111).

Infection with *H. pylori* is strongly linked with peptic ulcer disease; it is specifically associated with primary gastritis in children and epigastric pain and vomiting are the most common symptoms. When found in the duodenum it is at sites of gastric metaplasia. Under the microscope the organism has a Gram-negative spiral form (Figure 7.2). The role of *H. pylori* in duodenal ulceration has yet to be fully clarified, but eradication appreciably reduces the chances of ulcer disease relapsing. The organism is sensitive *in vitro* to the number of different antibiotics including ampicillin and metronidazole. It is also sensitive to bismuth salts and a combination of these three agents offers the best chance of eradication.

Asymptomatic colonization is common in siblings of children with *H. pylori* associated gastritis. Intrafamilial clustering suggests spread of the organism from person to person. Although clearing of *H. pylori* from the gastric mucosa and resolution of gastritis may lead to improvement in symptoms, this is mainly seen in those with duodenal ulcer disease. The exact symptomatology of *H. pylori* infection in children and indications for treatment therefore remain controversial.

Central pain, usually morning	Epigastric pain
Normal growth	Night pain
Normal examination	Family history of peptic ulcer
No other gastrointestinal symptoms	Vomiting
Long history	Blood in vomit/stools
No urinary symptoms	Diarrhoea
Paroxysmal pain and pallor	Growth failure
Family history migraine	Weight loss
Family history of irritable bowel	Misguided attempts in past to explain symptoms as psychogenic

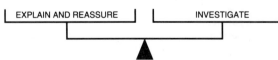

EXPLAIN AND REASSURE	INVESTIGATE

Figure 7.1   Recurrent abdominal pain: balancing explanation and reassurance against investigations.

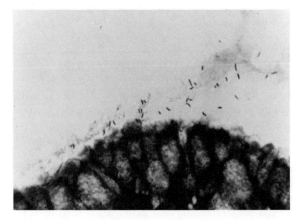

Figure 7.2   Gram-negative spiral *Helicobacter pylori* seen in the mucus layer above gastric mucosa. Photograph courtesy of Dr Gillian Batcup.

Irritable Bowel Syndrome

Irritable bowel syndrome affects older children, starting typically in late adolescence. Predominant symptoms may be those of lower abdominal pain with diarrhoea, constipation, or bloating. Rather than embarking upon exhaustive investigation to exclude other conditions, symptom patterns (Table 7.3) should allow a positive diagnosis to be made (Weber and McCallum 1992). It is now recognized that it is commonly associated with a disorder of gastroduodenal motility.

Pain is usually intermittent and in the right or left lower quadrants, often getting worse 60–90 min after meals. Patients have a lower pain threshold to gastro-intestinal distension than controls. There is a characteristic disturbance in stool frequency, form or passage with diarrhoea, constipation or both alternating. Loose stools may be passed frequently but are of small volume. Early morning, postprandial or stress-related urgency is common, followed by feelings of incomplete evacuation and up to 50% of patients report the passage of mucus. Feelings of abdominal distension are common and worsen during the day, improving overnight. The passage of blood represents a need for colonoscopy. Sometimes the history reveals a specific cancer phobia, perhaps as a result of a missed colonic carcinoma in a close relative. In these cases a normal colonoscopy is very helpful.

Physical examination should reveal normal growth and nutritional status, and if otherwise, an alternative diagnosis must be considered. A palpable sigmoid colon and some tenderness on palpation are commonly found non-specific signs. If a positive diagnosis can be made on clinical grounds extensive investigation is to be avoided. Dietary factors may be implicated by keeping a food and symptom diary for several weeks. A history suggestive of lactose or sucrose intolerance can be investigated by appropriate challenge tests using breath hydrogen measurements. Ultimate proof rests on the demon-

stration of low disaccharidase activity in a jejunal mucosal biopsy. If symptoms prove intractable, investigation should procede as for chronic diarrhoea, constipation, or recurrent pain.

First-line Investigations for Recurrent Abdominal Pain

In patients with a typical history of functional pain or irritable bowel syndrome, and absence of physical abnormality, a minimum number of investigations should be performed: full blood count, urine culture and microscopy. Abdominal ultrasound has a low diagnostic yield, although normal scans may be reassuring to all concerned. Once the diagnosis of functional pain has been made the pathophysiology and prognosis should be explained to the patient. Further follow-up is unnecessary and may reinforce anxieties about serious underlying disease.

Although an organic cause for recurrent abdominal pain can only be found in around 7% of cases, further investigation to exclude specific conditions is necessary if pain is atypical in nature or associated with other signs or symptoms (Table 7.2).

Imaging

There are pitfalls in performing and interpreting pae-diatric imaging and detailed investigation is most appropriately carried out in a paediatric unit experienced in the radiological and ultrasonic investigation of children. To maintain the necessary paediatric expertise, a radiologist should be performing frequent barium meals and abdominal ultrasound examinations in young children.

Radiological examination will demonstrate anatomical abnormalities of the small bowel such as malrotation or stenosis. In Crohn's disease there may be diffuse localized mucosal abnormality, ulcer craters, stenoses, oedematous loops of bowel and fistulae. Ultrasound can be used to detect cholelithiasis, renal tract anomalies, pancreatic disease and gynaecological disorders. Although calcified renal stones often show up on plain abdominal X-ray, an intravenous pyelogram may be required for certain diagnosis.

Other Investigations for Recurrent Abdominal Pain

Enzyme linked immunosorbent assay (ELISA) systems are available to detect serological responses to *H. pylori*. IgG antibody is highly sensitive (96%) and specific (99%) in identifying children with *H. pylori* associated gastritis. IgG antibody titres fall with eradication of

Table 7.3 Diagnostic criteria for irritable bowel syndrome

Continuous or recurrent symptoms for at least 3 months of abdominal pain relieved by defaecation or associated with a change in frequency or consistency of stool

and

Disturbed defaecation at least 25% of the time: three or more of
- Altered stool frequency
- Altered stool form (hard or loose/watery)
- Altered stool passage (straining, urgency, tenesmus)
- Passage of mucus
- Abdominal distension

infection and rise with recurrence. The finding of anti *H. pylori* antibodies in a child with symptoms is an indication for proceeding to upper gastrointestinal endoscopy.

Lead poisoning, porphyria and C1 esterase inhibitor deficiency (C1-INH) are other causes of chronic recurrent abdominal pain. In porphyria, vomiting and constipation are also prominent symptoms; urine should be tested for an excess of porphobilinogen, and may turn brown or red on standing. In C1-INH deficiency plasma concentrations may be low (around 15% of normal) or normal, but functionally deficient.

Referral Centre Investigations

Endoscopy

The indications for upper gastrointestinal endoscopy are shown in Table 7.4. This investigation is best performed in a paediatric gastroenterology or surgical unit (Cadranel and Rodesch 1988).

In *H. pylori* infection a nodular gastritis (Figure 7.3) is the most common finding in infected children. The gross appearance on endoscopy may be normal so that antral biopsy specimens for histological examination are essential. This may reveal both the organism and clear evidence of gastritis. *H. pylori* can be reliably identified using a Giemsa stain although more complex techniques (e.g. Warthin–Starry silver stain) are also employed. Antral biopsy material is ground and used to innoculate blood or chocolate agar, or Skirrow's medium, within 60 min of being taken. The plates are incubated at 37°C

Table 7.4 Indications for upper gastrointestinal endoscopy

Abdominal pain if associated with:
- Nocturnal pain
- Haematemesis
- Epigastric tenderness
- Family ulcer disease
- Positive *H. pylori* antibody

Haematemesis

Assessment of oesophagus if suspected:
- Oesophagitis
- Oesophageal stenosis
- Caustic burns
- Foreign body

Assessment/sclerotherapy of oesophageal varices

Endoscopic placement of feeding gastrostomy

Endoscopic retrograde cannulation of pancreatic duct in recurrent obstructive pancreatitis

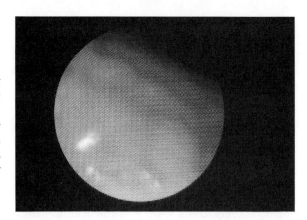

Figure 7.3 Nodular gastritis due to *Helicobacter pylori* infection of the gastric antrum. Photograph courtesy of Dr Stephen Murphy.

under microaerophilic conditions for up to 7 days. *H. pylori* is positive for urease, catalase, and oxidase and produces a negative reaction for hippurate hydrolysis and nitrate reduction. Alternatively, the biopsy specimen can be placed on a Christensen's urea slope. A positive test is when the medium changes from a tan to a pink colour. Commercial tests for urease production identify *H. pylori* in about 90% of biopsies from colonized children.

In some children with suspected Crohn's disease a histological diagnosis can be made by examining upper gastrointestinal biopsies even when macroscopic appearances are normal, and in the absence of any specific upper gastrointestinal symptoms. Similarly, colonoscopy may be useful in making a tissue diagnosis of Crohn's disease in the absence of symptoms suggesting colitis since characteristic histological appearances can be found in macroscopically normal colonic mucosa, and biopsies from the terminal ileum may also be obtained.

Breath Test for Suspected *H. pylori* Infection

Breath tests are highly sensitive and involve ingestion of urea labelled with ^{13}C or ^{14}C. Breakdown of urea by the bacterial urease results in expiration of labelled carbon dioxide which can be quantified using mass spectroscopy. ^{13}C should be used in children, but is very expensive.

Visually Evoked Responses

Abdominal migraine (periodic syndrome) presents in some children with paroxysmal abdominal pain, often associated with facial pallor or flushing, and malaise. Vomiting and headache may occur and there is frequently a family history of cranial migraine. Symptoms last for 1 or 2 days and subside spontaneously, although vomiting may be severe enough to cause dehydration. Visually evoked responses may be helpful in diagnosis, being similar to those in children with cranial migraine and showing a higher fast wave amplitude than in controls. In some cases, children and parents find it helpful to know that there is a demonstrable abnormality in the visually evoked response, particularly if they have been exposed to misguided attempts to convince them of a psychogenic basis.

Motility Disorders

Disorder of gastrointestinal motility can present with abdominal pain. Investigation of such problems is considered together with vomiting.

CHRONIC DIARRHOEA

Chronic diarrhoea is defined as the passage of four or more loose stools per day persisting for more than 2 weeks in a child who is either not growing or is losing weight. A detailed clinical history will help distinguish between the many causes (Table 7.5). For example, watery diarrhoea from birth together with a history of polyhydramnios points to congenital brush border transport abnormalities such as chloride diarrhoea or a defect in sodium/proton exchange. Onset following introduction of formula milk or gluten suggests cows' milk protein intolerance or coeliac disease. There may be a family history of diarrhoea in cystic fibrosis or with congenital transport defects. An algorithm for investigating watery diarrhoea is shown in Figure 7.4.

Toddler Diarrhoea

This condition presents typically during infancy, with frequent foul-smelling loose stools in a child who is clearly thriving. Stool frequency and consistency are remarkably variable and sometimes diarrhoea and constipation alternate. Vegetables such as peas, carrots and baked beans usually appear in the stool several hours after ingestion, indicating a rapid bowel transit time. In the majority of cases it is self-limiting and rarely persists beyond 6 years of age. Sucrose intolerance must be excluded (see below) and reassurance given to parents.

First-line Investigations for Protracted Diarrhoea

Infection

Stool culture for both bacterial and viral pathogens is essential and non-enteric infection such as empyema or

Table 7.5 Causes of protracted diarrhoea in infancy and childhood

Inborn errors of transport	Congenital chloridorrhoea Transcobalamin II deficiency Acrodermatitis enteropathica Defective sodium/proton exchange
Protein intolerance	Coeliac disease Cows' milk protein intolerance Soy protein intolerance Other protein intolerance
Carbohydrate intolerance	Secondary lactose intolerance Secondary monosaccharide intolerance Lactase deficiency Glucose–galactose malabsorption Sucrase–isomaltase deficiency
Surgical	Malrotation Hirschprung's disease Stenoses Blind loops
Extraintestinal infection	Empyema Mastoiditis
Intestinal infections	Enteropathogenic *Escherichia coli* Giardiasis Dysenteric infections Cryptosporidia
Antibiotics	Pseudomembranous colitis
Pancreatic insufficiency	Cystic fibrosis Shwachman syndrome
Immunodeficiency	Severe combined immuno-deficiency Hypogammaglobulinaemia Acquired immunodeficiency
Tumours	Ganglioneuroma Lymphoma Histiocytosis X
Inflammatory bowel disease	Ulcerative colitis Crohn's disease
Other	Post necrotizing enterocolitis Addison's disease Lymphangiectasia Autoimmune enteropathy Congenital microvillous atrophy a-β-Lipoproteinaemia Idiopathic Munchausen's syndrome Munchausen's syndrome by proxy

mastoiditis may also cause diarrhoea. Microscopic examination of fresh stool is necessary to identify amoebic infection or parasitic infestation. *Giardia lamblia* in children is a cause of diarrhoea, intestinal malabsorption

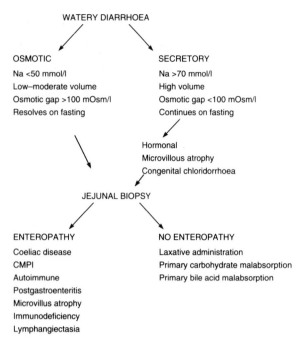

WATERY DIARRHOEA

OSMOTIC

Na <50 mmol/l
Low–moderate volume
Osmotic gap >100 mOsm/l
Resolves on fasting

SECRETORY

Na >70 mmol/l
High volume
Osmotic gap <100 mOsm/l
Continues on fasting

Hormonal
Microvillous atrophy
Congenital chloridorrhoea

JEJUNAL BIOPSY

ENTEROPATHY

Coeliac disease
CMPI
Autoimmune
Postgastroenteritis
Microvillus atrophy
Immunodeficiency
Lymphangiectasia

NO ENTEROPATHY

Laxative administration
Primary carbohydrate malabsorption
Primary bile acid malabsorption

Figure 7.4   Algorithm for investigating chronic watery diarrhoea. CMPI, cow milk protein intolerance.

and growth failure. *G. lamblia* cysts and trophozoites can be detected in stools, although the latter are only present when there is profuse diarrhoea and heavy infection. Three stool specimens on separate days will detect about three-quarters of cases. Otherwise, trophozoites can be seen in jejunal fluid obtained by intubation. Jejunal biopsy examination may also show trophozoites in the mucus layer above the epithelium. *G. lamblia* antigen can be detected in faeces by an ELISA, using a specific anti-*Giardia* antibody as the probe.

Haematology, Plasma Biochemistry, Serology and Immunology

Assessing the effects of diarrhoea by measurement of electrolytes, calcium, phosphate, plasma proteins and liver function should be part of the initial investigations. Malabsorption is suggested by iron deficiency, prolonged clotting, low vitamin B_{12} and folate, or reduced plasma concentrations of carotene and vitamins A and E. Trace elements such as zinc, copper, magnesium and selenium may also be low in chronic diarrhoea. In a,β-lipoproteinamia, vitamin E deficiency produces acanthocytosis on blood film, whilst plasma cholesterol and triglyceride concentrations will be low and β-lipoprotein (LDL) absent.

IgG antigliadin antibodies are nearly always present in serum at presentation of coeliac disease but lack specificity as they also occur in other gastrointestinal disorders (Guandalini et al 1989). IgA antigliadin antibodies are present in only about 90% of coeliacs at presentation but have a better specificity than IgG. Anti-endomysium antibodies have even better specificity (98%), and as with IgA antigliadin antibodies, disappear in most patients with coeliac disease on a gluten-free diet, reappearing following gluten challenge or in non-compliance. These tests cannot replace jejunal biopsy in definitive diagnosis, but in combination provide a useful screening test.

Differential white count and immunoglubulin measurement may indicate the need for more comprehensive investigation of immune status as an underlying cause for diarrhoea.

Blood in the Stool

Bloody stools suggest colitis. Even if blood is not visible, consistently positive (three samples) tests for faecal occult blood should be an indication for colonoscopy if an infective cause has been excluded.

Faecal Fat

Characteristically, stools containing excess fat are large, often greasy, and usually offensive. Offensiveness is difficult to grade – stools rarely smell of lavender! A positive "front door test" is useful. In this, parents faces light up with comprehension when asked if it is possible to tell that the child's dirty nappy has recently been changed as soon as they enter their front door. Children whose parents accept that they need a gas mask to change a nappy, usually have truly offensive stools.

Assuming an adequate fat intake, more than 5 g/day of fat excretion at any age is abnormal. A 72-h stool collection should be made using carmine red marker at the beginning and end of the study. Many laboratories have given up this test and looked towards more simple non-quantitative tests for steatorrhoea. Staining stool with Sudan III demonstrates fat on microscopy and is, for example, used as a way of monitoring response to enzyme replacement therapy in cystic fibrosis (Walters et al 1990). The steatocrit method relies on homogenizing a stool sample with water and a fat stain before spinning down in a capillary haematocrit tube. The length of the stained lipid and solid phases are measured by micrometer, and the lipid expressed as a percentage of the solid phase (D'Agostino and Orsi 1988). Although these are both simple tests, processing of faecal material presents the biochemistry department with practical problems. If either of these tests is abnormal, further investigation into causes of maldigestion or malabsorption should follow.

Stool Electrolytes

If the diarrhoea is watery, measurement of stool electrolytes in a single specimen of liquid stool can be helpful in distinguishing between osmotic and secretory diarrhoea. The osmolality of stool water is assumed to be the same as plasma. That part of the osmolality which can be accounted for by the stool electrolytes is calculated by doubling the sum of potassium and sodium concentrations. A difference between measured and calculated osmolality of more than 100 mOsm/l suggests an osmotic diarrhoea, whilst a level below this points to a secretory cause. During 24 h of intravenous fluids and complete enteral starvation an osmotic diarrhoea would be expected to stop, in contrast to a secretory diarrhoea which continues. Laxative administration (Munchausen syndrome or Munchausen syndrome by proxy) is an important exception.

Osmotic diarrhoea is caused by osmotically active substances within the bowel lumen. These may be malabsorbed nutrients such as lactose, or laxatives such as magnesium sulphate. In congenital chloridorrhoea the sum of stool sodium and potassium is less than the chloride concentration, whilst plasma sodium, potassium and chloride are low. This is an autosomal recessive condition in which there is defective gut exchange of chloride and bicarbonate. Severe watery diarrhoea and failure to thrive date from birth.

Carbohydrate Malabsorption

Lactose intolerance is usually secondary to mucosal damage from acute infection but may occasionally be a congenital autosomal recessive disorder. Glucose–galactose malabsorption is a rare disorder presenting in the neonatal period with watery diarrhoea. Sucrase–isomaltase deficiency is also an autosomal recessive disorder. Symptoms may be mild and intermittent, without failure to thrive.

Stool Reducing Substances

Unabsorbed carbohydrate will be present in the liquid phase of stool which must be collected on a plastic nappy liner (or inside-out disposable nappy), separately from urine. Stool pH alone is not a reliable indicator of carbohydrate malabsorption. Stools should be tested immediately or frozen at −20°C until later analysis. Dilute five drops of stool fluid with ten drops of water and add one Clinitest (Ames) tablet. All carbohydrates ingested by children are reducing substances with the excep-

tion of sucrose. If testing for sucrose, the liquid stool should first be boiled with hydrochloric acid to hydrolyse the disaccharide to glucose and fructose. The test can be read as for urine; more than 0.5% reducing substances suggests carbohydrate malabsorption. Abnormal findings can be confirmed by thin layer chromatography.

Carbohydrate Challenge

Oral loads of mono- or di-saccharides can be performed together with the above test. The sugar under investigation (2 g/kg body weight, to a maximum of 50 g) is given to a fasted patient, together with carmine red as a stool marker. Loose stools marked with carmine red are tested with Clinitest and sent for chromatography if carbohydrate is present.

Breath Hydrogen Testing

Carbohydrate escaping small intestinal absorption enters the colon and is fermented by colonic organisms producing hydrogen, which under normal circumstances is only found in traces in expired air. Increased hydrogen excretion occurs when there is malabsorption of sugars allowing abnormal quantities to pass into the colon, and where there is bacterial small bowel overgrowth as in a stagnant loop (Figure 7.5). Immediately before and then at half-hourly intervals following the administration of the chosen sugar (2 g/kg body weight), the breath hydrogen is measured using an automated hydrogen analyser which gives a digital read out in several minutes. End-expiratory air is sampled manually using a syringe with nasal prong, or by bag and face mask. The subject should be breathing regularly, co-operative and not crying. A hydrogen level of 20 ppm or an increase of 10 ppm or more above baseline are abnormal.

Jejunal Biopsy

Small intestinal biopsy is the investigation of choice when an enteropathy is suspected. Characteristic morphological abnormalities are found in coeliac disease, intestinal lymphangiectasia, a-β-lipoproteinaemia and, on electron microscopy, microvillous inclusion disease (microvillous atrophy). Mucosal disaccharidases can be measured in suspected sugar malabsorption. Crosby or Watson capsules contain a spring-loaded knife block which fires by suction to cut off a mucosal biopsy specimen. Although complications are very rare, clotting studies should be normal before proceeding. A dissecting microscope allows examination and orientation of the biopsy. If mucosal enzymes are to be measured the specimen should be quickly wrapped in aluminium foil

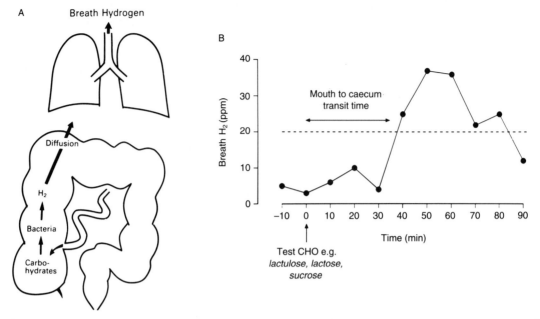

Figure 7.5   (A) Principles of breath hydrogen testing: non-absorbed carbohydrates enter the colon where they undergo fermentation by colonic flora. A fraction of the generated hydrogen is exhaled in the breath and measured. (B) A positive breath hydrogen result: a concentration of hydrogen in the breath of more than 20 ppm represents a positive response.

and frozen in dry ice. Poor orientation of specimen leading to misinterpretation of appearance can lead to the mistaken diagnosis of coeliac disease in inexperienced hands. Enterocyte vacuolation seen in a-β-lipoproteinaemia may be unrecognized if a fat stain is not performed.

Tests of Pancreatic Exocrine Function

The simplest test for pancreatic exocrine insufficiency is faecal chymotrypsin (Puntis 1993). The enzyme is assayed using a kinetic, potentiometric method, in which the rate of hydrolysis of enzyme specific substrate is recorded with an automatic titrator and recorder. A proprietary test kit (Boehringer-Mannheim C-system) is available and relies on an automated colorimetric assay. Mean chymotrypsin concentration in three stool specimens shows good correlation with chymotrypsin and trypsin duodenal secretion during hormonal stimulation testing of exocrine function using the "gold standard" pancreozymin–secretin intubation test.

Pancreatic exocrine function may also be assessed indirectly using fluorescein dilaurate (pancreolauryl) (Dalzell and Heaf 1990). Given by mouth in a dose of 0.25 mmol it is cleaved by pancreatic cholesterol ester hydrolase to give lauric acid and fluorescein. The latter is excreted in a 10-h urine collection and can be assayed using spectrophotometry or fluorimetry; less than 30% recovery is an abnormal result. A second-day test with unesterified fluorescein improves test specificity since malabsorption but not pancreatic exocrine failure will be associated with a low recovery.

Urine Toxicology Screen

In the child with unexplained diarrhoea urine should be examined for evidence of laxative administration.

Referral Centre Investigations

Measurement of enzymes in duodenal juice following hormonal stimulation with pancreozymin and secretin is indicated when non-invasive tests suggest pancreatic disease, for detailed assessment of conditions known to involve the pancreas such as cystic fibrosis, or for suspected single enzyme defects. Using a jejunal biopsy capsule with outer aspiration tube, duodenal juice is collected for 20 min following 2 u/kg body weight of intravenous cholecystokinin (pancreozymin) and 30 min after 2 u/kg secretin. Although reference ranges have been published, problems with standardizing analysis of enzymes makes comparisons between laboratories extremely difficult.

Supraregional Laboratory Investigations in Chronic Diarrhoea

Congenital watery diarrhoea without the biochemical features of congenital chloride diarrhoea suggests a functional defect of sodium/proton exchange. This can be investigated in specialized laboratories using an enterocyte brush border membrane vesicle preparation. Profuse diarrhoea with steatorrhoea from soon after birth is seen in congenital malabsorption of bile salts; plasma and urine bile salt profiles are abnormal. Some children with protracted idiopathic diarrhoea of infancy are now recognized as having an autoimmune enteropathy. There may be other autoimmune disorders in the patient or family. Enterocyte antibodies found in serum confirm the diagnosis. Increased secretion of some gastrointestinal hormones can cause watery diarrhoea and fasting blood samples need to be sent to a reference laboratory which can perform a hormone profile including vasoactive intestinal peptide (VIP), gastrin and calcitonin.

CONSTIPATION AND SOILING

Most children present around 3–4 years of age with a history of constipation for some 6 months to 2 years. Causes are shown in Table 7.6. The majority of cases are idiopathic and may have started during a short period of acute illness, or following an anal fissure.

First-line Investigations for Constipation

The commonest and most important organic causes of chronic constipation are Hirschprung's disease and hypothyroidism. In general, organic causes usually have additional signs and symptoms and are more likely to be found if problems start in early infancy (see Table 7.7). In

Table 7.6 Constipation

Idiopathic
Poor fluid intake
Hirschprung's disease
Anal stenosis
Hypothyroidism
Renal tubular acidosis
Diabetes insipidus
Irritable bowel syndrome
Lead poisoning
Hypercalcaemia
Coeliac disease
Cows' milk protein intolerance

Table 7.7 Features suggestive of Hirschprung's disease which require a rectal biopsy

Delayed passage of meconium
Onset of constipation from birth
Symptoms/signs of recurrent subacute obstruction
Marked abdominal distension
Severe, intractable constipation with minimal soiling
Episodes of severe unexplained diarrhoea suggestive of Hirschprung's enterocolitis
Failure to thrive

addition to measurement of serum thyroxine and thyroid stimulating hormone, full blood count, calcium, creatinine, and urine testing should be performed at the outset.

Radiology

A plain abdominal radiograph is usually not required but may be useful to exclude constipation in the child with encopresis. A barium enema is rarely, if ever, indicated and is unreliable in the diagnosis of Hirschprung's disease, for which rectal biopsies are required.

Measurement of Colonic Transit Time

Constipation is hard to define and some objective method of measurement is required. Whole bowel transit time can be assessed by recovery of coloured, radioactive, or radio-opaque markers from the stool. The ingestion of solid markers followed later by plain abdominal radiography can be used to measure colonic transit time, and some normal reference data are available (Casanovas et al 1991). This technique is useful in severe constipation for investigating the effect of therapy.

Paediatric Referral Unit Investigations

Rectal Biopsy

Chronic constipation dating from birth, a history of failure to pass meconium in the first 24 h of life, abdominal distension and failure to thrive suggest the diagnosis of Hirschprung's disease. A suction biopsy can be obtained without the aid of a proctoscope and should cause no discomfort. The instrument's operating principle is the same as for a peroral jejunal biopsy capsule. Suction biopsies should be taken at 2 and 5 cm and stained for ganglion cells and acetylcholinesterase. The former are absent in Hirschprung's disease, whilst nerve fibres may show increased amounts of the latter.

Anorectal Manometry

Anorectal manometry was originally developed for the diagnosis of Hirschprung's disease but has also been used to study children with other causes of chronic constipation in an attempt to shed some light on pathophysiology. The apparatus consists of a rectal balloon connected to a probe bearing a number of pressure-sensitive balloons connected to a chart recorder. These pressure-sensitive balloons are sited in the anal canal. Anorectal manometry can be divided into a number of phases: the resting phase before rectal distension occurs, the early inflation responses when aliquots are added to the rectal balloon, and then the point of maximal rectal distension when there is complete inhibition of the anal canal, or the child has the sensation of needing to defecate urgently. When the rectal balloon is deflated the annal canal closes spontaneously.

Normally, rectal distension causes relaxation of the internal sphincter with contraction of the external sphincter. In Hirschprung's disease external sphincter contraction follows rectal distension as usual, but the internal sphincter contracts instead of relaxing. However, anorectal manometry without rectal biopsy is not sufficiently reliable as the sole test for diagnosis of Hirschprung's disease.

VOMITING

Assessment of the vomiting child often presents a difficult problem; causes vary from the trivial to the life-threatening (Table 7.8). History taking will determine the nature of the vomit (including the presence of bile),

Table 7.8 Causes of regurgitation/vomiting

Gastro-oesophageal reflux
Achalasia
Oesophagitis
Foreign body
Retropharyngeal abscess
External compression (tumour)

Duodenal diaphragm
Annular pancreas
Malrotation
Volvulus
Duplication
Pseudo-obstruction
Protein intolerance
Coeliac disease

Raised intracranial pressure
Cyclical vomiting (periodic syndrome)

its relation to meal times, precipitating factors and the duration of symptoms. The effect on hydration or growth, and the presence of associated problems such as respiratory symptoms, neurological signs or evidence of infection will indicate the subsequent pattern of investigation.

Cyclical Vomiting (Periodic Syndrome)

This term refers to recurrent episodes of severe vomiting which may be either short lived or prolonged, causing dehydration and metabolic disturbance. Episodes can start acutely or build up gradually and emergency treatment focuses on rehydration and correction of metabolic imbalance. Although this condition appears to resolve spontaneously in most cases, careful psychosocial investigation may reveal family-based problems.

First-line Investigations for Vomiting

These include an assessment of the effects of vomiting on serum electrolytes and acid–base status and, particularly during infancy, evidence of infection or inborn error of metabolism should be sought (urine for amino acids and organic acids).

Radiology

In an acute situation where symptoms suggest possible obstruction to the bowel a plain abdominal radiograph should be performed. Contrast studies are needed to demonstrate anatomical causes for vomiting such as hiatus hernia or malrotation; gastroesophageal reflux may also be diagnosed but the severity cannot be assessed accurately. Central nervous system disorders should always be considered in intractable vomiting and computerized tomography (CT) or magnetic resonance imaging (MRI) brain scanning may be indicated.

Gastric emptying can be studied radiographically using a test meal to which barium sulphate has been added. This technique is both unphysiological and difficult to quantify and is not recommended. Only the time of complete disappearance of barium from the stomach can be measured.

24-h pH Monitoring

Whilst endoscopy is the only reliable way to detect oesophagitis, oesophageal pH monitoring (Tappin et al 1992) will both confirm the presence and indicate the severity of gastro-oesophageal reflux. Intraoesophageal pH monitoring is the best way of discriminating between physiological and pathological gastro-oesophageal reflux and can be regarded as the gold standard in the diagnosis of reflux disease. However, the technical expertise required to produce reliable results can only come with experience of the technique. Clinical indications for 24-h oesophageal pH monitoring are shown in Table 7.9. The threshold for performing the study in children with chronic neurological disease, cerebral palsy in particular, should be low. About half such children will have gastro-oesophageal reflux.

Glass or antimony electrodes (usually < 3 mm diameter) are used as pH sensors and require an external reference electrode. Slightly larger electrodes combined with an internal reference are also available. Electrodes may be disposable, or to a limited extent reusable. The tip is positioned proximal to the lower oesophageal sphincter and can be located fairly accurately using measurement of height and a nomogram. Precise placement requires use of manometry, endoscopy, or radiology. Recorders are digital and solid state, pocket size and portable, and include an event marker to record symptoms. Anti-reflux treatment is usually withdrawn 24 h prior to monitoring and studies should be performed under as near normal conditions as possible including access to feeds or meals. Recordings are analysed using a personal computer and a detailed printed record produced. Automated analysis produces a summary of frequency and duration of reflux and the amount of time pH < 4.

When the above investigations fail to explain the basis of intractable vomiting, disorders of gastrointestinal motility such as chronic idopathic pseudo-obstruction need to be excluded. Such investigations are best performed in a paediatric gastroenterology unit.

Referral Centre Investigations

Scintigraphy

Gastro-oesophageal reflux may also be investigated using a radionuclide scan which permits more prolonged assess-

Table 7.9 Indications for 24-h oesophageal pH monitoring

Vomiting
Oesophagitis
Peptic oesophageal stricture
Aspiration pneumonia
Apnoea in the preterm resistant to standard therapy
Near-miss sudden infant death
Patients being considered for anti-reflux surgery
Failure to thrive
Feeding difficulties

ment than radiological methods. Infants are fasted for 4 h before a scan and then fed freshly prepared ^{99m}Tc sulphur colloid mixed with a small amount of normal feed. Monitoring with a γ-camera over 2 h will detect reflux and allow some assessment of severity.

Scintigraphic gastric emptying tests involve consumption of a radioactively labelled test meal. Images of the distribution of radioactivity within the abdomen are obtained with an anteriorly placed γ-camera. Emptying of solid and liquid meals are different and should be studied separately. Different test meals and analytical techniques make comparison of results between centres difficult.

Electrogastrography

Electrogastrography is the recording from surface electrodes of electrical activity generated by the stomach. The technique allows prolonged non-invasive recording of gastric electrical activity and is useful for demonstrating arrhythmias of the electrical control activity of the stomach.

Impedance

The electrical resistance (impedance) of the upper abdomen is influenced by the contents of the stomach and this can be used to measure gastric emptying. A 100–200 kHz current is passed through surface electrodes and the impedance recorded. There is a sudden change when a liquid meal with a resistivity different from that of the human body is ingested. The slope of the curve following this sudden change is a measure of gastric emptying.

Gastrointestinal Manometry

Manometry of the stomach and small intestine may be useful in children with gastroparesis and intestinal pseudo-obstruction. Once again it is a technique which demands a high standard of expertise to perform reliably. The standard manometric perfusion system is a multi-lumen tube connected to pressure transducers and perfused with water by a pneumohydraulic pump. It is possible to record contractile activity in various regions of the gut. The presence of these fine tubes does not seem to cause any significant stimulus. In older children a triple or quadruple lumen tube of 2.5–3 mm outer diameter is used, with each lumen 0.9 mm and with ports 5 cm apart perfused at a rate of 0.2 ml/min through each catheter. Motility recordings are usually interpreted visually, although quantification is possible with the aid of computer software programs.

In the oesophagus, swallow-induced peristalsis and the relaxation of the lower oesophageal sphincter can be studied. Antroduodenal motility during fasting can be compared with motility following an age-appropriate meal. The disruption of fasting activity and the establishment of postprandial activity provides information regarding the humorally mediated response to food and clarifies whether enteroenteric reflexes are intact. Myopathic processes give rise to low amplitude, poorly propagated contractions, whilst neuropathic processes are associated with contractions of normal amplitude which are often both unusual in waveform and abnormally propagated. Rectosigmoid motility during feeding can give information regarding the gastrocolonic reflex.

Histological Examination

For full investigation of chronic idiopathic intestinal pseudo-obstruction a full thickness piece of bowel (2 cm × 2 cm) should be taken for histology, histochemistry, immunocytochemistry, electron microscopy and silver staining. Careful planning between physician, surgeon and pathologist is essential before the biopsy is taken.

GASTROINTESTINAL BLEEDING

The causes of gastrointestinal bleeding are shown in Table 7.10. Investigation commonly requires specialized techniques available only in referral centres.

First-line Investigations of Gastrointestinal Bleeding

A blood count and film together with clotting studies will exclude a blood dyscrasia, bleeding diathesis or thrombocytopenia. Stool culture is necessary for identifying enteric pathogens causing bloody diarrhoea. These include entroinvasive *E. coli*, *Shigella*, *Campylobacter jejuni* and *Yersinia enterocolitica*. Paroxysmal abdominal pain, pallor and crying in the young infant suggests intussusception. In this condition barium or air enema may be both diagnostic and therapeutic. Massive painless rectal bleeding suggests peptic ulcer of the ileum adjacent to a Meckel's diverticulum; almost 60% of cases occur before 2 years of age.

Referral Unit Investigations

Upper Gastrointestinal Haemorrhage

The diagnostic value of radiology and endoscopy are dependent upon the experience of the operators. The

Table 7.10   Gastrointestinal (GI) bleeding

Upper GI bleeding
Idiopathic
Oesophagitis
Ulcerated hiatus hernia
Mallory–Weiss
Oesophogastric varices
Gastric ulcer
Acute ulceration
Haemorrhagic gastritis
Duodenal ulcer
Duodenitis

Lower GI bleeding
Anal fissure
Protein intolerance
Dysentery
Intussusception
Volvulus
Meckel's ulcer
Juvenile polyps
Ulcerative colitis
Crohn's disease
Henoch–Schonlein
Vascular malformation

Upper and lower GI bleeding
Blood dyscrasia
Bleeding diathesis
Thrombocytopenia
Hereditary telangiectasia
Vasculitis

superiority of endoscopy has been shown in studies of both adults and children and barium studies should no longer be the investigation of first choice (Cadranel and Rodesch 1988). Examination is best undertaken during the 24 h following haemorrhage; the nature of the lesion can then be established in about 70% of cases, but this proportion decreases as time between bleed and endoscopy increases. If no cause can be found and bleeding recurs, a second examination should be performed.

Lower Gastrointestinal Haemorrhage

Dietary protein intolerance may present with severe colitis and bloody diarrhoea within the first 2 years of life (Hill and Milla 1990). Colonoscopic appearances are those of patchy colonic erythema, whilst histological examination reveals inflammatory cell infiltrates in the lamina propria in which eosinophils and plasma cells predominate. Rectal bleeding from 1 to 6 years of age is most commonly due to a juvenile polyp. Colonoscopy is the investigation of choice when either polyps or inflammatory bowel disease are expected (Howdle et al 1984); barium studies are rarely indicated.

Radio-isotope Studies

Should upper and lower endoscopy fail to identify the cause of bleeding, intravenous injection of ^{99m}Tc sulphur colloid may be diagnostic. This isotope tracer is taken up by the reticuloendothelial system and remains within the vascular compartment for only a short time (half-life < 2.5 min). When there is active bleeding greater than 0.1 ml/min the tracer is concentrated at the bleeding site (Figure 7.6). Less brisk bleeding sites may be identified using injection of ^{99m}Tc labelled red cells.

Intravenously administered [^{99m}Tc]pertechnate is excreted by gastric mucosa and can be used to show gastric mucosa in a Meckel's diverticulum. A negative result, however, does not completely exclude this diagnosis.

Angiography

When the origin of haemorrhage has not been identified and massive bleeding continues, angiography is indicated. Selective arteriographs are performed of the superior and inferior mesenteric arteries and the coeliac axis. The cause of bleeding such as tumour or angioma may be demonstrated. If all investigations are negative yet bleeding persists, an exploratory laporotomy must be considered. Colonoscopy at the same time may help identify vascular anomalies.

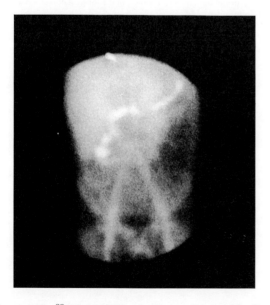

Figure 7.6 ^{99m}Tc labelled red cell scan showing bleeding from the small intestine in a boy with tuberculous ileitis. Photograph courtesy of Dr Stephen Chapman.

REFERENCES

Apley J (1959) *The Child with Abdominal Pains*. Blackwell Scientific Publications, Oxford.

Cadranel S, Rodesch P (1988) Fiberendoscopy of the upper gastrointestinal tract. In: Gans SL (ed) *Pediatric Endoscopy*, pp. 67–86. Grune & Stratton, New York.

Casasnovas AB, Cives RV, Jeremias AV et al (1991) Measurement of colonic transit time in children. *J Pediatr Gastroent Nutr* 13: 42–45.

D'Agostino S, Orsi M (1988) The steatocrit. *J Pediatr Gastroent Nutr* 7: 935–936.

Dalzell AM, Heaf DP (1990) Fluorescein dilaurate test of exocrine pancreatic function in cystic fibrosis. *Arch Dis Child* 65: 788–789.

Drumm B (1990) *Helicobacter pylori*. *Arch Dis Child* 65: 1278–1282.

Farrell MK (1993) Dr Apley meets *Helicobacter pylori*. *J Pediatr Gastroent Nutr* 16: 118–119.

Guandalini S, Ventura A, Ansaldi N et al (1989) Diagnosis of coeliac disease: time for a change? *Arch Dis Child* 64: 1320–1325.

Hill SM, Milla PJ (1990) Colitis caused by food allergy in infants. *Arch Dis Child* 65: 132–140.

Howdle PD, Littlewood JM, Firth J, Losowsky MS (1984) Routine colonoscopy service. *Arch Dis Child* 59: 790–793.

Puntis JWL (1993) Tests of pancreatic exocrine function. *Arch Dis Child* 69: 99–101.

Tappin DM, King C, Paton JY (1992) Lower oesophageal pH monitoring – a useful clinical tool. *Arch Dis Child* 67: 146–148.

Vandenplas Y, Goyvaerts H, Helven R, Sacre L (1991) *Paediatrics* 88: 834–839.

Walters MP, Kelleher J, Gilbert J, Littlewood JM (1990) Clinical monitoring of steatorrhoea in cystic fibrosis. *Arch Dis Child* 65: 99–102.

Weber FW, McCallum RW (1992) Clinical approaches to irritable bowel syndrome. *Lancet* 340: 1447–1452.

Appendix: Reference Ranges for Investigations

Blood

Carotene	1.9–5.6	µmol/l
C1 esterase inhibitor	0.15–0.35	g/l
C1 esterase functional	70–130	U/ml
Cholesterol	3–5.2	mmol/l
Copper	11–22	µmol/l
Folate	2.5–20	µg/l
Red cell folate	>100	µg/l
Lead	<1.21	µmol/l
Magnesium	0.7–1.0	mmol/l
Selenium	0.6–1.8	µmol/l
Triglycerides	<1.7	mmol/l
Vitamin A	300–1000	µg/l
Vitamin B12	180–800	ng/l
Vitamin E	5–33	mg/l
Zinc	12.6–22.0	µmol/l

Stool

Chymotrypsin	>120	µg/g stool

Testing Stool for Carbohydrate

Use a plastic nappy liner to collect fluid stool. Immediately mix 5 drops of liquid stool with 10 drops of water and add 1 Clinitest (Ames) tablet. If sucrose malabsorption is suspected, boil first with dilute hydrochloric acid. Read sugar concentration from colour chart as for urine testing. More than 0.5% reducing substances suggests carbohydrate malabsorption.

24-h Oesophageal pH Monitoring

Percentiles for four parameters* in healthy infants up to 1 year of age ($n = 509$)

Percentile	Reflux index*	No.	No. >5	Long
1	0	1	0	0
5	0	6	0	1
10	1	9	0	2
25	2	16	1	5
50	4	27	3	12
75	7	41	5	22
90	10	56	7	34
95	10	71.5	8.5	41
99	13.9	99.7	16.4	63

Data from Vandenplas et al (1991).
*Reflux index is the percentage of time for which the pH is <4; number of episodes with a pH <4; number of episodes with pH <4 lasting longer than 5 min; duration of the longest episode with a pH <4 (in minutes).

8

Hepatology

D A Kelly

INTRODUCTION

The investigation of a complex organ such as the liver relies on a multidisciplinary approach including: clinical chemistry, haematology, radiology and histopathology. It is essential to understand the many functions of the liver and to recognize the effects of hepatic dysfunction on other body systems (Table 8.1). An overview of useful investigations will first be given.

The approach to investigation of paediatric liver disease will then be considered in two parts:

- The investigation of the neonate or child of less than 2 years with prolonged jaundice.
- The investigation of older children (over the age of 2 years) with hepatomegaly and/or encephalopathy.

USEFUL INVESTIGATIONS IN THE ASSESSMENT OF LIVER DISEASE

Standard Liver Function Tests

Standard liver function tests (Table 8.2) usually reflect the severity of hepatic dysfunction (i.e. the more abnormal the test the worse the liver damage), but rarely provide diagnostic information on individual conditions. The best tests of liver "function" are the assessment of plasma albumin concentration and coagulation time. Hypoglycaemia, in the absence of other causes, indicates poor hepatic reserve and may have prognostic implications.

Imaging

A number of radiological techniques provide useful information in the investigation of paediatric liver disease.

Table 8.1 Functions of the liver

Function	Effect of dysfunction	Assessment
Metabolism/storage		
Carbohydrate	Loss of glucose homeostasis	Hypoglycaemia on fasting/stress
Fat	Accumulation of fat in hepatocytes ↓ Oxidation of fatty acids	High/low cholesterol. High BOH, FFA organic aciduria
Protein	↓ Catabolism	Low BCAA, urea, ammonia
Synthesis of:		
Albumin	Loss of muscle bulk, PEM	Low albumin
Coagulation proteins	Coagulopathy	Prolonged PT/PTT
Degradation of:		
Drugs	Prolonged drug effect, e.g. sedation	Clinical
Hormones	Telangiectasia Gynaecomastia	Clinical
"Waste products"	Encephalopathy	Abnormal EEG
Bile synthesis and excretion		
	Cholestasis Fat malabsorption Fat soluble vitamin deficiency Failure to thrive	↑ Conjugated bilirubin, GGT, ALP

ALP, alkaline phosphatase; BCAA, branched-chain amino acids; BOH, β-hydroxybutyrate; EEG, electroencephalogram; FFA, free fatty acids, GGT, γ-glutamyltranspeptidase; PEM, protein energy malnutrition; PT, prothrombin time; PTT, partial thromboplasmin time.

Table 8.2   Liver function tests

Reference range of test	Abnormality
Conjugated bilirubin, <20 µmol/l	Elevated: any derangement of hepatocyte function or biliary obstruction
Aminotransferases: Aspartate (AST), <50 u/l Alanine (ALT), <40 u/l	Elevated: hepatitis, non-specific hepatocyte inflammation/damage
Alkaline phosphatase (ALP), <600 u/l* γ-Glutamyltransferase (GGT), <30 u/l	Elevated: biliary epithelial inflammation/damage/ obstruction
Albumin, 30–50 g/l	Reduced: chronic liver disease
Prothrombin time (PT), 12–17 s Partial thromboplastin time (PTT) 33–37 s	Prolonged: vitamin K deficiency; reduced hepatic synthesis
Ammonia <50 µmol/l Glucose >4 mmol/l	Elevated: abnormal protein catabolism/Urea cycle defect Low in: acute or chronic liver failure

*Age-dependent see p. 87.

X-rays

Plain X-ray of the abdomen will give an indication of liver size but is rarely of value diagnostically.

Chest X-ray may show a number of skeletal abnormalities, e.g. butterfly vertebrae in Alagille's syndrome, a dilated heart in end-stage liver disease, or evidence of congenital heart disease which is commonly associated with liver disease.

Wrist and knee X-ray will identify bone age and/or the development of osteoporosis or rickets.

Abdominal Ultrasound

The development of Doppler ultrasound has been an important recent advance in the investigation of liver disease. Ultrasonic investigation of the abdomen provides information on the size and consistency of both liver and spleen, and may identify tumours, abscesses and cysts within the liver. It is usual to visualize the gallbladder (especially after fasting) and extrahepatic bile ducts, although intrahepatic bile ducts are rarely seen unless dilated.

Doppler ultrasound will identify whether the portal vein, hepatic and splenic vessels are patent. Portal hypertension is suggested by the presence of splenomegaly, especially if abdominal or gastric varices are visualized in the presence of ascites.

Radioisotope Scanning

Soluble radioisotopes (technetium DISIDA, HIDA or more recently TEBIDA)* which are taken up well by hepatocytes despite elevated bilirubin levels, are utilized to demonstrate:

- *Hepatic uptake* which is an index of hepatic function. This is of particular value in the diagnosis of hepatic vein obstruction (Budd–Chiari syndrome), as poor uptake of isotope is demonstrated in most of the liver except for the caudate lobe which has a separate venous drainage.
- *Biliary excretion of radioisotope.* Radioisotope scanning is most useful in the assessment of biliary excretion and in the differential diagnosis of neonatal cholestasis and biliary atresia.

Pretreatment with phenobarbitone (5 mg/kg) for 3–5 days prior to the investigation improves hepatic uptake of the isotope.

Endoscopic Retrograde Cholangiopancreatography (ERCP)

In this endoscopic technique a fibre-optic duodenoscope is passed into the first part of the duodenum, the pancreatic and biliary ducts are cannulated, and radiolucent dye injected. The technique has an 80% success rate in skilled hands and is invaluable for the assessment of extrahepatic biliary disease in older children, e.g. choledochal cysts or primary sclerosing cholangitis, or for the assessment of chronic pancreatitis. Its value in the differential diagnosis of neonatal cholestasis has still to be established.

Percutaneous Transhepatic Cholangiography

This technique is useful for the identification of biliary disease when intrahepatic bile ducts are dilated and an ERCP is impossible or unsuccessful. A thin needle (Shima) is passed through the liver and the bile ducts or gall bladder are punctured and radiolucent dye is injected.

Angiography

Visualization of the coeliac access, hepatic and splenic blood vessels, is obtained by femoral artery catheterization and injection of radiolucent dye. This technique has two parts. The arterial phase provides information on the coeliac axis, hepatic and splenic artery abnormalities,

*DISIDA: 99 M Technetium Diisopropyl-Imino Diacetic Acid
HIDA: 99 M Technetium Diethyl-Imino Diacetic Acid
TEBIDA: 99 M Technetium Trimethylbromo-Imino Diacetic Acid

vascularization and anatomy of hepatic tumours, hepatic haemangiomas or detection of hepatic artery thrombosis. The venous phase of the investigation provides information about the patency of the portal and splenic veins and the presence of portal hypertension by identification of mesenteric, oesophageal or gastric varices. In skilled hands the investigation can be performed in infants with little risk. Femoral artery spasm or thrombosis is an occasional side-effect, but rarely requires surgical treatment.

These radiological techniques are mostly only available in specialized centres. Although abdominal ultrasound is available at most district general hospitals, the interpretation of findings in infants may require specialist expertise.

Computerized Tomography (CT)

CT scanning of the liver is useful for the identification of hepatic tumours or space-occupying lesions of the liver. Intravenous contrast medium causes enhancement of vascular lesions and the walls of abscesses, and may be helpful in differentiating tumours from other solid masses.

Magnetic Resonance Imaging (MRI)

MRI scanning is probably the best way to stage or diagnose hepatic tumours and identify their vascular supply.

Histopathology

The diagnosis of most liver diseases requires histological confirmation and liver biopsy is a routine procedure in specialist centres. An aspiration technique, using a Menghini needle, has a complication risk of 1 : 1000 liver biopsies and may be performed under sedation with local anaesthesia. In fibrotic or cirrhotic livers a Tru-cut needle, which removes a larger core, may be necessary. Transjugular liver biopsies, in which the liver is biopsied through a special catheter passed from the internal jugular vein into the hepatic veins, are not routinely available for children as yet. The complications of this potentially dangerous procedure are much reduced if performed in expert hands in specialized units under controlled conditions. It is essential to have information about liver size from ultrasound and accurate information about coagulation parameters. Prothrombin time should be within 3 s of control values; platelet count should be at least 60×10^9/l. It is prudent to cross-match a unit of blood prior to the procedure. Biopsy specimens should be obtained for routine histopathology, microbiology, electron microscopy and copper (if appropriate), and frozen

for enzymatic or metabolic investigations. The interpretation of the histology is difficult and requires considerable specialist expertise.

Metabolic Investigations

Many inborn errors of metabolism present with hepatomegaly and/or liver disease. It is essential to screen for these diseases as part of the investigation of liver disease as detailed below (Table 8.3) and in Chapter 4.

Table 8.3 Investigation of liver disease

Baseline investigations
Bilirubin – conjugated; unconjugated
Aspartate aminotransferase
Alanine aminotransferase
Alkaline phosphatase
γ-Glutamyltranspeptidase
Albumin
Glucose
Full blood count and platelets
Prothrombin time
Partial thromboplastin time

Second-line investigations
Bacterial culture of blood and urine
TORCH screen
Hepatitis A, B, C
α_1-Antitrypsin level and phenotype
Abdominal ultrasound

Metabolic investigations
Plasma lactate, BOH, FFA
Serum iron and ferritin
Plasma amino acids
Urine: reducing sugars; organic acids; amino acids

Neonate
Galactose-1,6 phosphate uridyl transferase
Free T4, TSH
Chromosomes

Older child (> 2 years)
Copper, caeruloplasmin, urinary copper, C3, C4, ANF, SMA, LKM

If indicated
Liver biopsy: with or without endoscopy, ERCP, PTC

ANF, antinuclear factor; BOH, β-hydroxybutyrate; C3, C4, complement; ERCP, endoscopic retrograde cholangiopancreatography; FFA, free fatty acids; LKM, liver kidney microsomal antibodies; PTC, percutaneous transhepatic cholangiography; SMA, smooth muscle antibodies; T4, free tyroxine; TORCH, toxoplasma, rubella, cytomegalovirus, herpes simplex; TSH, thyroid stimulating hormone.

Bone Marrow Aspiration

Bone marrow aspiration should be performed in all babies with undiagnosed neonatal hepatitis to exclude Niemann Pick disease type C, or other storage disorder.

Skin Biopsy

This procedure should be considered if an inborn error of metabolism is being considered, and the specimen stored frozen for future culture.

Endoscopy

Upper gastrointestinal endoscopy (gastroscopy) using a flexible fibre-optic endoscope is useful to diagnose oesophageal and gastric varices secondary to portal hypertension. The technique is normally performed under sedation.

Neurophysiology

Electroencephalography will identify abnormal rhythms secondary to either acute or chronic liver failure.

Ophthalmology

A number of inherited conditions have associated occular lesions, e.g. Kayser–Fleischer rings in Wilson's disease and posterior embryotoxin in Alagille's syndrome.

NEONATAL LIVER DISEASE (see also Chapter 20)

Persistent Jaundice

As physiological jaundice may be present in up to 90% of babies, the diagnosis of liver disease may be difficult at this stage. In practice, if jaundice persists beyond 2 weeks after birth it should be investigated even in breast-fed babies. The differential diagnosis lies between breast milk jaundice, other causes of unconjugated hyperbilirubinaemia (Chapter 20), extrahepatic biliary disease and the neonatal hepatitis syndrome (Tables 8.3 and 8.4).

The first step is to confirm whether the prolonged jaundice is due to an elevation of conjugated or unconjugated bilirubin in the plasma and whether there is bilirubin in the urine. The presence of bilirubin in the urine is always abnormal and suggests obstructive jaundice.

If the estimation of bilirubin indicates that > 85% is in the unconjugated fraction, then breast milk jaundice

Table 8.4 Neonatal liver disease

Extrahepatic biliary duct disorders
Biliary atresia
Choledochal cyst
Gallstones
Caroli's disease

Neonatal hepatitis
Idiopathic

Intrauterine infection:
Cytomegalovirus
Toxoplasmosis
Rubella
Herpes simplex
Treponema pallidum
Coxsackie
Adeno and echo virus

Inborn error of metabolism
α_1-Antitrypsin deficiency
Galactosaemia
Hereditary fructose intolerance*
Tyrosinaemia type I
Niemann–Pick type C
Cystic fibrosis
Zellwegers/peroxisomal disorders
Infantile haemochromatosis
Bile salt metabolism

Urinary tract infection

TPN cholestasis

Chromosomal disorders:
Trisomy 13 and 18
Down's syndrome

Hypoxia/hypotension
Postcardiac surgery

*Presents on weaning.
TPN, total parenteral nutrition.

or another cause of unconjugated hyperbilirubinaemia is likely (Chapter 20).

However, if > 15% of the total bilirubin is conjugated or bilirubin is detected in the urine, liver disease must be excluded (Tables 8.3 and 8.4).

Immediate investigation for neonatal liver disease should include abdominal ultrasound and standard liver function tests to assess the degree of hepatic dysfunction and chronicity (Table 8.2). Immediate referral to a tertiary centre is mandatory if a neonate has two or more of the following:

- Conjugated hyperbilirubinaemia > 40 μmol/l.
- Pale stools.
- Bilirubin in urine.

- Bleeding tendency.
- Failure to thrive.
- Recurrent hypoglycaemia.

More specialized investigations, e.g. radioisotope scanning, biochemical investigations for metabolic disease and liver biopsy should distinguish between biliary atresia and the neonatal hepatitis syndrome and are best performed at a specialist centre.

As the clinical presentation of biliary atresia and neonatal hepatitis syndrome are similar most of the investigations listed in Table 8.3 are performed at presentation. Many specialized investigations require collection of fresh samples, and should be performed at a referral centre where there is appropriate laboratory support.

Table 8.5 Liver disease in older children (> 2 years)

Disease	Diagnostic investigations
Acute hepatitis	
Viral hepatitis A, B, C and E, EBV, CMV	Viral serology
Drugs: halothane, isoniazid	Halothane antibodies
Autoimmune hepatitis	IgG > 20 g/l, C3, C4, LKM, ANF, SMA
Chronic liver disease	
Chronic persistent/active hepatitis	Inflammatory infiltrate on biopsy
Hepatitis B, C and D, EBV, CMV	Serology
Autoimmune hepatitis	As above
Wilson's disease	Serum copper, caeruloplasmin, urinary copper
α_1-Antitrypsin deficiency	α_1-Antitrypsin level and phenotype
Cystic fibrosis	Sweat test, liver biopsy
Cryptogenic cirrhosis	Liver biopsy
Primary sclerosing cholangitis	ERCP and liver biopsy
Tyrosinaemia type I	Urinary succinylacetone
Hereditary fructose intolerance	Fructose-1,6-phosphate aldolase in liver

ANF, antinuclear antibodies; C3, C4, complement; CMV, cytomegalovirus; EBV, Epstein–Barr virus; ERCP, endoscopic retrograde cholangiopancreatography; LKM, liver kidney microsomal antibodies; SMA, smooth muscle antibodies.

Biliary Atresia

Biliary atresia is a rare disorder in which there is destruction and fibrosis of both intra and extra hepatic biliary ducts. The disease presents with obstructive jaundice in a baby of normal birth weight. Liver function tests demonstrate conjugated hyperbilirubinaemia > 100 μmol/l, elevated alkaline phosphatase, and a modest rise in transaminases (80–200 u/l). Coagulation times and plasma albumin are normal in the early stage. There is no pathognomonic test but the diagnosis is suggested by the combination of:

- Abdominal ultrasound which indicates either a small or absent gallbladder after a 4 h fast.
- Delayed biliary excretion of radioisotope (DISIDA or TEBIDA) after 24 h.
- Liver histology which demonstrates extensive biliary fibrosis with biliary ductule proliferation.

If the above diagnostic tests are equivocal it is necessary to proceed to an operative cholangiogram which is performed at laparotomy. If extrahepatic biliary obstruction is confirmed a Kasai portoenterostomy may be performed.

The operation has an 80% success rate *only if performed within 60 days of birth*; hence the urgent need for early diagnosis and treatment in babies with prolonged jaundice.

Choledochal Cysts

Choledochal cysts are cystic dilatations of the extrahepatic biliary tree which are more common in females (3 : 1). The cysts may present with obstructive jaundice in infancy or with abdominal pain or cholangitis in the older child.

Liver function tests will indicate conjugated hyperbilirubinaemia (80–200 μmol/l);

- Alkaline phosphatase raised for age (see p. 87).
- Transaminases 80–200 u/l.
- Plasma albumin and coagulation may be normal.

The diagnosis is made by identifying a biliary cyst on ultrasound and confirmed by ERCP or PTC. Biliary fibrosis or cirrhosis may be present on histology, and may be reversible following successful surgery.

Neonatal Hepatitis Syndrome

In contrast to biliary atresia, babies with the neonatal hepatitis syndrome may be small for gestational age, and present with hepatosplenomegaly, failure to thrive and a bleeding tendency. Stools are usually pigmented although the urine will be darker than normal. The diagnosis is confirmed biochemically with a rise in transaminases (100–300 u/l), and a modest rise of alkaline phosphatase; plasma albumin may be low and coagulation times may be abnormal.

Abdominal ultrasound may demonstrate hepatosplenomegaly but the gall bladder size is usually normal. A DISIDA or TEBIDA radioisotope scan will demonstrate poor uptake throughout the liver but biliary excretion is normal and should be complete within 4–6 h following injection.

Specific Causes of the Neonatal Hepatitis Syndrome

The known causes of the neonatal hepatitis syndrome are outlined in Table 8.4. It is important to exclude sepsis because, although infection may cause unconjugated hyperbilirubinaemia, urinary tract infection is associated with the neonatal hepatitis syndrome. Adequate treatment of the urinary tract infection produces rapid resolution of the hepatitis.

Intrauterine Infection

Cytomegalovirus is the commonest intrauterine infection to produce the neonatal hepatitis syndrome. Clinically the disease presents with hepatosplenomegaly, petechiae and failure to thrive.

Diagnostic tests are:

- Cytomegalovirus (CMV) IgM antibodies in serum.
- CMV early antigen in the urine.

CMV IgG antibodies may be due to maternal transfer and are non-diagnostic.

Hepatitis A, B or C are rare causes of neonatal hepatitis. The incidence of HIV hepatitis in this age is not yet established.

Inborn Errors of Metabolism

α_1-Antitrypsin deficiency is the commonest inborn error of metabolism to present with neonatal liver disease. The diagnosis is confirmed by detecting a low serum α_1-antitrypsin level (normal > 0.9 g/l) and identifying the phenotype of the protein. Phenotype PiMM is the commonest; PiZZ or PiSZ are known to be associated with liver disease. Although liver disease is usual in homozygotes, heterozygotes may develop liver disease with levels of α_1-antitrypsin in the low–normal range. It

is therefore necessary to measure the serum level and determine phenotype in all cases.

Liver histology varies from a giant cell hepatitis to biliary fibrosis, but hepatocytes will contain the characteristic PAS positive, diastase resistant granules of α_1-antitrypsin. Immunoperoxidase staining is an alternative method of demonstrating the granules.

Cystic fibrosis occasionally presents with cholestatic neonatal hepatitis. All babies with undiagnosed neonatal hepatitis should have a sweat test when old enough.

Tyrosinaemia type I is due to a deficiency of fumarylacetoacetase (FAA). It may present at any age. Clinical features in the neonate include hypoglycaemia and acute liver failure with coagulopathy. Diagnosis is based on:

- An elevated plasma and urinary tyrosine, methionine with or without phenylalanine.
- Detection of succinyl acetone in the urine.
- Elevated α-fetoprotein (> 800 ku/l).
- Deficiency of FAA in cultured skin fibroblasts.

Confirmation of tyrosinaemia type I by detection of succinyl acetone is essential to exclude:

- Transient neonatal hypertyrosinaemia.
- Tyrosine aminotransferase deficiency (tyrosinaemia type II).
- Non-specific elevation of tyrosine secondary to severe liver failure or other metabolic liver disease, e.g. galactosaemia.

Liver histology may show a non-specific neonatal hepatitis with an increase in fat in hepatocytes. The development of dysplastic hepatocytes may indicate the inevitable development of malignancy.

Galactosaemia

This should be excluded in any acutely ill infant with hypoglycaemia. The diagnosis is confirmed by assay of the red cell enzyme galactose-1-phosphate uridyl transferase (GAL-1-PUT) as detection of reducing sugars in the urine may be unreliable if there is not enough lactose or galactose in the feeds.

Hereditary Fructose Intolerance

The clinical features of this disease only present when sucrose or fructose is introduced into the diet, normally on weaning. The diagnosis is suspected by detection of reducing sugars in the urine following a feed containing sucrose and confirmed by measurement of fructose 1,6-diphosphate aldolase in liver or intestinal biopsy.

Note: babies with severe hepatic dysfunction may have a positive test for urine reducing sugars because of galactose in their urine which is non-specific.

Glycogen Storage Disease

Glycogen storage disease does not present with neonatal cholestasis but with hepatomegaly and occasionally hypoglycaemia with a raised lactate (> 3 mmol/l). There may also be hyperlipidaemia with elevated cholesterol and triglyceride (Type I). The diagnosis may be confirmed by:

- Liver histology which demonstrates glycogen storage in hepatocytes.
- Measurement of the appropriate enzymes in liver, leucocytes or muscle (Chapter 4).

Niemann Pick Disease Type C

Niemann Pick disease type C should be excluded in any baby with undiagnosed neonatal hepatitis, prolonged cholestasis and prominent splenomegaly.
   The diagnosis is confirmed by:

- Detection of the characteristic foamy storage cell in liver, bone marrow aspirate.
- Neurona storage in ganglion cells on rectal biopsy.

Niemann Pick disease types A and B do not present with neonatal cholestasis but with hepatosplenomegaly, neurological abnormalities and failure to thrive (Chapter 5).

Infantile Haemochromatosis

This rare inherited disease presents with acute liver failure in infancy. The diagnosis is confirmed by:

- Serum iron > 50 μmol/l.
- Serum ferritin > 1000 μg/l.
- Liver histology which demonstrates extensive hepatic necrosis with excess iron storage.

Bile Salt Disorders

These rare disorders should be suspected in a child with persistent unexplained cholestasis. Confirmation is by identifying the abnormal bile salt metabolite in urine which is only possible at specialist centres.

Zellweger's Syndrome and Peroxisomal Disorders

Zellweger's syndrome should be considered in any child

with liver dysfunction who is severely hypotonic with abnormal neurology. The diagnosis is confirmed by:

- Elevation of very long chain fatty acids (VLCFA) in plasma.
- Raised serum iron (> 50 μmol/l).
- Absence or presence of abnormal peroxisomes in liver tissue.

Endocrine Disorders

The neonatal hepatitis syndrome is associated with hypothyroidism and hypopituitarism. Hypothyroidism is confirmed by:

- Increased thyroid stimulating hormone (TSH) (normal < 5 mU/l).
- Low thyroxine (free T4) < 12 pmol/l.

   Hypopituitarism is confirmed by:

- Low random cortisol < 140 μmol/l.
- Low TSH, low T4.
- Normal response to thyrotropin releasing hormone.
- Poor response to growth hormone.

Cholestasis Secondary to Total Parenteral Nutrition

Liver damage is likely to develop in any infant fed for more than 4 weeks by total parenteral nutrition (TPN), particularly if there has been difficulty in enteral feeding. Diagnosis is confirmed by:

- Elevated transaminases (100–300 u/l).
- Rise in bilirubin (> 100 μmol/l).
- Rising alkaline phosphatase.
- Abdominal ultrasound may demonstrate a contracted gall bladder, gallstones or biliary sludge.
- Liver histology includes fatty change, canalicular and hepatocyte cholestasis, portal tract expansion with fibrosis and inflammatory infiltrate and bile duct reduplication.

The Acutely Ill Neonate

The differential diagnosis of liver disease in an acutely ill neonate includes sepsis or an inborn error of metabolism. If the clinical presentation is:

- Acute liver failure with hypoglycaemia, cholestasis and abnormal coagulation, then consider:
  (a) tyrosinaemia type I,
  (b) galactosaemia,
  (c) infantile haemochromatosis,

(d) fatty acid oxidation defects,
(e) electron transport chain defects (see Chapter 4).
- With encephalopathy without prominent cholestasis and neurological signs, consider:
  (a) urea cycle defect (see Chapter 4),
  (b) Zellweger's syndrome,
  (c) organic acid disorders.

The Dysmorphic Neonate

Many inborn errors of metabolism are associated with dysmorphic features. The best-known association with neonatal liver disease is Alagille's syndrome. The clinical picture is characteristic with hypertelorism, deep-set eyes and a triangular face. The diagnosis is confirmed by:

- Posterior embryotoxin in 90% of cases.
- Skeletal abnormalities such as butterfly vertebrae and short distal phalanges.
- Peripheral pulmonary stenosis detected by echocardiography or cardiac catheterization.
- Renal tubular acidosis or glomerulonephritis (increased urinary protein/creatinine ratio (> 20 mg/mmol) and aminoaciduria.
- Liver biochemistry indicates severe cholestasis with conjugated bilirubin (> 100 μmol/l), raised alkaline phosphatase, γ-GT (> 200 u/l), cholesterol (> 6 mmol/l) with normal triglycerides (0.4–2 mmol/l).
- Liver histology demonstrates reduction in the number of interlobular bile ducts within the portal tract, although this may be subtle and in early stages the biopsy resembles neonatal hepatitis.

LIVER DISEASE IN CHILDREN OLDER THAN 2 YEARS

In contrast to neonatal liver disease, older children may not be jaundiced despite advanced liver disease. The clinical presentation may vary from acute hepatitis to the insidious development of hepatosplenomegaly, portal hypertension and malnutrition. Initial investigations should concentrate on establishing evidence of hepatic damage and the extent of hepatic dysfunction with standard liver function tests (Tables 8.2 and 8.3) and then screening for the known causes (Table 8.5).

Acute Liver Disease

The commonest causes of acute liver disease in childhood are viral hepatitis, autoimmune hepatitis, or metabolic liver disease.

Table 8.6   Acute liver failure in children

Fulminant hepatitis	Diagnostic investigations
Infection	
Viral hepatitis A, B, C	Viral serology
Undefined, EBV, CMV	
Poison/drugs	
Paracetamol, isoniazide	Paracetamol level
Halothane	Halothane antibodies
Aminata phalloides	
Autoimmune hepatitis	Autoimmune screen
Metabolic	
Wilson's disease	Copper, caeruloplasmin
Tyrosinaemia	Urinary succinylacetone
Reye's syndrome	Microvesicular fat in liver

Acute Viral Hepatitis

The diagnosis of acute viral hepatitis may be made by demonstrating:

- Elevated transaminases aspartate aminotransferase, alanine aminotransferase (AST, ALT $\times$ 10–100).
- A moderate elevation in alkaline phosphatase.
- Specific viral serology.

Conjugated bilirubin may or may not be elevated. Plasma albumin levels are usually normal. Prolonged coagulation times which are unresponsive to vitamin K therapy indicate severe hepatitis or acute liver failure and immediate referral to a specialist centre.

Acute viral infection is indicated by detection of: IgM antibodies to hepatitis A (IgM HAV); hepatitis B IgM anticore; cytomegalovirus (CMV) IgM antibodies or polymerase chain reaction (PCR) of Buffy coat (PCR is only available in special centres); or Epstein–Barr virus (EBV) early antigen (EBNA).

Routine testing for hepatitis C depends on the detection of total antibody (HCV IgG) and thus diagnosis of acute infection is not possible. Identification of hepatitis C by PCR is only available at special centres.

Liver biopsy is not required for diagnosis of uncomplicated acute viral hepatitis. Histology demonstrates centrilobular liver cell damage and necrosis.

Acute Liver Failure

Acute liver failure may occur at any age and is fatal in over 70% of children without transplantation. The principal causes in childhood include acute viral hepatitis, metabolic liver disease or autoimmune hepatitis (Table 8.6).

Reye's syndrome or acute liver failure should be excluded in any child with encephalopathy and coagulopathy even if jaundice is not obvious.

First-line Investigations

- Bilirubin: jaundice may be a late feature, particularly in metabolic liver disease.
- Transaminases are grossly elevated ($\times$ 1–200).
- Coagulation is prolonged (prothrombin time $>$ 30 s).
- Albumin may be normal.
- Blood glucose (may be low).
- Ammonia ($>$ 100 μmol/l).
- Acid–base status.
- Plasma and urinary osmolality.
- Septic screen (but **not** lumbar puncture).
- EEG: a slow rhythm with triphasic waves is characteristic of an acute hepatic encéphalopathy.
- A CT scan may indicate cerebral oedema if encephalopathy is present.
- Specific investigations (Table 8.5).

A mortality of $>$ 70% and immediate referral for transplantation is indicated by:

- Prothrombin time $>$ 60 s.
- Decreasing transaminase levels are, of course, normally a sign of resolution indicate deterioration if associated with increased coagulopathy.
- Rising bilirubin ($>$ 300 μmol/l).
- Decreasing liver size as indicated either clinically or by ultrasound.
- Acid–base pH $<$ 7.3.
- Hypoglycaemia ($<$ 4 mmol/l with increasing dextrose requirement).
- Serum creatinine $>$ 300 μmol/l.
- Coma grade II–III (Glasgow Coma Scale).

Progress is monitored by measurement of 4-hourly glucose, prothrombin time and acid–base status.

Reye's Syndrome

This rare condition is probably a disorder of fatty acid oxidation (Chapter 4). The diagnosis is suggested by the clinical presentation of hypoglycemia, encephalopathy and convulsions which have been preceded by a prodromal illness. The diagnosis is confirmed by:

- Low blood glucose ($<$ 4.00 mmol/l).
- Raised ammonia ($>$ 100 μmol/l).
- Transaminases ($>$ 100 u/l).
- Prothrombin time $>$ 4 s greater than control.

- Microvesicular fatty infiltration in liver histology.
- Organic acids in urine (in those with an underlying metabolic disorder, see Chapter 5).

Chronic Liver Disease

Chronic Viral Hepatitis

Hepatitis A does not cause chronic viral hepatitis. Approximately 90% of infants infected with hepatitis B virus (HBV) at birth and 10% of those infected horizontally will become chronic carriers and develop chronic liver disease and cirrhosis. The diagnosis is confirmed by demonstrating chronic HBV:

- HBsAg-positive for more than 6 months with HBeAg positive, or HBe antibody positive.
- Liver histology will identify hepatitis B surface antigen by orcein staining in hepatocytes and a persistent inflammatory infiltrate in the portal tracts.
- Transaminases may be normal.
- Coagulation times and albumin are normal.

As there is a risk of hepatocellular carcinoma annual abdominal ultrasound and serial alphafetoprotein monitoring is essential.

Chronic liver disease and cirrhosis will develop in 30% of children with Hepatitis C. Diagnosis is confirmed by:

- Detection of HCV-IgG.
- Hepatitis C PCR.
- Fluctuating transaminases.
- Liver histology indicates persistent inflammatory infiltrate in portal tracts and fatty infiltration of hepatocytes.

Autoimmune Hepatitis

This disease of unknown aetiology is commonest in girls (female/male 3 : 1). The presentation varies from an acute hepatitis with classic autoimmune features, including skin rash, joint pain, fatigue and malaise, to the insidious development of cirrhosis and portal hypertension with malnutrion. Diagnosis is suggested by:

- Non-organ-specific autoantibodies (Table 8.6) are present in 70% of children, but may be negative in the early stages.
- Immunoglobulins are usually raised (IgG $>$ 20 gm/l).
- Complement levels (C3 and C4) may be reduced.

Children with positive liver/kidney microsomal antibodies (LKM antibodies) usually have a worse long-term prognosis than those with positive antinuclear factor (ANF) or smooth muscle antibodies (SMA).

Wilson's Disease

This rare disease is unusual before 3 years of age, and may present with any form of liver disease. It should always be excluded in children of this age.

Kayser–Fleischer rings may be visible on slit-lamp examination in children over the age of 7 years. Standard liver function tests may indicate chronic liver disease with a low albumin, minimal elevation of transaminases and an unusually low alkaline phosphatase. Evidence of haemolysis on blood film is usually present. The diagnosis is established by detecting:

- A low serum copper ($< 10\ \mu mol/l$).
- A low serum caeruloplasmin ($< 200\ mg/l$).
- Excess urine copper ($> 1.0\ \mu mol/24\ h$).
- Elevated hepatic copper ($> 250\ mg/g$ dry weight).

Approximately 25% of children may have a normal or borderline caeruloplasmin as this protein is also an acute-phase protein. All children will have an elevated urinary copper excretion, particularly after penicillamine treatment (20 mg/kg).

There are four characteristic histological patterns: fatty change in hepatocytes; chronic active hepatitis; cirrhosis; and massive hepatic necrosis with underlying cirrhosis.

An orcein stain to demonstrate copper storage will be positive except in the very early stages of the disease. If the diagnosis is equivocal, measurement of radioactive copper (^{64}Cu or ^{67}Cu) incorporation into caeruloplasmin may be helpful. If neurological symptoms are present, CT scan or MRI scan may show cerebral atrophy and lucencies in the basal ganglia.

Cystic Fibrosis

The spectrum of liver disease in cystic fibrosis includes fatty liver, focal biliary fibrosis and cirrhosis and portal hypertension. Early liver disease is particularly difficult to diagnose but suspicion may be raised by detecting transient increases in transaminases, alkaline phosphatase or γ-glutamyltranspeptidase (GGT). In practice, few children are diagnosed until overt liver disease with splenomegaly and portal hypertension have developed.

Diagnostic investigations are best performed at a specialist centre and include:

- Abdominal ultrasound which may identify an enlarged fatty liver ("bright" echos), dilated bile ducts or a small echogenic liver suggestive of cirrhosis with splenomegaly and/or varices.
- DISIDA or TEBIDA radioisotope scans may indicate abnormalities in biliary excretion which include the pooling of radioisotope dye in intrahepatic bile ducts or delayed biliary excretion ($> 4\ h$).
- Upper gastrointestinal endoscopy to identify oesophageal and gastric varices.
- Liver histology may demonstrate fatty change throughout the hepatocytes, areas of focal biliary fibrosis or established cirrhosis.
- Positive sweat test (see Chapters 5 and 13).

Jaundice is a late feature and liver synthetic function (as indicated by albumin and coagulation times) are well maintained until the terminal illness.

Cirrhosis and Portal Hypertension

Cirrhosis is the development of extensive fibrosis with areas of regeneration throughout the liver cells. It represents the end-stage of all forms of chronic liver disease irrespective of aetiology. Cirrhosis may be compensated (i.e. hepatic function is normal and complications are minimal) or decompensated, when hepatic dysfunction is severe with many complications.

Children with compensated cirrhosis may have normal liver function tests, normal coagulation and normal growth. Diagnosis may only be obvious on ultrasound which demonstrates a small shrunken echogenic liver or on liver histology.

As the cirrhotic process becomes decompensated, abnormalities in liver function are more easily identified, there is a reduction in growth veolcity and an increase in complications.

Confirmation of cirrhosis should be performed at a specialist centre and includes the following.

Biochemical Abnormalities

- Mild rise in transaminase levels (AST, ALT = 80–300 u/l).
- An increase in alkaline phosphatase and GGT ($\times 2$ normal).
- A gradual fall in albumin ($< 30\ g/l$).
- Low serum calcium and phosphate (development of rickets).

Haematological

- Anaemia (from bleeding varices, etc.).
- Prolongation of coagulation time (PT > 3 s greater than control).

Radiology

- Abdominal ultrasound, which will demonstrate a small shrunken echogenic liver with splenomegaly and/or ascites.
- Chest X-ray: fluid overload with enlarged heart; congenital heart disease.
- Wrist X-ray: delayed bone age; rickets.

Endoscopy

Upper gastrointestinal endoscopy to identify oesophageal or gastric varices and/or erosive gastritis.

Electroencephalography

Electroencephalogram (EEG) to determine presence of chronic hepatic encephalopathy (slow irregular low-frequency waves).

Histology

Liver biopsy will confirm extensive fibrosis with regenerative nodules. The aetiology of the liver disease may also be obvious, e.g. α_1-antitrypsin granules.

Microbiology

Sepsis is common in these children and a septic screen should be performed if pyrexial. Septic screen should include:

- Urine and blood cultures.
- Ascitic tap (if ascites is present).
- Lumbar puncture is omitted if coagulopathy is severe.

Renal function

Oliguria and renal failure are common. It is important to differentiate between: pre-renal failure, secondary to sepsis and dehydration; functional renal failure, secondary to hepatorenal failure; and acute tubular necrosis.

- An *elevated urea* with normal creatinine suggests pre-renal failure. (*Note*: creatinine may be low because of poor muscle mass secondary to malnutrition; urea may be low because of poor hepatic synthesis.)
- *Plasma and urinary sodium*. Hyponatremia (plasma sodium < 130 mmol/l) develops in end-stage liver disease and indicates a poor prognosis. In pre-renal failure urinary sodium is < 20 mmol/l and the urine/plasma osmolality ratio is > 1. In acute tubular necrosis, urinary sodium is > 20 mmol/l, and the urine/plasma osmolality ratio is 1 (see Chapter 6).

- *Urine protein/creatinine ratio* may be elevated (> 20 mg/mmol) with coexisting nephritis or renal tubular disorders.
- *Urinary pH* > 6. Renal tubular acidosis is common in certain metabolic liver diseases, e.g. tyrosinaemia type I and hereditary fructose intolerance. There is a generalized proximal tubular leak with aminoaciduria and glycosuria.

Malnutrition

Malnutrition is inevitable with chronic liver disease. Serial anthropometry may indicate a decrease in fat (measured by triceps skin fold) and protein stores (measured by calculation of the mid-arm muscle area (MAMA)). The effects of vitamin deficiencies are common whether or not there is cholestasis.

Biochemical Investigations

- Vitamin A (0.7–2.1 kIU/l).
- Vitamin E (6–40 mmol/l).
- Low calcium, phosphate.
- Cholesterol (< 2.0 mmol/l).

Monitoring Progress in Liver Disease

The aim in serial monitoring of liver disease is to assess the effect of a specific treatment (e.g. immunosuppression for autoimmune hepatitis, penicillamine for Wilson's disease) and to identify at which stage of the disease transplantation may be indicated. Monitoring includes:

- *Conjugated bilirubin*. Following an acute hepatic illness return to normality of bilirubin levels usually indicates recovery. However, bilirubin levels may be normal despite the development of fibrosis and cirrhosis.
- *Transaminases*. Fluctuating and transient increases in transaminases indicate continued hepatic dysfunction.
- *Protein synthesis*. A persistent decrease in albumin levels indicates the development of chronic liver disease.
- *Prothrombin time*. Increasing coagulation time, which is unresponsive to vitamin K administration, indicates deteriorating liver function.
- *Nutrition*. Serial anthropometry may indicate a reduction in fat and muscle stores despite intensive nutritional support, and is a poor prognostic sign.
- Persistence of hepatic encephalopathy is a poor prognostic sign.

Indications for Transplantation

Transplantation is indicated for either acute liver failure (see above) or chronic liver failure. There are no specific tests of hepatic function which will reliably indicate when transplantation should be considered. In general this operation should be considered if there is:

- Persistent elevation of conjugated bilirubin > 120 μmol/l.
- Prolongation of prothrombin > 4 s greater than control.
- Falling albumin < 30 g/l.
- Persistent encephalopathy.
- Recurrent hepatic complications, e.g. ascites. spontanous bacterial peritonitis, variceal haemorrhage and persistent encephalopathy unresponsive to medical therapy.
- Diminishing quality of life.
- Malnutrition.

It is mandatory to refer a child for consideration for liver transplantation before there is irreversible growth retardation and developmental delay.

Assessment for Liver Transplantation

Assessment for liver transplantation should only take place at a specialist centre. Investigations are based on establishing:

- Hepatic function (Tables 8.1 and 8.2).

- Vascular anatomy of the liver by abdominal ultrasound or angiography.
- Previous viral infection (CMV, EBV, measles, varicella, HIV, hepatitis A, B or C).
- Cardiorespiratory status ECG, echochardiography, and chest X-ray).
- Neurological status (EEG; CT scan if required).
- Nutritional status.

Donor organs are matched for blood group, size and, if possible, by CMV status.

REFERENCES

Clayton PT (1991) Inherited errors of bile acid metabolism. *J Inher Metab Dis* 14: 478–496.

Fernandes J (1990) The glycogen storage diseases. In: Fernandes J, Saudubray JM, Tada K (eds) *Inborn Metabolic Diseases*, pp. 69–88. Springer-Verlag, Heidelberg.

Gitzelmann R, Hansen RG (1980) Galactose metabolism, hereditary defects and their clinical significance. In: Burman D, Holton JB, Pennock GA (eds) *Inherited Disorders of Carbohydrate Metabolism*, pp. 61–101. MTP Press, Lancaster.

Heymans HSA, Wanders RJA, Shutgens RBH (1990) Peroximal disorders. In: Fernandes J, Saudubray JM, Tada K (eds) *Inborn Metabolic Diseases*, pp. 421–436. Springer-Verlag, Heidelberg.

Hull J, Kelley DA (1991) Investigation of prolonged neonatal jaundice. *Curr Paediatr* 1: 228–230.

Kelly DA (1993) Fulminant hepatitis in acute liver failure. In: Butts JP, Sokal EM (eds) *Management of Digestive and Liver Disorders in Infants and Children*, pp. 551–568. Elsevier, Oxford.

Kelly DA, Green A (1991) Investigation of paediatric liver disease. *J Inher Metab Dis* 14: 531–537.

Mowat AP (1994) *Liver Disorders in Childhood*, 4th edn. Butterworth, London.

Tanner S (1989) Paediatric hepatology. *Current Reviews in Paediatrics*, Vol. 4. Churchill Livingstone, London.

9

Neurology

S J Wallace

INTRODUCTION

After some consideration of the investigations themselves, a problem-orientated approach is taken. Further investigation of the child with a neurological complaint depends primarily on a full neurodevelopmental history. Physical examination is essential, likewise; but, without a good knowledge of the prior physical and cognitive development, it is usually impossible to determine whether investigation for a progressive disorder is appropriate. For most symptoms, clear definition of the accompanying neurological signs is essential if relevant tests are to be requested; and, in many cases, examination of other systems can be critical in guiding the investigator to the diagnosis. Sources of further information on the tests considered and disorders itemized are listed at the end of the chapter.

MODES OF INVESTIGATION

Some tests have age-dependent values. The two main areas involved are imaging and neurophysiology. There are also some biochemical investigations for which age is an important variable.

Imaging

Children with neurological disorders often have difficulty in keeping still enough for imaging of the central nervous system. Appropriate sedation or general anaesthesia is part of the preparation of the young or potentially uncooperative child for computerized tomography (CT) scanning or magnetic resonance imaging (MRI), both of which require complete immobility for 30 minutes or more.

Ultrasound Scanning (USS)

USS of the brain is possible only while the anterior fontanelle is at least 1 cm across; or it may be used during intracranial operations. Intracerebral haemorrhage, gross malformations or atrophy, enlargement of the ventricular system and intracerebral cysts can be identified.

CT Scanning

In the young infant's brain, as a result of incomplete myelination, the grey-white difference is not as marked as in adults. Thus cortical anomalies may be difficult to define. This problem resolves by about 3 months postnatally. In the first year of life, the temporal and frontal lobes often appear smaller than expected, giving an erroneous appearance of atrophy. CT can give information on acute trauma, haemorrhage, static cerebral lesions, gross malformation, cerebral atrophy, space-occupying lesions, hydrocephalus, tuberous sclerosis, cerebral abscess and vascular malformations. In association with myelography, examination of specific, localized areas of the spinal cord can be imaged using CT scanning.

Magnetic Resonance Imaging (MRI)

MRI gives pictures of greater sensitivity than USS or CT. Imaging depends on the different water contents of the various intracerebral structures, and secondarily on the maturation of myelination of the white matter. Myelination commences in the immature brain in the pons and medulla at about 12 weeks of prenatal life and is finally complete many years postnatally. Age-related references for MRI of the brain and spinal cord are necessary if interpretation of a young patient's imaging is to be correct. MRI is appropriately used for examination of the spinal cord; and, the brain, where tumours, degenerative disease, encephalitis, haemorrhage, vascular malformations, trauma, infarction, disorders of myelination or neuronal migration and enlargement of the ventricular system can be identified. Calcification is not shown by MRI.

Single Photon Emission Computerized Tomography (SPECT)

An isotope labelled tracer is injected, and gives images of regional cerebral blood flow allowing areas of hypo- or hyper-perfusion to be identified.

Positron Emission Tomography (PET)

Various substrates, including drugs, can be labelled with positron-emitters. In the brain, studies of local glucose and oxygen utilization, blood flow, protein synthesis and neurotransmitter uptake binding have been undertaken.

Angiography

The ability of MRI to define vascular lesions has largely superceded the need for angiography.

Myelography

Where MRI is available, it is the investigation of choice for spinal cord lesions; but, where there is considerable spinal deformity it may be easier to obtain an overall picture of the spinal cord with contrast myelography.

Miscellaneous

X-rays of the skull are now rarely performed, since CT can give better definition. Spinal X-rays still have a place as a first line investigation for congenital defects and acquired deformities. X-rays or other forms of imaging of areas other than the central nervous system can be crucial in directing the investigator to the diagnosis.

Neurophysiology

Electroencephalography (EEG)

Routine EEGs are from scalp electrodes only. Maturation of the EEG occurs throughout childhood, making it very important that request forms state the age of the child; and for premature infants, the gestation. EEGs recorded in infants of younger than 32 weeks gestation resemble, but are not identical to, the suppression-burst picture of severe cerebral dysfunction of older patients. More continuous activity is found as age increases; and from 36 to 40 weeks the EEG varies markedly with sleep states. On the whole, background rhythms are slower the younger the child, with frequencies of 3–4 Hz usual under 4 years, 4–7 Hz between 5 and 8 years, with α-rhythm at 8–12 Hz gradually becoming dominant after 9–10 years. The hallmark of an epileptic discharge is the spike. Sharp waves and other changes can be suggestive of epilepsy, but are not diagnostic. A slow wave focus should always be followed up by cerebral imaging. Sphenoidal, foramen ovale, and direct cortical recordings can give further information, but are the preserve of specialized centres.

With routine recording most information is gained during unsedated sleep, to include both REM and non-REM phases, in the neonate; and during the awake state with eyes open and eyes closed in older children. If sedation is required it is important not to use benzodiazepines, or other drugs which might significantly alter the EEG; droperidol is very useful for those who are overactive. Sleep EEGs and ambulatory monitoring, preferably with simultaneous video recording can add important additional information in equivocal or difficult cases.

Peripheral Nerve Studies

Measurement of conduction velocities (NCV) and the amplitudes of action potentials (AP) can be uncomfortable, but is not frankly painful. A small electrical stimulus is applied to the skin over a superficial peripheral nerve and the AP picked up at some distance, either distally or proximally, from the site of the stimulus, along the path of the same nerve. In infants and small children the distances involved are necessarily very short, making the margin of potential error greater. APs are of low voltage and NCVs slow in younger subjects with values approaching those of adults after the age of 3 years. Sedation should be avoided, since this may affect results.

Electromyography (EMG)

EMG is an invasive procedure and can be very uncomfortable. A bipolar needle is inserted into the muscle to be examined and muscle action potentials (MAP) recorded while the muscle is at rest, contracting maximally and contracting just sufficiently to produce single-fibre MAP. The MAP is of low amplitude in infants and young children. Comments on the findings during spontanous activity and maximal effort can be difficult when cooperation is less than ideal.

Evoked Potentials

All evoked potentials are generated by sensory stimuli.

Visual Evoked Potentials (VEP)

Responses to either repetitive flashes in younger children or pattern-reversal stimuli in those able to fixate are recorded by scalp electrodes placed over the occipital regions. Latencies of VEP depend on conduction of stimuli from the eye through the brain to the visual cortex, and thus can give valuable general, as well as specific information. They are normally longer in infants and young children; with gradual approach to adult values in the first 8 years. The form of the VEP and its amplitude is also age dependent.

Electroretinogram (ERG)

In childhood this is most easily measured by averaging the responses recorded by a surface electrode at the nasion to repeated light flashes. The normal ERG is well-formed at birth, but maturation proceeds through childhood to adult values at 11 years.

Brain-stem Auditory Evoked Potentials (BAEP)

BAEPs are measured as potential differences between the ear and vertex during a series of 60-dB clicks presented alternately to each ear. Maturation of the wave forms and latencies is complete at 2 years. Information on both brain-stem and auditory function is obtained.

Somatosensory Evoked Potentials (SEP)

Scalp recordings comparing contralateral parietal to ipsilateral frontal voltages are taken after stimulation of a peripheral, usually the median, nerve. Values are dependent on limb length as well as age. Measurement of cervical and cortical values as well as the central conduction time are possible; and SEPs are helpful in monitoring possible interference with long tracts during spinal operations.

Lumbar Puncture (LP)

LP can give information on cerebrospinal fluid (CSF) pressure, cellular content; microbiological and virological infection; and glucose, total and specific protein, lactate, pyruvate, amino acid, organic acid, succinyl purine and biogenic amine levels in the CSF. Before performing LP it is essential to consider which tests will be necessary and make certain with relevant laboratories how, and into which receptacles specimens should be collected.

LP should *not* be performed if intracranial or, intra-spinal space-occupying lesions including abscesses, brain swelling or obstructive hydrocephalus are suspected. Caution, and prior consultation with a neurosurgeon, should be exercised if a chronic meningitic process with possible secondary hydrocephalus could be present. Tonic attacks or opisthotonic posturing suggest hind brain herniation may be imminent and are an absolute contraindication.

Haematological Examination

In specific circumstances almost any aspect may be disturbed in association with diseases also affecting the nervous system. Evidence of infection, malignancy, vitamin deficiency, thrombosis or haemorrhage and storage disorders are the areas where examination of peripheral blood or marrow are most likely to be helpful.

Biochemical Tests

Investigations which demonstrate multisystem disease often assist in defining the cause of neurological problems. γ-Aminobutyric acid (GABA) in CSF and catecholamine exretion in urine are but two of the biochemical parameters that are age dependent. Magnetic resonance spectroscopy (MRS) allows non-invasive biochemical analysis of brain for specific inorganic and organic substances including phosphorus and N-acetylaspartate. MRS can monitor normal and abnormal cerebral biochemical development, but is likely to remain an investigative technique available only in limited centres for the foreseeable future. Toxicological studies can be relevant for both acute and chronic neurological problems.

Microbiology

Bacterial, viral, fungal and parasitic infections can all cause neurological disease. Culture of blood, urine, stool, swabs from the upper respiratory tract or skin lesions, or marrow can be as helpful as examination of the CSF. Antibody titres in serum, or, if appropriate, in CSF early in disease with subsequent convalescent levels, are more helpful than convalescent examination alone. Herpes virus encephalitis may be disagnosed early in the illness by identification of the specific DNA in CSF samples.

Immunology

When requesting immunological studies, the age-related values for serum immunoglobulins should be noted. If

CSF immunology is being examined, serum levels are also required.

Tissue Examination
Muscle Biopsy

It is usual, unless a specific muscle or muscle group is involved to biopsy the lateral quadriceps. Biopsy may be either open, usually under general anaesthesia, or performed by wide bore needle. USS can help to identify the site of maximal involvement. Muscle must be sent immediately to the laboratory, entirely fresh and unfixed, so that appropriate histochemical techniques and electron microscopy can be arranged, in addition to routine histology.

Peripheral Nerve

In a generalized peripheral neuropathy, the sural nerve is chosen. Prior consultation with the neuropathologist should ensure that handling of the nerve is optimal during removal and transportation. Biopsy of conjunctiva or skin, or in the neuronal ceroid lipofuscinoses, the rectum, may identify the characteristic intraneuronal changes of specific disorders.

Skin

Characteristic inclusions may be found in some degenerative disorders. Skin biopsy, with subsequent fibroblast culture can be important for further elucidation of lysosomal, peroxisomal and medium and long-chain fatty acid disorders. In addition fibroblasts may be frozen and used for enzyme estimation at a future date, should further examination appear indicated, particularly when a genetic condition is suspected.

Liver

Biopsy can be helpful in the confirmation of Wilson's disease.

Brain

Biopsy of the brain for progressive disease is rarely indicated, now that biochemical definition is likely to be possible. For generalized disorders, the frontal lobe is preferred.

Genetic Investigations

The most important of these is the family history. Routine chromosomal analysis may not identify impor-

tant causes of neurological dysfunction. It is usually necessary to request specifically for fragile X, deletions on chromosome 15 (Prader–Willi or Angelman's sydromes), etc., if these are suspected.

Specific examination of DNA is increasingly being used in both disease identification and prediction, whether prenatally or presymptomatically. Contact with a department of medical genetics may be necessary for up-dating. Blood, skin or chorionic villi are the tissues usually examined.

Cognitive Assessment

Standard measures of cognitive skills can be used both to give an indication of current ability and to monitor whether deterioration, developmental arrest or recovery of skills are occurring.

SYMPTOMS OR SIGNS REQUIRING INVESTIGATION
Alterations in Behaviour, Mood and Intellectual Status
Behavioural and Mood Changes

Important points in the history are shown in Figure 9.1. Children with situation-related non-stereotyped behavioural/mood changes are unlikely to have an underlying organic problem and further neurological investigation is not indicated if these are the only symptoms. Anxiety can provoke both cardiac and epileptic seizures. If the behavioural changes are stereotyped and consciousness is impaired and/or there are motor symptoms an EEG is indicated. If consciousness is unimpaired, at least initially, an ECG should be ordered.

Behavioural and mood changes which are non-situation related may be non-specifically secondary to illness, particularly pain, which a young or handicapped child cannot express; or to organic brain disorders. Full neurological and general physical examinations are indicated. Further investigation of overactive behaviour is usually unrewarding. Catastrophic rage outbursts suggest a temporal lobe abnormality – EEG and CT or MRI scanning are indicated. If consciousness is impaired there are three main possibilities: epileptic seizures, ingestion of toxic or pharmacologically active substances, and metabolic disturbance. Acute or subacute encephalitis, especially if due to herpes simplex or chronic measles infection can also present in this manner.

The EEG is the most helpful general investigation, recording spike or spike/wave discharges if an ictal trace

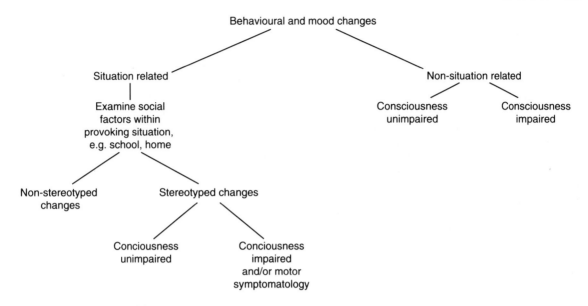

Figure 9.1   Behaviour and mood changes – assessment of history.

is obtained, but less reliably positive interictally; fast activity with barbiturates or benzodiazepines; and slow activity with many other drugs and with metabolic or infective disease. Full details of appropriate metabolic tests can be found in Chapter 4. Blood and urine should be sent for toxicological screening, or more specific tests if these can be identified. If an encephalitic illness is suspected the organism should be sought in blood, CSF, urine, stools and swabs of the upper respiratory tract; in particular, CSF should be examined for herpes DNA in addition to cells, protein, glucose and evidence of other infections.

Coma and Impaired Consciousness

Coma can be due to traumatic and non-traumatic causes. If secondary to trauma, either CT or MRI are indicated. Causes of non-traumatic coma are listed in Table 9.1. Additional points in the history are likely to be helpful in directing investigation. Prior headaches, vomiting and subacute loss of motor skills make a space-occupying

Table 9.1   Non-traumatic coma: causative groups

Metabolic
Infective
Toxic
Vascular
Post-ictal
Associated with raised intracranial pressure due to mass
lesion

lesion likely and CT/MRI would be the initial test. Sudden loss of consciousness with the abrupt onset of neurological signs is suggestive of a vascular cause: CT/MRI is indicated. A history of a prior epileptic seizure may be enough to cause coma, but failure to regain consciousness between seizures, particularly in an infant or young child, should raise the possibility that seizures are complications of metabolic or infective illness, or secondary to ingestion of a toxic agent. Non-convulsive status epilepticus can seriously impair consciousness, and is diagnosed on EEG. Medication given to control seizures may also impair awareness for some hours.

Metabolic causes of coma are dealt with in more detail in Chapter 4. As a minimum the following should be requested:

- Blood: urea, electrolytes including bicarbonate, glucose, lactate, arterial pH and gases, creatine kinase, ammonia, amino acids.
- Urine: organic acids, amino acids.
- CSF (provided LP is not contraindicated by suspected cerebral swelling): glucose, protein, amino acids, organic acids.

Out of routine laboratory hours, specimens should still be collected and frozen for future examination. Failure to obtain specimens for, in particular, glucose and organic acid estimation before therapeutic intervention may make diagnosis of a metabolic cause of acute neurological dysfunction very difficult.

Specimens for toxicological examination must also be obtained as soon as possible. Sedative drugs, antidepressants and analgesics are most likely to be causative. Solvents and other substances of abuse are further possibilities. A full history of therapy prescribed to parents, siblings and others in close contact can help to direct investigation. Samples of both blood and urine are essential. Examination of gastric contents may be relevant. Intracranial infection, regardless of the organism, is likely to be associated with impaired consciousness. In children who are obtunded and febrile the following are indicated: blood count; cultures for bacteria and viruses from blood, upper respiratory tract swabs, stools, urine, skin lesions; serum for viral titres (acute and convalescent); and CSF for microscopy (cells and organisms), culture for bacteria, glucose, total protein. If a viral illness is suspected, CSF culture and titres for viruses, and, in suspected herpes simplex infection, herpes DNA should be requested. Full investigation of immunological competence can be relevant. Acute metabolic derangement in children with underlying inborn errors may be precipitated by minor infections. It is often appropriate to investigate for both infective and metabolic disease.

Epileptic Seizures

The initial approach to the child with epileptic attacks is given in Figure 9.2. A complete witness account of the seizure is a highly desirable starting point. Identification of epileptic syndromes requires definition of the seizure type, neurological and cognitive assessment and EEG. For primary generalized tonic–clonic, typical absence and myoclonic absence seizures, and juvenile myoclonic epilepsy, EEG is the only investigation necessary. In addition, those presenting with simple partial seizures involving the face and oral structures, and whose EEG shows typical centrotemporal spikes, do not require neuroimaging. Otherwise, whenever seizures are partial, CT or MRI is essential. In temporal lobe epilepsy, specific views should be requested. Unclassified and secondarily generalized seizures can be secondary to a very wide variety of disorders, including those caused by acute or chronic metabolic, infective, toxic, malignant, degenerative or vascular diseases. Consideration of the general and specific disease histories should determine which line of investigation is likely to be fruitful. Causes of seizures in the neonate are given in Table 9.2; and of infantile spasms in Table 9.3. Intravenous pyridoxine given under EEG control can confirm pyridoxine dependency in the neonate. In both neonatal seizures and infantile spasms, but particularly with infantile spasms, clinical examination and early neuroimaging may obviate time-consuming and expensive metabolic studies. Examination for depigmented patches using a Wood's light facilitates an early diagnosis of tuberous sclerosis. Chromosomal analysis can be relevant. For example, Angelman's syndrome may present with early intractable epilepsy; epilepsy is much commoner in children with abnormal complements of sex chromosomes than in the general population; and many other children with learning difficulties and epilepsy have definable chromosomal abnormalities. The causes of the Lennox Gastaut syndrome are similar to those of infantile spasms. When persisting focal seizures are a problem, very careful MRI, SPECT, or preferably PET, may be necessary for definition of localized lesions which might be amenable to surgery.

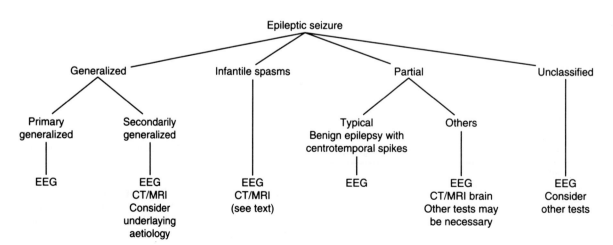

Figure 9.2   Epileptic seizures – clinical assessment.

Table 9.2 Causes of neonatal seizures

Before birth
Genetic – benign familial neonatal convulsions
Cerebral dysmorphism
Prenatal vascular occlusion leading to porencephalic cysts
Prenatal infection: toxoplasmosis, cytomegalovirus, other viral infections
Maternal drug ingestion
Pyridoxine dependency

During birth
Hypoxic-ischaemic encephalopathy

Intracranial haemorrhage

Birth trauma

After birth
Perinatal infection – bacterial, viral

Local anaesthetic intoxication

Temporary metabolic disturbance – hypoglycaemia, hypocalcaemia, hypomagnesaemia

Inborn errors of metabolism:
Pyridoxine dependency

Hyperammonaemia/urea cycle disorders

Amino acid disorders including non-ketotic hyperglycinaemia, maple syrup urine disease, etc.

Organic acidurias

Pyruvate dehydrogenase deficiency

Sulphite oxidase deficiency – molybdenum cofactor deficiency

Peroxisomal disorders – Zellweger's disease

Table 9.3 Causes of infantile spasms

Neurocutaneous disorders – tuberous sclerosis

Cerebral dysmorphism, including:
Aicardi syndrome
Immature dendritic development
Hydranencephaly
Down syndrome
Miller–Dieker syndrome (characteristic facies, digital and retinal abnormalities)

Pre- and post-natal vascular and ischaemic events

Postinfective:
Bacterial meningitis
Viral encephalitis

Metabolic disorders:
Abnormal amino acids
Organic acidurias
Lysosomal enzyme dysfunction
Any metabolic condition giving rise to gross generalized brain disturbance

Table 9.4 Progressive myoclonic epilepsy: principal causes

Metabolic
Non-ketotic hyperglycinaemia
Branched-chain amino acid disorders
Biopterin deficiency
D-Glyceric aciduria
Hexosaminidase deficiencies
Sialidoses (types I and II)
Juvenile Gaucher's disease (type III)
GM_1 gangliosidosis
Niemann–Pick C disease
Mitochondrial cytopathies (especially MERFF and MELAS)
Molybdenum cofactor deficiency
Menkes disease

Degenerative, metabolic cause undetermined
Ceroid lipofuscinoses
Juvenile neuroaxonal dystrophy
Alpers disease
Hallervorden–Spatz disease

Specific myoclonic syndromes
Ramsey–Hunt syndrome
Baltic/Mediterranean myoclonus epilepsy
Lafora body disease

MELAS, myoclonic epilepsy, lactic acidosis, stroke; MERFF, myoclonic epilepsy with ragged red fibres.
Adapted from Aicardi (1992).

With the exceptions of benign myoclonic epilepsy in infants, myoclonic–astatic epilepsy and juvenile myoclonic epilepsy, myoclonic seizures are usually indicative of severe brain disorder which is likely to be progressive. Possible aetiologies are listed in Table 9.4. Depending on the concomitant clinical picture, serum and urinary amino acids, urinary organic acids, lysosomal enzymes, lactate, pH and gases, serum uric acid, urinary sulphite excretion, serum copper and caeruloplasmin, EEG, VEP, ERG, rectal, skin, conjunctival, muscle or brain biopsy could be appropriate. Baltic/Mediterranean myoclonus is identifiable by DNA analysis.

Estimation of blood antiepileptic drug (AED) levels is indicated if a patient on treatment goes into status epilepticus. Routine monitoring is required only for phenytoin. Levels of other AED should only be measured if intoxication or non-compliance is suspected. The effects of valproate and vigabatrin are not related to plasma levels.

EEGs do not give useful information in children presenting with febrile seizures, and are unnecessary.

Global or specific learning difficulties should be recognized and fully assessed.

Non-epileptic Seizures

Breath-holding spells, reflex anoxic seizures, benign paroxysmal vertigo, benign paroxysmal torticollis, stimulus-bound myoclonus, cataplexy and vasovagal attacks are diagnosed on the basis of the history and further investigation is not indicated. Cardiac dysrhythmias such as the prolonged Q–T syndrome can be confused with epilepsy, if suspected, an ECG with specific attention to rhythm is indicated.

Pseudo-epileptic seizures are part of the spectrum of conversion disorders, and most often simulate generalized tonic–clonic attacks. Ambulatory EEG during the attack and serum prolactin within 2 h will distinguish major seizures from pseudoepileptic ones. Partial seizures are not always identifiable by the limited montages available on monitors and may not cause a rise in the prolactin level.

Headache

Factors in the history and examination, useful in guiding investigation are given in Table 9.5. Most headaches are

Table 9.5   Headache

Characteristics	Investigation
Continuous, unvarying during waking hours, no vomiting, no physical signs	Full history of family, school and social circumstances
Associated with upper respiratory or other infections and fever	Tests appropriate for infections
Paroxysmal, lateralized, visual symptomatology, vomiting, various sensory/motor symptoms	Neuro imaging *only* if: (a) *no* family history of migraine; (b) sensory or motor symptomatology; (c) persisting physical signs
Early morning, or after daytime recumbancy; associated vomiting; worse on coughing, straining; with/without motor symptoms	Neuroimaging urgent; do *not* LP
Accentuated by exercise, no signs raised intracranial pressure	Check blood pressure; consider metabolic problem
Associated with alteration in consciousness or confusion	EEG; toxicological screen; metabolic studies

not due to significant organic disease, but nevertheless cause great parental concern. Headaches are common symptoms in conversion disorders, but when otherwise non-organic are most likely to be secondary to stressful circumstances at home or school. Usually a close family member acts as a role model. Migraine can present in young children, but a confident diagnosis is possible only in those with classical symptomatology and a positive family history. Cluster headaches also occur. Early morning headaches with accompanying effortless vomiting readily suggest raised intracranial pressure, but some children with space-occupying lesions have additional headaches throughout the day. Irritability, anorexia, associated changes in motor ability and torticollis are some of the additonal features which indicate urgent CT/MRI is needed. Metabolic problems particularly likely to cause headache are those secondary to mitochondrial disease or partial defects of the urea cycle: creatine kinase, lactate and ammonia levels at rest and on exercise are indicated. Toxicological screening in blood and urine should be at the time of symptoms. Severe headache can follow epileptic seizures, particularly in benign epilepsy with occipital paroxysms.

Alterations in Special Senses

Investigation of disorders primarily of sight and hearing are dealt with fully in Chapters 16 and 17. However, visual and auditory disturbances may be the first symptoms of more generalized neurological problems. Investigations relevant to conditions in which acquired loss or alteration of vision is an early feature are given in Table 9.6. Often a combination of tests will be helpful. In particular, the reduced ERG, accentuated VEP and abnormalities on EEG can be highly suggestive of late infantile lipofuscinosis, which may be confirmed by rectal biopsy.

Acquired hearing loss, as part of a generalized neurological problem is most commonly reported in peroxisomal abnormality, diagnosed on estimation of very long chain fatty acids in blood; or, in mitochondrial cytopathy, when estimations of blood, and possibly cerebrospinal fluid, lactate and pyruvate levels, supplemented by muscle biopsy, searching for ragged red fibres and abnormal mitochondria, are appropriate. "Loss" of vision or hearing can be symptomatic of conversion disorders. Evoked potentials can be helpful in investigation of these problems.

Abnormal Movements

Involuntary movements are considered in this section. It is essential that the movements are characterized cor-

Table 9.6 Investigation when acquired alteration of vision is part of neurological disorder

Investigations	Disorders
Metabolic	
Lysosomal enzyme screen	Lysosomal storage
Very-long chain fatty acids	disorders
Cobalamin screen	Peroxisomal disorders
Lactate, pyruvate	Lebers optic atrophy
Lipoproteins	Mitochondrial dysfunction
	A-β-lipoproteinaemia
Imaging	
Optic nerves: MRI	Optic nerve glioma in
Brain: CT or MRI	neurofibromatosis I
	Any condition affecting
	optic tracts and occipital
	lobes
Neurophysiology	
ERG	Peroxisomal disorders
	A-β-Lipoproteinaemia
	Lipofuscinoses
	Mitochondrial cytopathy
	Hallervorden–Spatz
	disease
VEP	Optic neuritis
	Multiple sclerosis
	Leukodystrophies
	Lipofuscinoses
EEG	Any condition affecting
	occipital cortex
	Generalized cerebral
	dysfunction
	Lipofuscinoses

rectly. All children with acquired chorea, athetosis, dystonia or myoclonus should have neuro imaging, preferably MRI. Causes of calcification demonstrable on CT or lucency shown by CT or MRI in the basal ganglia are extensively reviewed by Aicardi (1992). Those conditions for which other investigations complement CT or MRI are listed in Table 9.7. The diagnosis of Segawa syndrome may be made in children with dystonia, usually with marked diurnal variation, by giving a trial of small doses of L-dopa. Attention to physical signs other than disturbed movement will help to indicate which tests are the most relevant.

Likewise, acquired cerebellar ataxia should always be investigated by neuro imaging, preferably MRI. Other relevant investigations are summarized in Table 9.8. Only those conditions for which a positive test is found are listed. Other disorders with associated cerebellar ataxia are described in Harding (1984), Brett (1991) and Aicardi (1992).

A confident diagnosis of tic or habit spasm does not require further investigation.

Abnormal Gait

Abnormality of gait may be secondary to spasticity, involuntary movements, weakness or a conversion disorder. Causes of involuntary/abnormal quality of movement are considered in the previous section. Pathology of the pyramidal tract results in spasticity. Neuroimaging is the major investigation, as follows: upper and lower limbs involved with an upper motor neurone facial weakness – CT/MRI of the brain; no cranial nerve abnormality, upper and lower limb spasticity – MRI of the upper cervical cord; spasticity at lower levels – MRI of the spinal cord at the level identified by the clinical findings. Many hereditary disorders with prominent spasticity are diagnosed by the cluster of physical signs, rather than specific investigations, but lysosomal storage diseases should also be considered. Nicotinamide–adenine dinucleotide oxidoreductase is deficient in skin and leucocytes in Sjögren–Larsson syndrome.

Weakness associated with hypotonia may be due to a recent-onset upper motor neurone lesion; but, if chronic,

Table 9.7 Investigation of involuntary movements associated with midbrain pathology

Disorder	Predominant movement abnormality	Investigation
Sydenham's chorea	Chorea	ASO titre
Huntington's chorea	Rigidity (in childhood)	DNA
Postencephalitic abnormality	Chorea, dystonia	Viral tests
Multiple sclerosis	Variable	MRI brain VEP CSF oligoclonal bands
Systemic lupus erythematosis	Chorea	LE cells Autoimmune investigation

Table 9.7   *continued*

Disorder	Predominant movement abnormality	Investigation
Moya-moya disease	Chorea	MR vascular imaging Angiography
Glutaric aciduria type I	Chorea, dystonia	Glutaric acid in urine, glutaryl Co A dehydrogenase in lymphocytes, fibroblasts or liver
Choreoacanthocytosis	Chorea	Blood film for acanthocytes
Leigh's disease	Chorea, jerky eye movements, dystonia	Lactate in serum and CSF. MRI. Respiratory chain enzymes, biotinidase
Mitochondrial cytopathy	Chorea, dystonia, myoclonus	Lactate in serum and CSF Muscle biopsy
Drug-induced	Chorea, athetosis, dystonia	Toxicological screen
Tumours of basal ganglia	Dystonia, chorea, athetosis (unilateral)	CT/MRI
Wilsons disease	Dystonia	Serum copper and caeruloplasmin. Urinary copper. (Liver biopsy)
Gangliosidoses	Dystonia	Hexosaminidases, beta-galactosidase
Segawa syndrome	Dystonia ($\pm$ diurnal variation)	Trial of L-Dopa
Metachromatic leukodystrophy	Dystonia	Arylsulphatase A
Lipofuscinoses	Dystonia, myoclonus	VEP, ERG, EEG, rectal biopsy
Lesch–Nyhan syndrome	Dystonia, athetosis	Uric acid. Hypoxanthine–guanine phosphoribosyl transferase in blood or skin fibroblasts
Homocystinuria	Dystonia	Homocystine in urine. Cystathionine β-synthase in lymphocytes, fibroblasts
D-Glyceric acidaemia	Dystonia	Urinary D-glyceric acid. Fructose loading test
Sulphite oxidase deficiency	Dystonia	Serum uric acid, sulphite in urine, sulphite oxidase and molybdenum cofactor in lymphocytes and fibroblasts
Ataxia-telangectasia	Dystonia	Serum α-fetoprotein and carcinoembryonic antigen. Chromosomes
Neuraxonal dystrophy	Dystonia	Conjunctival or skin biopsy
Myoclonic encephalopathy	Myoclonus, dancing eyes	Urinary catecholamines, VMA. EEG. CT body scan
Epilepsies with myoclonic component	Myoclonus	EEG (see Table 9.4)
Neuraminidase deficiency	Myoclonus	Neuraminidase in lymphocytes
Subacute sclerosing panencephalitis	Myoclonus, spasms	Serum, CSF measles titres, EEG

Table 9.8 Investigation of cerebellar ataxia

Investigation	Disorder
Neuroimaging:	
CT/MRI	Cerebellar: tumour congenital malformations degeneration infarct abscess contusion
Toxicological:	
Benzodiazepines, antiepileptic drugs, antihistamines	Self-administration or child abuse (or wrong prescription)
Bacteriological/viral:	
Varicella. Epstein–Barr virus, enteroviruses, etc., mycoplasma	Parainfectious, cerebellar disorder
Neurophysiology:	
EEG	Non-convulsive status epilepticus, encephalitis
NCV	Ataxia with associated neuropathy
ERG, VEP, EEG	Ceroid lipofuscinoses
Metabolic:	
Very long chain fatty acids	Adrenomyeloneuropathy
Lipoproteins	A-β-lipoproteinaemia
Vitamin E	Vitamin E deficiency in chronic hepatic disease, etc.
Lysosomal enzymes	Lysosomal storage disorders, especially gangliosidoses
Lactate in blood and CSF, muscle biopsy	Mitochondrial disorders
Immunological:	
Immunoglobulins (immune screen): in blood, in CSF.	Infections, ataxia telangectasia, autoimmune disorders
Oligoclonal bands CSF	Multiple sclerosis
Miscellaneous:	
α-Fetoprotein	Ataxia telangectasia
Chromosomes: breakages,	Ataxia telangectasia
microdeletion 15	Angelman syndrome

Table 9.9 Preliminary analysis of weakness

Presentation	Probable location
Sudden, catastrophic	Brain, spinal cord
Subacute (hours, days): With UMN signs (brisk reflexes)	Brain, spinal cord
Mixed UMN + LMN signs	Spinal cord
LMN signs (absent or reduced tendon reflexes)	Anterior horn cell, peripheral nerve
Primary muscle problem (tendon reflexes retained)	Muscle
Variable, exercise related	Neuromuscular junction, muscle
Gradually progressive	Comparable to subacute (above) but much more slowly evolving picture
Chronic, stable or very slowly progressive	Mixed UMN + LMN signs suggest separate involvements

LMN, lower motor neurone; UMN, upper motor neurone.

Table 9.10 Investigation of lower motor neurone disease

Location of problem	Investigation
Intraspinal:	
Cauda equina	MRI spine
Anterior horn cell:	
Acute:	Virology LP
Chronic (spinal muscular atrophies)	NCV EMG Muscle biopsy DNA
Peripheral nerve:	
Acute	LP NCV Virology Toxicology
Chronic (with CNS signs)	NCV EMG Toxicology Nerve biopsy Lysosomal enzymes Very long chain fatty acids
Neuromuscular junction:	Edrophonium test Acetylcholine receptor antibodies (EMG with tetanic stimulation)

is more likely to be secondary to disorders either peripheral nerve or muscle. Investigation of weakness starts with identification of the most likely anatomical site or sites as in Table 9.9. Once localized to peripheral nerve or muscle, further investigation is itemized in Tables 9.10 and 9.11. Chronic hereditary peripheral

Table 9.11   Investigation of muscle disease

Categories	Investigations
All	Creatine kinase Chest X-ray ECG EMG Muscle biopsy
Limb-girdle weakness	DNA Dystrophin in muscle
Metabolic/ mitochondrial disorder suspected	Blood and CSF lactate Urinary organic acids Specific metabolic investigation of muscle (e.g. carnitine, α-glucosidase, mitochondrial enzymes, etc.) Urinary myoglobin
Inflammatory	ESR Virology, especially Coxsackie Urinary myoglobin
Autoimmune	ESR Autoantibodies Immune screen
Toxic	Drugs especially in relation to predisposition to malignant hyperthermia

neuropathies are usually categorized by the accompanying physical signs. Nearly all neonatal, early childhood or more chronic muscle diseases require biopsy for definitive diagnosis; but dermatomyositis and toxic and inflammatory myopathies can be recognized by accompanying symptomatology and signs. Confirmation of predisposition to malignant hyperthermia needs specific immediate examination of muscle and is available only in highly specialized centres.

Conversion disorders often mimic gait abnormalities. Inconsistencies between physical signs and function are suggestive. Observation of inappropriate simultaneous isotonic contraction of both agonist and antagonist muscles; holding the hand over the face and releasing it (the hand is likely to miss the face); and sensory mapping, revealing failure to keep to anatomically acceptable borders, are highly indicative of a conversion disorder.

Stiff Neck

Acquired torticollis or neck stiffness, with associated irritability but without systemic illness, are suggestive of expanding lesions in the posterior cranial fossa or cervical spine. Urgent CT/MRI is indicated. Neck stiffness with fever and obtunded awareness suggest infective menin-

gitis, for which full details of investigation are available in Chapter 12. Non-infective meningitis can be secondary to malignant disease, sarcoidosis, Behçet's syndrome, autoimmune arteritis, Kawasaki disease and multiple sclerosis. Appropriate tests for these conditions could be indicated.

Stroke

A sudden unilateral hemiparesis is most likely to be due to a primary vascular occlusion or rupture. Investigation is by CT with contrast enhancement, MR vascular imaging or angiography. Angiography is reserved for cases where surgical intervention might be relevant, or to confirm Moya-moya disease. Exclusion of a cardiac source of embolus is indicated. Clotting and infection screens, including toxoplasmosis titres should be performed if there is no vascular malformation demonstrable. Tests for autoimmune arteritis can be relevant.

Incontinence

Dribbling incontinence suggests a lower spinal cord or cauda equina lesion. MRI is indicated. Retention with overflow suggests a higher lesion; MRI is needed, with the level to be examined determined by additional localizing signs. Incontinence can be symptomatic of generalized disorders associated with polyuria; difficulties with mobilization, making visits to the toilet too much trouble; dementia; brief non-convulsive seizures; and behaviour difficulties. Investigation along one of these lines could be indicated. Examination of renal and bladder and/or bowel function should not be ignored.

Large Head

Large heads may be familial or secondary to pathological problems. Measurement of occipitofrontal circumferences (OFC) in parents and siblings gives norms. If the OFC is growing excessively in infancy, USS may be sufficient to demonstrate ventricular enlargement. Where the fontanelle is closed, or clearer definition is required, CT/MRI is indicated. Poor developmental progress or developmental regression with a large OFC and no evidence of obstructive hydrocephalus can be due to Canavan disease (test urinary N-acetylaspartate and fibroblast aspartoacylase); Alexander disease (no diagnostic test); or a variety of disorders associated with organic aciduria. Young children presenting with intracranial space-occupying lesions demonstrable by neuroimaging often have large OFC.

Dysmorphism with Neurological and/or Cognitive Problems

Two main lines of investigation are appropriate. Miller–Dieker, Angelman and fragile X syndromes are but a few of the conditions where there is presentation of a chromosomal disorder with neurological or cognitive symptomatology. Cytogenetic analysis is indicated whenever external malformations accompany neurological and cognitive problems.

Characteristic dysmorphic features can point to appropriate biochemical tests in the mucopolysaccharidoses, sialodoses, gangliosidoses, peroxisomal disorders, pyruvate dehydrogenase complex deficiencies, carbohydrate deficient glycoprotein syndrome, Menkes disease and many other disorders itemized in the age-related diagnosis (ARD) index (1993).

Dementia

Loss of cognitive skills can be the initial symptom of more pervasive neurological disease. Slow viral infection, particularly with measles, should be considered. Dementia with myoclonic jerks is investigated by EEG and blood and CSF measles titres. Other viral tests and brain biopsy may be indicated, rarely.

Non-convulsive status epilepticus, confirmed by EEG, can produce reversible dementia.

Juvenile or adult onset of lysosomal storage disorders is often with cognitive loss, rather than physical disability. Lysosomal enzyme estimations are indicated when dementia presents in childhood or in early or mid-adulthood.

CONCLUSIONS

Neurological and cognitive symptomatology is most often just part of a more generalized disorder. Full examination of all systems, and localization of the part of the nervous system involved are important prerequisites before investigation is planned. When requesting a test, the child's age and as full a physical description as possible should be given to the laboratory.

REFERENCES

Aicardi J (1992) *Diseases of the Nervous System in Childhood*. Mac-Keith Press, London.

Barnes PD (1992) Imaging of the central nervous system in pediatrics and adolescence. *Pediatr Clin N Am* 39: 743–775.

Baumann N, Federico A, Suzuki K (eds) (1991) Late onset neurometabolic genetic disorders. *Dev Neurosci* 13(4–5): 185–376.

Brett EM (1991) *Paediatric Neurology*. Churchill Livingstone, Edinburgh.

Chugani HT (1993) The application of PET and SPECT imaging in pediatric neurology. In: Fejerman N, Chamoles NA (eds) *New Trends in Pediatric Neurology*, pp. 13–21. Elsevier, Amsterdam.

Editorial (1991) Neurological conversion disorders in childhood. *Lancet* 337: 889–890.

Harding AE (1984) *The Hereditary Ataxias and Related Disorders*. Churchill Livingstone, Edinburgh.

Harkness RA, Harkness EJ (1993) Introduction to the age-related diagnosis index (ARD): an age at presentation related index for diagnostic use. *J Inher Metab Dis* 16: 161–170.

Roger J, Bureau M, Dravet C, Dreifuss FE, Perret A, Wolf P (eds) (1992) *Epileptic Syndromes in Infancy, Childhood and Adolescence*, 2nd edn. John Libbey, London.

Steinberg A, Frank Y (eds) (1993) *Neurological Manifestations of Systemic Diseases in Children*. Raven Press, New York.

Stephenson JBP, King MD (1992) *Handbook of Neurological Investigations in Children*. Butterworth, London.

10

Development

I McKinlay

INTRODUCTION

The purpose of this chapter is to describe the investigations of developmental delay and disorders and their associated impairments, with reference to other chapters where appropriate. The principal developmental delays or disorders affect movement, language, vision, hearing, cognitive function, including educational attainments and/or social behaviour. Delay may be transient, often familial, phenomena or may be persistent. It may be global or specific. Disorders from the same condition may be isolated or multiple. In each section, clinical examination is discussed and medical tests are considered. There is also discussion of medical investigations which assist in decisions about treatment.

MOVEMENT

Feeding Difficulties

It is not unusual for the first indication of developmental delay or disorder to declare itself in the neonatal period. Feeding difficulties may require tube-feeding and a number of specific conditions should be considered in consequence. Examine the mother for signs of myotonic dystrophy. Large head circumference in the infant may suggest Soto syndrome. Short babies may turn out to have Prader–Willi syndrome for which chromosome investigation, especially chromosome 15, is indicated. Other short children with feeding difficulty include those with Turner syndrome (chromosomes XO) or Noonan syndrome. Extreme hypotonia and feeding difficulties are early signs of Down syndrome or spinal muscular atrophy in which fasciculation of the tongue is seen. Some children who have experienced perinatal asphyxia have feeding difficulty as a consequence – this is one of the common features of "symptomatic asphyxia". It may be of such a degree as to require tube feeding. Often an ultrasound scan will show some degree of abnormality – either signs

of brain swelling or multifocal areas of abnormal density. These may resolve spontaneously or with treatment and the feeding pattern may improve or remit.

Feeding problems in the early months of infancy may lead to failure to thrive. This may be due to insufficient feeding through maternal inexperience, illness or depression, lack of organization and relaxation or due to oral motor dysfunction in the baby. There may be problems with sucking, swallowing, oral sensitivity (high or low) or recurrent aspiration.

It is appropriate to think of medical causes of failure to thrive e.g. congenital heart disease, malabsorbtion, renal failure, hypothyroidism, pulmonary insufficiency or chronic infection. These should be considered at the same time as social enquiry and observation of feeding. It is helpful for hospital doctors to discuss the child's home circumstances and feeding behaviour with someone (e.g. a nurse) who has observed these at first hand before committing the child to uncomfortable and expensive investigations unless clinical signs indicate a clear physical cause. Speech therapists make helpful observations of feeding behaviour and may be able to make practical suggestions as to how to improve the process. Sometimes a video recording of feeding may allow multidisciplinary discussion.

Among causes of early infant feeding problems presenting after the neonatal period are cerebral palsy (look for other motor signs), oral motor dyspraxia (sometimes in small for dates babies, also seen with fragile X), fetal alcohol syndrome (look for the other stigmata and obtain a maternal alcohol consumption history), and submucous cleft palate (nasal regurgitation, grooved or bifid uvula, notched hard palate).

When there are clear physical difficulties in the feeding process the first steps are advice about head and seating positions, food texture and oral sensitivity. Video-fluoroscopy with collaboration between an experienced paediatric radiologist and a speech therapist can be most helpful in locating and quantifying the problem. If repeated aspiration occurs and food or liquids pool in the pharynx in a dangerous way, gastrostomy should be considered and discussed with the parents.

If children are distressed after meal times and/or vomit or regurgitate more than usual, some degree of gastro-oesophageal reflux may be responsible. A full barium meal procedure will be helpful. This is sometimes preceded by oesophageal pH studies though their validity and reliability are questioned. If a gastrostomy is being planned, a barium meal with some inversion during the study will demonstrate whether there is any reflux. This will determine whether or not a fundoplication procedure is needed at the same time to avoid deterioration after surgery for gastrostomy.

Another cause of distress in infants during or soon after eating is constipation. The meal stimulates peristalsis which turns into inspissated faecal material and colonic gas. Clinical examination will indicate hard faeces in the colon/rectum and treatment for this will make the child more comfortable. Only if the problem is persistent or recurrent is radiological or histological investigation needed (see Chapter 7).

Delayed Motor Development

There is a wide range of normal development but concern may be expressed if a child is not sitting by a year or walking by 18 months. A number of factors should be considered. The general level of the child's development may indicate a specific motor delay or global delay. If the latter applies, investigation for the cause of learning disability may be appropriate, although there should be enquiry into the general level of care and possible neglect. If failure to thrive or recurrent injuries have been found there are grounds for considering social causes for delay. Boys are more at risk of delay than girls. Breech presentation carries a greater risk of motor delay (and cerebral palsy), irrespective of method of delivery suggesting pre-natal fetal factors. Difficulties with eyesight are considered in Chapter 17. These are associated with delayed motor development which is transient but will profit from physiotherapy advice.

When the motor delay is specific, then observation of poverty of movement, abnormal tone, stereotyped postures or abnormal movement suggest cerebral palsy. More commonly the child will be found to have normal movements and lax muscle tone. A family history of delayed motor development, bottom shuffling, creeping, rolling or walking without having crawled will indicate a benign normal variation with a good prognosis. That history may not be available at once. Parents may have to consult their families, especially when the child concerned is the firstborn.

For boys with delayed motor (or language) development with no family history of benign hypotonia, Duchenne muscular dystrophy should be considered because of genetic implications for future children. A family history of muscular dystrophy may be elicited but more commonly there is none because the gene mutation has occurred in the mother or in the affected boy. A serum creatine kinase is the simplest diagnostic test. If there is any question of a recent fall with muscle injury or a recent intramuscular injection the creatine kinase may be raised transiently and the test should be repeated. In future more emphasis will be placed on specific gene probes. Boys with Duchenne dystrophy are not able to run or jump and proximal weakness can be demonstrated by asking the child to stand unassisted from a supine lying position and observing the boy rolling to a prone position then pushing up by stages with the hands on the floor then the legs (Gower's sign). Climbing steps is difficult for them.

Dyspraxia and Clumsiness

One or two children in a hundred show difficulties with co-ordination as they grow up without a specific cause. There may be associated moderate learning difficulty or epilepsy, there may be a history of extremely low birthweight or intra-uterine growth retardation, including the effects of heavy maternal smoking, drug addiction of fetal alcohol syndrome. More commonly there is no relevant history. One or both parents may have been unathletic or poor at handwriting. When the difficulty is with complex movements or sequences of movements the child may be described as showing dyspraxia – an organizational difficulty without other specific neurological signs. There may be general clumsiness or poor balance. Visual impairment such as short-sightedness should be checked for. There may also be immaturity in visual or kinaesthetic perception. Assessment by a clinical psychologist will clarify this in the school child. A history of early feeding problems and/or speech difficuties (expressive language and articulation problems) is common and a speech therapy assessment for such children is valuable.

Population based studies indicate a 50% excess of boys with motor learning difficulty. However, clinic based studies show a four-fold male excess. The explanation is that it is common for motor problems to be associated with anxiety. Girls are more likely to respond by withdrawal whereas boys tend to be more demanding and difficult. Psychological help with the associated emotional features may be more beneficial than specific physical remediation. Often it is behaviour problems which have led to referral. However, therapy advice is appropriate when the child wants help to learn specific tasks. Full co-operation with teachers is essential, especially in relation to handwriting and physical education.

Although medical investigations are unrewarding in general, a neurological examination by the general practitioner, school doctor or paediatrician is helpful. Occasionally children with clumsiness show early signs of a degenerative neuromuscular disorder, e.g. Friedreich's ataxia. They show abnormal reflexes when the condition is still at an early stage. If these are diminished or absent referral to a neurologist and nerve conduction studies are indicated.

Cerebral Palsies

Reference has been made to children with abnormal signs in the neonatal period following clinical asphyxia – so-called symptomatic asphyxia. Many of these children show abnormal muscle (hypotonia and hypertonia) and feeding difficulties. However, three-quarters of them will outgrow their motor abnormalities and will not turn out to have cerebral palsy.

Likewise, it is common for premature babies to go through a phase of increased muscle tone around the time of 40 weeks postconceptional age: the dystonia of prematurity. Though such infants feel stiff and are hard to handle, nine-tenths of them grow out of this without cerebral palsy. Nonetheless, as more extremely low birthweight premature babies survive there has been an increase in incidence of cerebral palsy, especially spastic quadriparesis associated with cortical visual impairment and learning disability, of about 2 babies per 10 000 live births in the last decade (Nicholson and Alberman 1992). These extremely premature infants have abnormal ultrasound brain scans in the perinatal period with extensive signs of periventricular leukoencephalopathy and show abnormalities which persist on CT scan in later infancy and childhood. However, most premature children with abnormal brain scans, especially milder abnormalities, grow up with normal motor development. Prognosis should be cautious with regular review.

Most children with cerebral palsies have normal birthweights and no significant perinatal illness. Their disorder may be symmetrical or asymmetrical and it is usual for detection to occur in the second part of the first year unless it is very severe or associated with other signs, e.g. microcephaly. Most early postural movements occur at a subcortical level. It is only when cortically controlled activities such as reaching, grasping and manipulating begin that the abnormal signs become clear.

The signs of cerebral palsies are diverse. Feeding difficulties, sometimes associated with drooling have been referred to. Children with spastic cerebral palsies show poverty of movement, stereotyped postures and increased tone, sometimes following a period of hypotonia. The increased tone becomes evident distally before proximal signs evolve – persistent plantigrade posture of the feet and fisting of the hand(s). In severe forms of spastic quadriparesis increased adductor tone ("scissoring" of the legs) evolves in the early months but in less severe forms it develops later.

Children who later show ataxia or athetoid cerebral palsies are often hypotonic throughout the early months of life, even into the second year, before more specific signs appear. Usually ataxia affects truncal posture more than causing the dysmetric features associated with acquired ataxia. In athetoid children difficulties with conjugate eye movements have been seen before limb dyskinesia is evident. The child may have such difficulty with gaze as to be thought to have visual impairment in early life.

The timing of investigations depends on the confidence of the clinician in the abnormal signs elicited. Most children thought to have cerebral palsy at 12 months grow out of their motor abnormalities, though many turn out to have learning difficulty later (Nelson and Ellenberg 1982). Another consideration is the pressure of time for genetic counselling. If the parents are anxious to add to their family quickly there is greater need to consider early investigation than when there is time to see how the presenting child turns out (Hughes and Newton 1992).

The commonest causes of severe spastic quadriparesis with microcephaly are periventricular leukoencephalopathy and congenital cytomegalovirus infection, although congenital rubella and syphilis should not be forgotten. In some places congenital human immunodeficiency virus infection is of increasing importance as a cause. CT scans often show characteristic abnormalities. Blood and urine samples for virological testing are also indicated.

Children with a congenital spastic hemiparesis usually show a CT scan abnormality, most commonly infarction and brain reabsorbtion in anterior or middle cerebral artery territory or both. Other lesions include a porencephalic cyst, subdural haematoma, cerebral malformation, large ventricle or small hemisphere. Occasionally a cerebral tumour is found.

In children with ataxic cerebral palsy the CT scan may show underdevelopment of the cerebellum, especially midline structures. Athetoid children may show abnormalites of the basal ganglia.

It is exceptional for the CT scan to show evidence of pathology which influences treatment. Sometimes the scan is normal. The main benefits of the scan are in counselling parents and in clarifying genetic implications. When acquired pathology is present, especially when this is asymmetrical, or when there is a developmental brain abnormality, the genetic recurrence risk is low. There may be increased recurrence risk through premature delivery which requires advice in its own right. When cerebral palsies are symmetrical and the scan shows symmetrical under development, or is normal, the recurrence risk is high – between 1 : 8 and 1 : 10. Unfortunately we lack genetic markers for antenatal testing.

Children with cerebral palsies have a high risk for associated conditions and these should be checked for. Vision may be affected through refractive errors, retinal or cortical pathology. Hearing may be affected through associated sensorineural loss, cortical pathology or conductive loss with chronic secretory otitis media. One-third of children with cerebral palsies develop epilepsy, especially those with hemiparesis or acquired asymmetrical spastic quadriparesis. Electroencephalography is indicated as the presence of abnormalities implies higher risk of the development of epilepsy, albeit the relationship is not precise. Although parents are concerned to learn about the risk of epilepsy and this may increase the anxiety in their attachment to their child, they prefer to know about it. When parents have not been prepared and the child develops seizures they may be devastated and think that the child has died. In addition they may not understand what is going on when the child has a seizure and this may delay obtaining help. They may gain some confidence from the advice that the longer the child continues to be seizure-free, the better the prospects are of remaining so.

Musculoskeletal abnormalities evolve in many children with cerebral palsies, especially those with spasticity. The most important are the risks of hip subluxation (and dislocation if not prevented) and of scoliosis. The hips and spine should be X-rayed when the diagnosis is made. Regular clinical examination should be made every 3 months until 18 months and every 6 months until age 5 years. Repeated radiological investigation is required but the frequency depends on the severity of the child's condition. Ultrasound examination of the hip joint will reduce the dose of radiation used. However it is difficult to judge the degree of subluxation of the hip from clinical examination alone in children with moderate or severe spasticity and X-rays may be required every 6–12 months if there is any doubt. Physiotherapy advice on handling and seating helps to protect the hips by maintaining an abducted position of the child's hip as much as possible.

Scoliosis develops when the child has poor trunk control and is the consequence of posture and the effects of gravity over time rather than the inevitable consequence of spasticity. It is especially a risk when the child has a strong preference for lying on one side and, when sitting, to turn to that side also. The tendency is for children with severe poverty of active movement to develop a "windswept" posture which includes scoliosis concave towards the side of the head turn, chest deformity and turning of the hips in the direction of head turn. The contralateral hip is adducted and at special risk of subluxation or dislocation.

While every effort is made by therapists to ensure that parents and others involved in the child's care understand the importance of varied position using aids and appliances when appropriate, promotion of active movement and provision of suitable seating, it is difficult to control development of scoliosis. Repeat X-rays of the spine is a way of monitoring progress and should be considered at regular intervals, depending on severity of the clinical condition. The growth spurt during puberty is a time of particular risk of deterioration. In children who are severely affected, spinal X-ray is appropriate every 2 years in childhood and annually during puberty.

Progressive deformities of the ankles (equinovarus with spasticity, calcaneovalgus with low tone) can be judged clinically, as can flexion contractures of the wrist. Regular examination is required with advice on suitable splinting and footwear during growth. Wrist deformities may also require splinting. It is beyond the scope of this chapter to review gait analysis as a means of investigation of leg muscle and joint function as a precursor to appropriate surgery. A wide range of methods has been developed at a wide range of costs. No doubt the benefits of such investigations will become clear in future (e.g. Sutherland et al 1988, Gage 1991).

Spasticity and contracture of the masseter muscles compounds the effects of bulbar palsy by leading to mandibular retraction and an increasingly open bite leading to increasing feeding difficulties and greater tendency to drooling. The most hopeful solutions lie in the development of orthodontic appliances (e.g. Limbrock et al 1990). If they are introduced gradually and used at night they can become increasingly sophisticated and can be tolerated even by children with severe learning disability.

Difficulties with bowel function especially constipation, sometimes with overflow, are common in children with cerebral palsies and should be investigated, at least by history and examination at each regular review. The main causes for this are the problems in swallowing sufficient liquid, in tolerating a diet conducive to good bowel function and less efficient voluntary muscle activity during defecation. However, with good dietary advice, development of a regular bowel habit and good access to toilet facilities (adapted if need be) which can be used by the child independently as far as possible, problems of bowel incontinence can be reduced.

Urinary incontinence and recurrent bladder infection can be a problem for children and adolescents with severe cerebral palsy. Bladder dysfunction can occur (Reid and Borzyskowski 1993) and should be investigated by cystometric studies when careful bladder-training problems have failed. More commonly bladder dysfunction is secondary to chronic constipation with a persistently loaded bowel so this should be investigated and treated as a priority. Teaching children to communicate their toileting needs and ensuring ready access to suitable toilet facilities are important means of minimizing urinary incontinence.

Communication difficulties are common in children with cerebral palsies because of bulbar palsy, difficulties with gestures and associated language problems. Investigation of their capacity to use augmented communication by signing, symbols or use of switches to access communication aids require help from an experienced speech and language therapist.

LANGUAGE DELAY AND DISORDER

From very early in infancy there are signs of recognition of voice, especially the mother's voice. Infants will quieten and try to locate the voice when spoken to. In early months there is the beginning of reciprocal turn-taking with phonation leading on to babble in the second half of the first year. Babble is produced spontaneously, even in children with severe learning impairment. It fades at the end of the first year, being replaced by prespeech with more direct imitation of adult speech sounds in succeeding months. However, in the child with hearing impairment the babble fades and is not replaced by speech sounds. All children should have had their hearing tested by 8 or 9 months but some slip through the net or are tested but parents do not follow up subsequent appointments and there is a false negative risk for hearing tests. So fading babble without replacement should always prompt investigation of hearing.

There are other children for whom neonatal early hearing tests are a particular priority. These include those with a family history of hearing impairment, very low birthweight infants, those who have suffered prenatal infection (rubella, cytomegalovirus), perinatal asphyxia, significant jaundice, aminoglycoside therapy or meningitis, those with orofacial malformations or other neurodevelopmental disorders. Distraction testing may give satisfactory results but if there is any doubt there should be referral to a specialist audiology clinic for more sophisticated investigation, e.g. brain stem evoked response testing. In all population studies (e.g. review by Peckham 1986) the prevalence of hearing loss in excess of 50 dB in the better ear at 500, 1000 and 2000 Hz is in the range of 1–2 per 1000 children. When sensorineural loss of this degree is detected, genetic counselling should be offered. Most genetically determined causes are autosomal recessive with six main types though dominant forms and rare sex-linked recessive forms also occur.

Loss of reciprocal social communication can occur in other conditions such as pervasive developmental disorders (forms of autism in the first 30 months of life) and early degenerative conditions (see Chapter 9). This is not to be confused with shyness towards strangers which is a normal developmental feature of the latter part of the first year. In addition to hearing tests there should be investigation of vision (e.g. cataract, refractive error, retinopathy or cortical defects) (see Chapter 17). In girls with slowing of growth of head circumference and reduced hand function with regressed mobility the diagnosis of Rett syndrome suggests itself but there are, as yet, no confirmatory investigations. Children with fragile X chromosome lesions are often aversive about eye contact. They tend to have average or large head circumferences. The DNA test is worth considering – 5 ml of blood in an EDTA tube is required. An EEG sometimes shows left-hemisphere spikes even when the affected child has had no seizures in children with acquired asphasia.

When speech and language development are delayed (e.g. inability to make three-word phrases appropriately by age 3 years) the explanation is likely to be pathological in a fifth and idiopathic, or developmental, in most. Among the pathological explanations are chromosome abnormalities, especially of the sex chromosomes, associated cerebral palsy or orofacial malformations, acquired aphasia in association with seizures or EEG abnormalities, forms of more global learning disability, hearing impairment and elective mutism. Also boys with Duchenne dystrophy may present with language delay. Thus investigations include chromosome testing, EEG, hearing tests and in boys, creatine kinase.

The children for whom there is no pathological explanation are twice as likely to be male as female and are often children from large families with parents who were not successful academically at school. They usually have mixed receptive and expressive problems and commonly have problems with speech articulation as well as language. Assessment of language reception, expression and speech articulation should be done by a speech therapist using standardized test instruments, e.g. Reynell Developmental Language Scales (Revised), language assessment, remediation and screening procedure (LARSP), test for reception of grammar (TROG), and Edinburgh Articulation Test (Lees and Urwin 1991). The majority of children with language delay catch up so far as spoken language is concerned, but they are likely to have literacy problems in school.

In addition to language delay, children may show deviant or disordered language. They may use words without proper understanding of their meaning (semantic disorder), in the wrong context (pragmatic disorder), without proper grammatical structures (syntactical disorder) and may, incidentally, utter speech without the normal melodic variations of speech (prosodic disorder). Such children are unlikely to grow out of their language disability and require regular review by speech therapists in order to advise families and school. Chromosome and EEG testing are worth pursuing.

Articulation problems are common in young children. Strangers may find at least 1:10 children aged 4 years difficult to understand. Even by the age of 7 years children are not fully understood by teachers or doctors. Yet by the end of primary school, aged 10–11 years, there are few children who are difficult to understand. Speech therapy investigation is helpful in early years. Usually children are found to have phonological problems which are immature omissions, substitutions or reversals. When there are inconsistent phonological disorders, including disrupted syllable sequences, it is sometimes described as articulatory dyspraxia. In such children it is worth investigating hand function as a manual dyspraxia is commonly associated. However, when particular speech sounds cannot be made, e.g. "k" or "g", and there is consistent palatal escape it is important to examine the palate carefully for signs of submucous cleft and to consider palatal function tests such as anemometry.

LEARNING DISABILITY

Learning disability (mental handicap) may be moderate or severe. Most children with learning disability are ascertained following months or years of increasing concern about developmental delay (McKinlay and Holland 1986). However, some diagnoses are made antenatally (e.g. chromosome abnormalities, neural tube defect) which make it likely that children will have learning disability in future. Parents may opt for termination of pregnancy but, if they do not, the child's birth and early care require particular preparation and sensitivity. The degree of learning disability is not predictable from the biological diagnosis alone. Thus some children with trisomy 21 can cope with a mainstream curriculum and obtain leaving certificate examination passes. Others have profound and multiple disabilities and never walk or talk.

About a third of children with severe learning disability are diagnosed at birth. Much the commonest single diagnosis is trisomy 21 (Down syndrome). These neonates show profound hypotonia as the single most reliable feature. Other signs include brachycephaly, white Brushfield spots on the iris, marked tongue protrusion, single transverse palmar creases and short in-curved 5th fingers. It is always appropriate to carry out investigation of the karyotype, however typical the physical features. About 5% show a 14/21 translocation which may be carried in balanced form by a parent which has implications for genetic counselling. Also some children show a mosaic karyotype with only a proportion of cells showing trisomy 21. The prognosis is better for such children. Investigation *must* be preceded by appropriate counselling.

Other children with learning disability present with malformation of the face, limbs, heart or other systems, often associated with microcephaly indicating another chromosome abnormality, e.g. trisomy 13 or trisomy 18. It is justified to investigate the karyotype of any neonate with appreciable dysmorphic features, provided that the reasons for investigation have been discussed with both parents by an experienced doctor in an unhurried, undisturbed fashion. The parents may agree to allow a nurse or social worker to sit in to facilitate subsequent counselling. The doctor should offer further counselling arranged similarly to the above as soon as the test result is available.

Microcephaly at birth may be associated with other dysmorphic features such as cataracts, auricular abnormalities, enlargement of the liver or spleen or skin rashes, suggesting intrauterine infection with cytomegalovirus, rubella virus, syphilis or toxoplasma. Blood for IgG and IgM antibodies for virus infection and serological tests for syphilis and toxoplasma together with urine culture for cytomegalovirus and rubella virus are appropriate. It is likely that investigation for congenital HIV infection will be required more commonly in future. The reason for investigation must be explained fully to the parents and the results will be discussed with them when they become available.

An abnormality affecting a newborn baby causes shock and distress to parents. The birth of a baby with such problems is unpredictable and fairly infrequent in the experience of doctors and nurses in training. There needs to be a clear policy for management and continuing education programme to ensure that staff are prepared for the challenge.

Part of the early counselling includes explanation of future prognosis, sources of help and further investigations to find remediable associated conditions, e.g. visual or hearing impairments. Detailed investigation of the family history will assist genetic counselling which should be offered to all families. Even if the parents do not intend to add to their own family there may be other family members who wish to be advised or who could be affected. In any case most parents are anxious to know as much as possible about the cause of their son or daughter's disability, including genetic aspects, as part of the process of learning to come to terms with their new family responsibilities. Even though they had no reason to anticipate their child's condition there is some comfort from going through the family history and a physical examination without finding any abnormality.

Most children with learning disability are thought to be normal at birth but show some early motor delay. Of those with severe learning difficulty five out of six will be late to walk. All will show slow development of language comprehension and expressive language though some parents may not notice this at first. ("He understands everything doctor".) Also professionals can err on the side of reassurance, aware of the wide range of normal but sometimes playing down justified concern on the part of parents. There comes a time, however, when parents and professionals agree that there is a problem to solve.

The first investigation may be a formal developmental assessment by a clinical psychologist, often using the Griffith's test, though Bayley and Denver scales are also used quite widely. Assessment of receptive and expressive language by a speech therapist is often requested. It may be thought at first that the child's "only problem is speech". Demonstrating that this does not appear to be so, but that the language delay is part of a global cognitive impairment leads to discussion about the next step.

Detailed physical examinination is appropriate, including height, weight and head circumference related to standard up-to-date charts. Any changes in growth velocity are noted. Dysmorphic features or unusual skin lesions are measured and recorded. Unusual behaviour such as hand-wringing or flapping, mouth tapping, hyperventilating, self-hugging, spot picking, screaming or autistic features are noted as there may be clues to the diagnosis.

Occasionally children slip through the net of neonatal screening because their families are travellers or move home before the result comes through. Especially if the child is fair haired and no screening test result for phenylketonuria is available, it is worth requesting urine amino acid chromatography. If more than one child is born into a family with developmental delay or learning disability for no discoverable reason it is worth testing the mother's urine for phenylketonuria. Likewise if a child is short and developmentally delayed and no thyroid function test result is available from screening, thyroid function tests are justified. Though neither of these investigations is likely to be positive and the lack of a previous result in the records is usually an administrative hitch, they do have treatment implications if abnormal.

Chromosome testing is sometimes helpful though the

"strike rate" is lower for children than for neonates. Fragile X is underdiagnosed in boys and girls so the new DNA tests will be helpful. This is particularly worth considering when the child's head is bigger than the 50th centile, the skin feels velvety, the joints are lax, there is a history of early feeding difficulty or speech articulation problems and when the social manner is excessively shy or slightly autistic. The large pinna and testicular enlargement are present in prepubertal boys with Fragile X but are more obvious after puberty as is the long jaw (Hagerman and Silverman 1991). Trisomy 8 may be underdiagnosed as a cause of moderate learning disability. A thickened lower lip, club feet, brachydactyly and contracture are common. All cases described have arisen "de novo".

When chromosome testing is negative but the child looks unusual it is worth involving a paediatric geneticist (Super and Donnai 1986), ideally through a joint appointment, and using the dysmorphology database. This undergoes regular updating so, if one approach has failed, it is worth consulting it again after an interval of 2 or 3 years.

When a child is found to have a learning disability it is important to investigate vision and hearing as associated sensory impairments are common (Ellis 1986). If there is a need for visual or hearing aids the way in which these are introduced affects their continued use. They should be used for short periods under experienced adult supervision while developmentally appropriate tasks are undertaken.

When children with learning disability become ill there are particular difficulties in investigating the cause and in following treatment through to a successful conclusion. A common example is the investigation of recurrent episodes which may be a form of epilepsy. It is difficult for such children to describe their symptoms. Often their concentration is brief, they have limited comprehension, dislike restraint and find the context of investigations trying. When medication starts they may have difficulty in letting it be known whether they feel better or worse and especially whether they experienced side effects. Thus the responsibility is greater for parents, teachers and other caretakers to observe and report signs accurately. It is important that nursing staff, doctors and lab staff involved in tests have experience of communication with youngsters of limited ability. If behavioural changes or developmental regression occurs after medication has started, professional staff should be alert to the possibility of drug side-effects.

The need to inform children with learning disability about the purpose of examinations, investigations and treatments in a developmentally appropriate fashion is stressed. The outcome is most likely to be successful when they, and their parents, understand what is being done and why.

REFERENCES

Ellis D (1986) *Sensory Impairments in Mentally Handicapped People*. Croom Helm, Beckenham.

Gage JR (1991) Gait analysis in cerebral palsy. *Clinics in Developmental Medicine*, 121: MacKeith Press/Blackwell Scientific, London.

Hagerman RJ, Silverman AC (1991) *Fragile X Syndrome: Diagnosis Treatment and Research*. Johns Hopkins University Press, Baltimore.

Hughes I, Newton R (1992) Genetic aspects of cerebral palsy. *Dev Med Child Neurol* 34: 80–86.

Lees J, Urwin S (1991) *Children with Language Disorders*. Whurr, London.

Limbrock GJ, Hoyer H, Scheying H (1990) Drooling, chewing and swallowing dysfunctions in children with cerebral palsy: treatment according to Castillo-Morales. *J Dentist Child* 57: 445–451.

McKinlay I, Holland J (1986) Mentally handicapped children. In: Gordon NS, McKinlay I (eds) *Neurologically Handicapped Children: Treatment and Management*. Blackwell Scientific, Oxford.

Nelson KB, Ellenberg JH (1982) Children who "outgrow" cerebral palsy. *Paediatrics* 69: 511–514.

Nicholson A, Alberman E (1992) Cerebral palsy – an increasing contributor to severe mental retardation? *Arch Dis Child* 67: 1050–1055.

Peckham CS (1986) Hearing impairment in childhood. *Br Med Bull* 42: 145–149.

Reid CJD, Borzyskowski M (1993) Lower urinary tract dysfunction in cerebral palsy. *Arch Dis Child* 68: 739–742.

Super M, Donnai D (1986) Genetic counselling in the management of children with neurological disease. In: Gordon NS, McKinlay I (eds) *Neurologically Handicapped Children: Treatment and Management*. Blackwell Scientific, Oxford.

Sutherland DH, Olshen RA, Biden EN, Wyatt MP (1988) The development of mature walking. *Clinics in Developmental Medicine*, 104–105. MacKeith Press/Blackwell Scientific, London.

11

Child Abuse

C Hobbs

INTRODUCTION

The Children Act 1989 provides a new framework for the care and protection of children. This is reflected in "Working Together", a guide to arrangements for inter-agency co-operation for the protection of children from abuse (HMSO 1991).

The philosophy of the act is that at all times the child's welfare is paramount. Parents are given full opportunity to be involved and to work in partnership with local authorities.

Child abuse includes:

- *Physical* – injury inflicted or not prevented and includes deliberate poisoning, suffocation, and Munchausen's syndrome by proxy.
- *Sexual* – the sexual exploitation of a dependent and/or developmentally immature child or adolescent.
- *Neglect* – persistent failure to protect a child from exposure to any kind of danger, failure to carry out important aspects of care resulting in significant impairment of the child's health and development, including non-organic failure to thrive.
- *Emotional* – persistent or severe psychological ill-treatment or rejection leading to an adverse effect on the emotional and behavioural development of the child.

In reality children are often the victims of more than one form of abuse – emotional abuse is often central and physical and sexual abuse may occur together.

The investigation of suspected child abuse involves medical, social and police (forensic) inputs which must be co-ordinated through a process of information sharing and decision-making. The medical role in investigation includes:

- To recognize probable abuse and report to an agency with statutory responsibilities for child protection

(social service department of the local authority or NSPCC).
- To include abuse, where appropriate, within the differential diagnosis of a child's problems.
- To undertake a full paediatric assessment of the child in terms of a full history, the child's health, growth and development and any specific or non-specific signs of abuse.
- To consider causes other than abuse for the child's symptoms and signs and to be able to differentiate these from abuse.

To fulfil these functions the doctor must:

- Know the important patterns and clinical features of child abuse.
- Be able to undertake a detailed medical examination looking for evidence of injury, signs of neglect, and physical signs of sexual abuse as well as to assess the child's growth and development.
- Know how and when to use specific laboratory and radiological investigations.
- Know how to interpret investigations within a legal context.
- Provide a report which will be available to the court.
- Present evidence in court and respond to cross-examination.

Important Points to Remember

- Child abuse is an important diagnosis and influences the whole of the child's and the family's life.
- Strong denial by the family is usual and this may be reflected in a reluctance by professionals to accept the diagnosis.
- Wrong diagnosis may harm the child and family, but equally a missed diagnosis leaves the child and family at continuing risk.

- Complete certainty of diagnosis is not required for reporting or to achieve protection. Cases are proved on "the balance of probability".
- The doctor must demonstrate that other explanations have been considered and excluded where possible.

Consent to Investigations

Investigations are usually part of a wider assessment of the child in suspected abuse. It is important that the doctor considers:

- Who has the right to consent to this examination or assessment?
- Is the child subject to any court order?
- What are the directions of the court, if any, in relation to the order?
- Who has parental responsibility?
- Will the assessment be used in court proceedings?
- What are the views of the child, has a Guardian ad Litem been appointed?
- Does the child have any difficulty in communicating for which special arrangements need to be made?

Consent to hospital admission normally covers a number of routine procedures. It is better not to presume that, for example, skeletal survey, clinical photography or tests for sexually transmitted diseases, should be done without further informing the parents and obtaining their agreement. Therefore it is appropriate that proper informed consent (which may be verbal) is obtained for investigations of this kind in child abuse cases. Refusal is unusual but must be respected. A court order (usually an emergency protection order or child assessment order) should enable the doctor to complete the necessary assessment with the agreement and direction of the court.

PHYSICAL ABUSE

Physical abuse (non-accidental injury) includes injuries which result from deliberate actions or from a failure to prevent injury. The injuries include bruises, fractures, burns and scalds, internal injuries (brain, abdomen, eye), suffocation and poisoning. The usual task for the paediatrician is to distinguish abuse from accident. In addition, the paediatrician will need to consider other possible diagnoses when examining a suspected injury, particularly when no history of injury is given (Table 11.1).

Bleeding Disorders and Non-accidental Injury (see also Chapter 1)

It is often stated by parents who have injured their child that "he bruises easily". Where the child presents with bruises which are inadequately explained it is reasonable to undertake tests to exclude a bleeding disorder. It is important to recognize that inflicted injury and bleeding disorder may co-exist (16% of tests undertaken in one study (O'Hare and Eden 1984) were positive) and that the diagnoses are not mutually exclusive. Children who are being physically abused and who also have a disorder of coagulation are at increased risk from their injuries. Investigations to exclude a bleeding disorder are detailed in Table 11.2 and include those minimum tests used as a screen, and additional tests required for a complete and more comprehensive assessment where history indicates (see also Table 11.3).

Investigation of Skeletal Injury

An important part of the diagnosis and assessment of suspected physical abuse is the detection of skeletal injury. A radiological skeletal survey is not required in every case of suspected physical abuse and may be undertaken selectively.

Indications for Skeletal Survey

- Presence of a fracture which suggests abuse.
- Physically abused child under 3 years of age.
- Severe inflicted soft tissue injury in an older child.
- Localized pain, limp or reluctance to use limb in abused child.
- Previous history of skeletal trauma in child suspected of abuse.
- Unexplained neurological presentation.
- Child dying in suspicious or unusual circumstances.

A screening skeletal survey beyond 5 years has little use.

The following radiographs are required when searching for occult trauma (Carty 1989):

- Skull, anteroposterior and lateral (still required if CT obtained).
- Chest, spine and pelvis anteroposterior.
- Anteroposterior view of long bones, including hands.

All the films must be on separate plates, "babygrams" are

Table 11.1 Differential diagnosis in physical abuse – skin lesions

Presentation	Differential diagnoses	Features	Investigations
?Bruise	Blue spots, haemangioma, café au lait spots, prominent veins	Static lesions, no evolution with time	Follow-up, re-examine
?Bruise	Bleeding disorder, e.g. I.T.P., haemophilia, haemorrhagic disease of newborn, platelet disorder	Bruising with minimal trauma, sites – usual accidental ones. Family history, prolonged bleeding	Haematological investigations (Tables 11.2 and 11.3)
?Bruise	Infection, vasculitis: meningococcal septicaemia, disseminated intravascular coagulation	Ill child, rapidly developing purpuric rash	Blood culture, lumbar puncture, haematology
	Henoch–Schöenlein disease	Distribution of purpura, joint, abdominal, renal features	Urine microscopy, urine dipstick for protein
?Bruise	Allergy – periorbital swelling	History of allergy, contact, appearance, evolution	IgE, eosinophilia
?Bruise	Skin disease: Ehler's Danlos syndrome, erythema nodosum, other skin disease	Low elasticity, poor wound healing, easy bruisability painful, warm, erythematous, pretibial, joint pain	Seek dermatology opinion Biopsy
?Bruise	Ink, paint, dye, dirt	Removable	Soap and water
?Scald or burn (cigarette)	Infection – impetigo	Irregular, golden crusts, tend to spread, prompt response to antibiotics	Skin/nasal swab: *Staphylococcus aureus* or β-haemolytic *Streptococcus*
?Scald or burn	Staphylococcal scalded skin syndrome	Erythematous, painful lessions, + ve Nikolsky's sign	*S. aureus* phage group II, types 70 or 71 from skin/nasal swabs
?Scald or burn	Nappy rash, with or without infection	Distribution, pattern, blisters	—
?Scald or burn	Photodermatitis	Sensitization by contact with certain plant/fruit substances. Burn produced by light	History. Sensitivity testing of small areas
?Scald or burn	Folk medicine practice – cupping, coin rubbing or rolling	Red lesions, erythema, bruises. Middle East, Latin America, S.E. Asia, E. European	History
?Scald or burn	Fixed drug eruption	Purple/red plaque clearly demarcated border in same site repeatedly follows drug ingestion	History – usually salicylate, tetracycline, sulphonamide

not acceptable. These minimum radiographs must be supplemented with local views of any suspicious areas. Modern paediatric imaging systems use special films, cassettes and intensifying screens to minimize exposure. Subtle injuries such as metaphyseal, rib and other unusual injuries require modifications to the usual systems (Haller et al 1991).

Radionucleotide Bone Scans

These (Chapman 1993) provide increased sensitivity for showing rib fractures, subtle shaft fractures and areas of early periosteal elevation. Their use is supplementary to conventional radiology. Problems include:

• Missed fractures – some skull, vertebral and bilateral

Table 11.2 Tests to exclude a bleeding disorder in non-accidental injury (O'Hare and Eden 1984)

Comprehensive list:
Full blood count, film
Platelet count, size and shape
Partial thromboplastin time
Prothrombin time
Thrombin time
Fibrinogen
Bleeding time

List commonly abbreviated to include:
Platelet count
Prothrombin time
Partial thromboplastin time

Notes:
A bleeding time may be added to exclude platelet function disorders. A vasculitis can only be diagnosed by means of skin biopsy. Remember to take a drug history, e.g. salicylates can induce a platelet disorder.

metaphyseal fractures; completely healed fractures.
- Missed metabolic and congenital disease.
- Need for meticulous technique/high-quality images.
- Check all positive findings with conventional radiology.

Intracranial Injury

The majority of these injuries occur in the first 2 years of life and account for the greatest morbidity and mortality in physical abuse. It is important to remember that infants suffering from the effects of acute head injury do not always have a history of injury. Careful and detailed examination of the child for signs of external trauma to the head and elsewhere, for retinal haemorrhages, frenulum tears and anal/genital injury is essential in such cases.

Investigations of intracranial injury involves:

- Skeletal survey which includes skull films (antero-posterior and lateral).
- Cranial computerized tomography (CT) is suitable in the acute situation to identify trauma and any acute treatable conditions. Subarachnoid haemorrhage is better detected by CT than by magnetic resonance imaging (MRI).
- MRI scanning (where available) is substantially more sensitive at identifying and characterizing most intracranial sequelae of abusive assaults. This includes subdural haematomas, cortical contusions, cerebral oedema and white matter injuries (Haller et al 1991). Follow-up examinations may allow for dating of fluid collections and the detection of deep cerebral injuries, for example in cases where the child continues to show neurological signs.
- Cranial sonography is not recommended for a full evaluation of intracranial injury (Haller et al 1991).

Differential Diagnosis of Skeletal Injury

It is vitally important that paediatricians are fully conversant with the possible diagnoses (Table 11.4) which it may be suggested account for the child's skeletal findings. This is particularly relevant in the medico-legal arena where the defence may have few options other than to persuade that a child's multiple fractures are really the result of a pathological process rather than the actions of violent parents.

Table 11.3 Results of haematological investigations in four bleeding disorders

Bleeding disorder	Platelet count	Bleeding time	PTT	PT	Factor VIII level	Factor IX level
Idiopathic thrombocytopenic purpura	Low	Normal	Normal	Normal	Normal	Normal
Haemophilia	Normal	Normal	Prolonged	Normal	Low	Normal
von Willebrand's disease	Normal (defective platelet aggregation	Prolonged	Normal or prolonged	Normal	Low	Normal
Factor IX deficiency	Normal	Normal	Prolonged	Normal	Normal	Low

From Harvey et al (1991).
PTT, partial thromboplastin time; PT, prothrombin time.

Table 11.4 Differential diagnosis of skeletal disorders

Condition	Features	Radiology	Investigations
Normal variant pseudo-fracture	E.g. aberrant skull suture, symmetrical periosteal reaction, minor abnormality	Often symmetrical, identical to changes of trauma	Consult specialist, or large textbook
Birth trauma	Clavicle, humerus, femur, rib, depressed skull, etc.	Absence of callus after 2 weeks means not birth trauma	Check history at birth
Osteogenesis imperfecta* Heterogenous rare condition types I–IV	Fractures with minimal trauma, blue sclerae, deafness, family history, wormian bones, dental changes, easy bruising, growth retardation, scoliosis	Osteopenia, thin cortices, angulation and bowing of fractures	Diagnosis on clinical and radiological features. No laboratory test routinely available
Osteoporosis	Heparin, disuse, osteogenesis, copper deficiency	Poor mineralization	History, clinical and radiological diagnosis identified cause
Copper deficiency†	Rare, temporary features: sideroblastic anaemia, neutropenia, hypotonia. Occurs in preterm, low-birth-weight, fed by TPN	Osteoporosis, cup shaped and frayed metaphysis, sickle-shaped spurs, symmetrical fractures	80–90% Hb < 10.0 gm/dl. Neutropenia $< 1.0 \times 10^9$/l. Plasma copper < 40 µg/dl. Caeruloplasmin < 13 mg/dl
Osteomyelitis, congenital syphilis	Systemic signs and symptoms variable in early infancy. Local signs may predominate	Multifocal metaphyseal lesions, periosteal reaction, no corner fractures, bone destruction	Blood cultures, aspirates positive for *S. aureus*, coliforms, group B. *Streptococcus meningococcus*, syphilis serology positive, mother and baby
Caffey's disease	Rare disease of infants painful periosteal thickening in multiple bones	Any bones, especially mandible, clavicle and ulna. No fractures or metaphyseal irregularity	Clinical diagnosis, course of disease
Rickets	Premature infant, TPN confusion after discharge from neonatal unit older child-fractures unusual	Cupping, fraying costochondral junctions and metaphyses. Decreased bone density, looser's zones	Low serum calcium, low or normal phosphate, raised alkaline phosphatase. Low 25-hydroxy vitamin D
Scurvy, vitamin A intoxication	Rare, related to bizarre feeding practice	Periosteal and metaphyseal changes	Vitamin A or C levels in blood

*Albin et al (1990), Taitz (1987), Carty (1991).
†Shaw (1988).
TPN, total parenteral nutrition.

Differentiation of Child Abuse from Osteogenesis Imperfecta

Osteogenesis imperfecta (OI) is an inherited disorder of connective tissue resulting from abnormal quality and/or quantity of type I collagen (Albin et al 1990). The incidence is estimated to be between 1/15 000 and 1/60 000 births. There are four major types (I–IV) as well as various subtypes (A, B, etc.), reflecting the complexity of the collagen molecule.

Types II and III are severe: type II with multiple fractures at birth; type III is similar but less severe with progressive deformity and growth retardation. Confusion with abuse is very unlikely.

Type I is the most common type and has normal teeth (subtype A) or dentinogenesis imperfecta (subtype B).

Presence of blue sclera at all ages almost universally should avoid confusion with abuse (Taitz 1987).

Type IV is rare (5% of all OI), but sporadic cases occur. Sclera are normal or pale blue (compared with normal infants). Discussion of this differential diagnosis is important in medico-legal cases and the reader is referred elsewhere (Taitz 1987, Ablin et al 1990) for full detail and discussion.

Copper Deficiency

Copper deficiency (Shaw 1988) is a rare condition which, it has been claimed, is responsible for a temporary tendency to fractures which clears up when the child is removed to a safe home. The skeletal manifestations are part of a wider picture following impairment of various enzyme systems. Sideroblastic anaemia, neutropenia hypotonia and psychomotor retardation are also described. Predisposing factors include:

- Low birth weight (low body stores).
- Dietary deficiency (total parenteral nutrition (TPN) with deficient copper in solutions, with cows' milk including, occasionally, formula milk. Breast milk is rarely deficient).
- Antecedent malnutrition (malabsorption, starvation diet, coeliac disease etc.).
- Peritoneal dialysis (only one case).

Chapman (1993) suggests it would be unlikely to occur:

- In a full-term infant aged < 6 months, breast or modern formula fed.
- In a preterm infant < 2.5 months of age.
- In a term infant with rib or skull fractures.
- In the absence of the above predisposing factors.
- In the absence of anaemia or neutropenia.
- In the absence of osteoporosis, abnormal metaphyses or retarded bone age.

Abdominal and Thoracic Injuries

After head injury, thoracoabdominal injury is the next major cause of death in physical abuse. These injuries are uncommon, occurring in 1–5% of cases. They are important to recognize because of the potential for treatment. Thus a high index of suspicion is required as the history may be unhelpful. Overlying soft tissue injury, if present, may be an indicator to investigate further, but it is often absent. A blow or kick to the abdomen may produce serious internal injury with little external bruising. The presentation may be non-specific gastro-intestinal (hollow viscus) or with lethargy or coma following haemorrhagic shock (solid viscus) (Cooper 1992).

Investigations

Clinical Abdominal Examination

- Is there distension?
- Insert nasogastric tube and empty stomach. Is blood, food or bile obtained? Does distension remain?
- Is rectal examination required? Are there signs of injury (sexual abuse can perforate the rectum in infancy), blood or anterior tenderness?

Laboratory Investigations

- Serial haematocrit for blood loss.
- Serum amylase (raised in pancreatic and in some cases of splenic injury because the spleen lies close to the pancreas).
- Serum aspartate aminotransferase, alanine aminotransferase, and lactate dehydrogenase (raised in liver laceration) (Coant et al 1992).
- Urine: gross or microscopic haematuria (> 20 red blood cells per high-power field suggests damage to the kidney or urinary tract).

Radiology

- Chest X-ray: rib fracture, pneumothorax, and pleural fluid/haemothorax.
- Posteroanterior abdominal and chest radiographs, taken in supine and erect positions, allow visualization of free air and fluid levels following perforation of a hollow viscus. Plain X-rays of abdomen may reveal ground-glass appearance of intraperitoneal haemorrhage (or fluid from other cause).
- CT scanning is the most sensitive method of identifying injuries of the lungs, pleura and solid abdominal organs, including pancreatic injury and duodenal haematoma.

Note: urgent laparotomy is the most appropriate way to confirm the presence and site of a perforation.

Intramural Haematoma of Duodenum (sometimes Jejunum)

With the exception of the presence of a bleeding disorder, this finding indicates trauma (usually blunt) to the upper abdomen. A submucosal haematoma forms often slowly with the onset of unexplained bilious vomiting with or without a boggy epigastric mass. Ultrasonography or CT may detect the mass but they are not always reliable and a barium meal may be required and may demonstrate the "coiled spring" appearance.

Pancreatitis and Pancreatic Pseudocysts

There is a well-established association between pancreatitis, pancreatic pseudocysts and blunt upper abdominal trauma (abuse). Ultrasonography is the investigation of choice, and CT and MRI also contribute valuable information in both pancreatitis and pseudocyst.

Liver and Spleen

Ultrasonography, CT and isotope scanning can detect acute bleeding as well as scars. Splenic subcapsular haematoma has been detected by means of ^{99m}Tc sulphur colloid scan.

FAILURE TO THRIVE

Although traditionally difficult to define, failure to thrive (FTT) refers to children who are growth retarded secondary to malnutrition from whatever cause. These children fail to achieve their potential for growth.

Frank and Zeisel (1988) have described three aspects of FTT:

- *Organic* – ascribed to a major illness or organ system dysfunction (see Chapter 3).
- *Non-organic* – attributed to "maternal deprivation", an insufficiently nurturing environment in home or institution.
- *Mixed* – the effects of organic disease compounded by psychosocial difficulty.

The causes and effects of FTT are shown in Figure 11.1.

Existing studies show the prevalence rate of FTT to be between 1% and 9% of the child population, although the exact growth criteria chosen are likely to influence this figure. Of these children by far the majority will fail to thrive for non-organic reasons and only a small proportion (probably less than 5%) will have a primary medical cause.

For this reason, investigation into the reasons behind the FTT will often focus on the family, the feeding and the relationships, and medical investigations can be used selectively for those cases where the history and clinical assessment point toward an organic problem or where real concerns by the parents that the cause of the problem is to be found medically must be addressed.

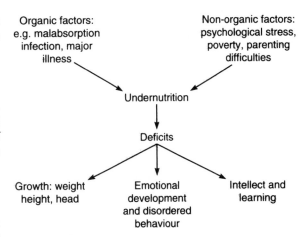

Figure 11.1   Causes and effects of failure to thrive. From Hanks and Hobbs (1993).

Various studies (Sills 1978, Berwick et al 1982) have agreed that clinical history and physical examination are the most valuable tools in the evaluation of FTT. In the cases described, many laboratory investigations had been carried out with poor yield of positive results.

It is emphasized that admission to hospital and laboratory testing is unlikely to lead to a specific organic diagnosis in a child whose FTT is unexplained after careful clinical assessment. Furthermore, inappropriate laboratory testing can prove a distraction from the important task of assessing the non-organic factors leading to the FTT. Each case will therefore need careful individual appraisal.

Plan of Investigation in FTT

It is useful to see both parents (to assess the family as a whole, the relationships within the family, the father's role, and to observe siblings). More than one session is usually needed. It is important to observe the parents with the child (Hobbs et al 1993b).

History

- *Feeding history*. Dietary recall, 3-day diet diary, video-taped meal in hospital/at home. How often, how much, what food? Difficulties, refusal, rumination, vomiting, spitting. Who (how many people) does the feeding? Has there been forcing or giving up?
- *Pregnancy and birth history*. Assess the emotional climate around child. Was the child planned, wanted? Previous miscarriage or cot death? How difficult is the child to care for?

- *Child's health*. Illnesses, admissions. Physical symptoms, e.g. diarrhoea, vomiting, respiratory symptoms. Behaviour (sleeping, crying, tantrums, hyperactivity, etc.); assess development, especially social and language development, and correlate history to the pattern revealed by the growth chart.
- *Full family history*. This includes parents' health (physical and psychological), eating patterns and weights and heights. Genetic disease, FTT in siblings or parents as children.
- *Parents' relationship and family structure and function*. Social and psychological assessment will be needed in non-organic and mixed cases. This will include financial information, employment, debt, expenditure on food.
- *Information from other professionals* (e.g. Health Visitor, G.P.) about the family. What support can they give?

Physical Examination

- *Anthropometric measures*. These include weight, height or length (< 2 years), mid-upper-arm circumference (MUAC), head circumference, and skin-fold thickness. Velocities and ratios can be calculated, if required, from these basic measurements.
- *Assess nutrition*. Skin-fold (e.g. abdomen) thickness; hair; wasting; prominent bones; musculature.
- *Posture*: persistent flexion, signs of withdrawal.
- *Hands and feet*: cold, red (deprivation) extremities.
- *Affect*: expression.
- *Teeth*: delayed eruption, neglected dental care (caries). Injuries, old or recent, to mouth, lips, teeth or frenulum.
- *Other injuries*: either inflicted or not prevented, indicating abuse or neglect.
- *Behaviour*. Variable and at opposite ends of the spectrum: lively and active, sad and quiet, over-friendly or shuns contact, etc.
- *Signs of organic disease*. These should be looked for and are usually obvious, e.g. renal, cardiac, liver, etc., disease.
- *More difficult (or hidden) organic diagnoses*. These should be considered. Malabsorption – e.g. coeliac disease, cystic fibrosis or hypothyroidism. Iron deficiency anaemia – may be associated with anorexia, recurrent urinary tract infections. Tonsillar-adenoidal hypertrophy interfering with feeding.

Clinical Assessment

Simple investigations in FTT are undertaken according to clinical assessment and include (as appropriate):

- Haemoglobin and full blood count including haematocrit.
- Urinalysis, microscopy and culture.
- Stools, for ova and parasites.
- Urea and electrolytes.

Other investigations include:

- Sweat test.
- Thyroid function tests.
- Screening investigations for malabsorption (see Chapter 7) and mantoux testing.

Hospital or Out-patient Investigation

The *clinical assessment* of an infant or child who is failing to grow adequately can usually be satisfactorily achieved in the out-patient clinic supplemented by information about the child's home from the health visitor, school nurse or GP.

A *home visit* at meal times can be most helpful too. The process of assessment and management in practice go hand in hand and it will often become apparent, even when the parents deny strongly any feeding inadequacies, what the nature of the problem is. Whilst this is happening it is not unusual for the child's growth to improve, although it is not always immediately clear why.

Admission to the hospital ward for "feeding" should be reserved for serious situations, for example where the child is consistently losing weight, where the parents are so anxious that they are not coping, or where other concerns place the child at serious risk (e.g. physical abuse, intercurrent illness).

Obviously a rapid gain in weight on feeding will confirm previous inadequate intake, but the reverse, i.e. continuing FTT, is common and does not signify the reverse (an organic cause). Therefore organic causes, if not indicated clinically, should not necessarily be vigorously pursued. Usually the reason for continuing poor weight gain lies in continued inadequate calorie intake, poor feeding pattern and emotional deprivation ("lack of a close relationship").

Very careful and detailed *monitoring* of food intake by individually allocated nursing staff is required. Adjustment of calorie intake to 1.5 to 2 times the expected intake for age should induce catch-up growth.

MUNCHAUSEN SYNDROME BY PROXY AND POISONING

The wide spectrum of this complex form of abuse has been recognized recently. It includes fabricated illness, non-accidental poisoning, some cases of suffocation, fictitious or exaggerated accounts of illness, doctor shopping, and false allegations of abuse. Within the spectrum there are varying degrees of severity with a fatal outcome recorded in some cases, e.g. 2 children out of 12 died following non-accidental salt poisoning (Meadow 1993). There are links with other forms of abuse.

Munchausen syndrome by proxy (MSBP) includes the following features (Rosenberg 1987):

- Illness in the child which is faked and/or produced by the parent (or carer).
- Presentation of the child for medical assessment or care, usually persistently and resulting in multiple medical procedures and multiple medical opinions.
- Denial of knowledge by the perpetrator of the cause of the child's illness.
- Acute symptoms and signs in the child abate when the child is separated from the perpetrator, although sequelae of the disorder may persist.

Warning Signals

These alert physicians to this possible diagnosis:

- An unexplained illness, prolonged over months or years, which has caused physicians to comment on the uniqueness of the case.
- A description of symptoms or signs that are inappropriate or incompatible.
- A history of previous therapies for the same illness that have been ineffective.
- The listing of numerous foods and drugs to which the child is allegedly allergic.
- A history in the family of previous unexplained infant deaths.
- A history of many family members also alleged to have serious but vague illnesses.
- A lack of parental concern while providing this dramatic, concerning history.

Common Clinical Presentations of MSBP

- Bleeding.
- Seizures.
- CNS depression (drowsy, coma).
- Apnoea.
- Failure to thrive.
- Diarrhoea.
- Vomiting.
- Fever.

- Rashes.
- Hypertension.

Investigations in MSBP

In fictitious illness, laboratory tests are often repeatedly normal despite continuing reported illness. This may result in additional investigations being ordered in a search for the diagnosis.

Alternatively, laboratory tests may vary from normal to grossly abnormal in the same child from day to day without appearent explanation, indeed this is another warning sign. This is due to tampering with specimens, e.g. adding blood to urine to create haematuria, or fat to stool to suggest malabsorption.

Finally laboratory tests may be abnormal on admission and revert to normal when the parent is not with the child, only to become abnormal again when he/she returns (e.g. feeding the child salt). Radiological investigations are usually normal as they are more difficult to interfere with. (See Table 11.5.)

Collection and Storage of Samples for Toxicological Analysis

It is important to note that such samples may form part of a criminal investigation and, therefore, the doctor who takes the blood must label the tube to which the blood has been added immediately with the child's name address or hospital number, date and sign his name on the tube. The attached label or form must also be signed. Hospitals usually have a limited biochemical screen of the commonly encountered drugs. In some cases the sample will be treated in the same way as a forensic swab in a sexual assault case, i.e. handed in person to the police officer. The officer will transport the sample to the regional forensic laboratory, which has a detailed toxicology screen. This will establish continuity of evidence.

Samples Required for Toxicological Analysis

It is always advisable to seek the advice of the laboratory which is to carry out the analysis. In general the following routine is satisfactory:

Blood
- 15 ml blood in plain tube to clot.
- 5–10 ml in anticoagulant, such as EDTA, heparin or oxalate.
- 5 ml in sodium fluoride, if alcohol assay required.

Urine
- 20–30 ml of urine is placed in a universal container. If

Table 11.5   Mechanisms for creating or simulating illness in MSBP

Substances and manouevres creating or simulating illness	Effects	Investigation
Drugs and poisoning (chloral, barbiturates, hypnotics phenothiazines, etc.)	Apnoea, lethargy, coma, poisoning, induced asphyxiation	Complex toxicology screens (blood and urine samples)
Drugs/substances altering fluid and electrolyte balance (salt, diuretics, excessive water, insulin)	Hypernatraemia (if given excess salt and water deprived), hypoglycaemia, hyponatraemia (these effects are often repeated)	High urine sodium excretion, normal kidney and endocrinological investigation (salt ingestion) C peptide levels (insulin-induced hypoglycaemia)
Foreign blood added to sample (parental or animal)	Haematuria, haematemesis, other bleeding	Radioisotope labelling of transfused blood, typing, etc.
Injection of faeces or contaminated fluids into intravenous line	Fever, polymicrobial bacteraemia	Bacteriological studies, covert video surveillance
Recurrent suffocation, production of seizures – pressure on neck, poisons	Acute life-threatening event, recurrent apnoea	Multichannel physiological recording of oxygen saturation, breathing movements, ECG, heart rate, nasal airflow. Covert video surveillance*
Administration of emetics	Vomiting	Toxicology
Withholding food, removing feed by nasogastric tube	Failure to thrive	Weight gain achieved away from parent. Disparity between apparent food intake and weight gain

*Samuels et al (1993).

there is delay in reaching the laboratory a small amount of sodium azide may be added.

Other samples
- Occasionally required. Include stomach contents, faeces (heavy metal poisoning – arsenic, mercury and lead) and *post-mortem* samples of liver.

Many cases of poisoning are chronic, and continued administration of poison occurs while the child is in hospital. Relapse after initial recovery of a condition thought to be due to administration of a substance will require that further samples are taken, sometimes even before the results of the first samples are fully worked out.

Household Substances used in Poisoning

These have included salt, pepper, pine oil, vitamin A, and water excess. In addition, drugs such as insulin or ipecac are not usually part of the toxicological screen.

SEXUAL ABUSE

Child sexual abuse (CSA) is increasingly recognized as a common and major morbidity in children of both sexes

and of all ages. Important recent published reviews include the report of the Cleveland Inquiry (Butler-Sloss 1987) and the report of the Royal College of Physicians (1991), *Physical Signs of Sexual Abuse in Children*. The diagnostic process in sexual abuse is similar to that in other clinical situations, although it is often more complex and involves information gathering from other agencies such as social services and the police. The diagnosis is built up gradually over time, starting with the history, the physical examination and including laboratory investigation. The child's growth, development and behaviour are also important. The pieces are then joined together (Hobbs and Wynne 1993, Hobbs et al 1993c).

The role of laboratory investigation in CSA is fourfold:

- To elucidate other differential diagnoses.
- To identify sexually transmitted diseases (STD).
- To identify forensically useful material.
- Pregnancy testing.

Differential Diagnosis

Whilst many of the symptoms reported in sexually abused children, e.g. abdominal pain, wetting, and dysuria, may have in themselves a wide differential diagnosis, it is more useful to consider the differential diagnosis of genital and anal signs seen in childhood.

Differential diagnosis of genital signs
- Recent trauma due to sexual interference.
- Accidental injury, e.g. straddle injury.
- Vulvitis, e.g. threadworms, irritants (detergents), or trauma.
- Skin disorder, e.g. lichen sclerosus, or eczema.
- Congenital abnormality, e.g. vascular lesion.
- Infection, e.g. *Candida*, associated with foreign body in vagina.
- Infection complicating trauma, e.g. CSA or STD.
- Previous trauma with scarring.
- Urethral carbuncle, haemangioma, prolapse, or polyp.

Differential diagnosis of anal signs
- Accidental trauma.
- Skin disorder, e.g. lichen sclerosus, or eczema.
- Congenital abnormality, e.g. midline raphe, or wedge-shaped midline area.
- Infection, e.g. candidiasis, or streptococcal cellulitis.
- Inflammatory bowel disease, e.g. Crohn's disease.
- Severe chronic constipation causing anal laxity.
- Single anal fissure, e.g. constipation.

- Neurological disorder, e.g. neurogenic bowel in association with spina bifida, or dystrophia myotonica.
- Rectal tumour.

Laboratory testing may assist in identifying various infective agents including threadworms (sellotape slide test), although the clinical examination will be critical in many cases.

Identification of Sexually Transmitted Disease

Children who have been sexually abused are at risk of acquiring a sexually transmitted disease. Accurate identification is required for treatment and forensic purposes (Lacey 1993). The presence of such an infection may be a marker for sexual abuse (Table 11.6).

Important points to note are:

- Where one STD has been found, others should be searched for.
- Modes of transmission vary between different infections and include: sexual; mother to fetus (vertical); mother to infant during parturition (perinatal); non-

Table 11.6 STD and the probability of abuse

STD	Incubation period	Vertical transmission – neonatal disease	Probability of abuse (after RCP 1991)
Gonorrhoea	3–4 days	Neonatal ophthalmia, neonatal vaginitis (rare)	++(+++ if child >2 years)
Trichomonas	1–4 weeks	Rare but occasionally seen, usually clears spontaneously	+++
Chlamydia	7–14 days	Neonatal conjunctivitis, neonatal pneumonitis	++(+++ if child >3 years and organism cultured is child's)
Condyloma acuminata (genital warts)	Several months	Laryngeal papillomata (HPV-II)	+
Herpes	2–14 days	Localized or disseminated	++
Bacterial vaginosis	2–14 days		+
HIV	Majority convert in 3 months	If maternal	Sexual assault
Hepatitis B	Up to 3 months	Infection	Recognized
Syphilis	Up to 3 months		+++

Notes:
+, Possible; ++, likely CSA; +++, almost certain CSA.
The previously presumed importance of fomites is decreasing (Clarke and Lacey 1990).
Full penetrative sexual intercourse (vaginal or anal) is not necessary for infection.
Orogenital sex and intercrural contact may transmit pathogens (Branch and Paxton 1965).

sexual adult or child to child (horizontal); and mechanisms within an individual (autogenous).

- Routine screening for STD in all children suspected of being sexually abused may reveal higher prevalance, but some children do not tolerate swab taking well.
- The commonest encountered infections are: gonorrhoea, chlamydia, genital warts, and genital herpes.
- Infections may be oral, anal, genital or systemic (combinations).

Investigations for STD (Table 11.7)

Gonorrhoea

Gonococci can be seen in Gram-stained preparations of vaginal, urethral or conjunctival material. Diagnosis must be confirmed by culture as the former can be unreliable.

Direct inoculation or use of transport media (e.g. Stuart's) with selective culture media is required. Cultured strains can be sent to the reference laboratory and occasionally be matched to that of alleged abuser.

Trichomoniasis

Diagnosis is made by phase-contrast microscopy of a wet mount of vaginal secretions. Culture (on Kupferburg medium) is probably more sensitive. A conjugated monoclonal antibody stain, both specific and sensitive, has also been described.

Chlamydia trachomatis

Because of the forensic implications of a positive diagnosis in CSA, care must be taken to note which test has been used:

Table 11.7   Protocol for screening for STDs (Hobbs et al 1993c)

1. *Kit comprises*:
   (a) 2 Gram film slides
   (b) 1 Microtrak slide (chlamydia screen)
   (c) 3 VCAT plates (GC culture)
   (d) 4 swabs (1 rectal, 1 throat, 2 vaginal)
   (e) 1 trichomonas bottle
   (f) 1 chlamydia media bottle
   (g) 1 bacteriology request form
   (h) 1 virology request form (chlamydia culture)

2. *Which swabs to do?*
   Depends on clinical situation.

   1st vaginal swab — Smear frosted side – Gram film
   — Inoculate VCAT plate (GC plate)
   — Cut tip of swab into trichomonas bottle

   2nd vaginal swab — Inoculate Microtrak (chlamydia)
   — Cut tip of swab into chlamydia culture
   — Smear frosted slide – Gram film

   Rectal swab ——— Inoculate VCAT plate (GC plate)

   Throat swab ——— Inoculate VCAT plate (GC plate)

3. *Other tests*:
   (a) *Candida* culture in vulvovaginitis
   (b) Herpes simplex culture if vesicles
   (c) Pregnancy test
   (d) Cervical cytology
   (e) Histology for condyloma acuminata and DNA typing (special techniques)
   (f) Serological tests for HIV, Syphilis, Hepatitis B as indicated.

4. *Forensic tests*
   Are these needed as well?

   Suggest local procedures are formulated with a specialist in genitourinary medicine

---

GC, gonococcus.

- Culture.
- Enzyme immunoassay (EIA) – Chlamidiazyme, Pathfinder, or Microtrak EIA.
- Direct fluorescent antibody (DFA) tests – Microtrak, or Pathfinder.
- DNA probe – Pace II.

EIA and DFA are 70–90% sensitive and 90% specific, compared with culture (Hammerschlag and Rawstron 1992).

Therefore EIA and DFA tests are not recommended in child sexual abuse investigation and a specimen should only be considered positive if a culture has been obtained.

Condyloma Acuminata (Genital Warts)

Whilst up to 70 different genotypes of human papillomavirus have been described over 90% of genital warts are caused by types 6 and 11, with fewer by 16, 18 and others (Lacy 1993). Diagnosis is usually clinical; histological confirmation can also be linked with DNA HPV typing.

Herpes Simplex Virus (HSV)

Both HSV 1 and HSV 2 infections can be sexually transmitted. Diagnosis is confirmed by culture with typing (confer with virologist).

Bacterial Vaginosis

This polymicrobial infection is due to an interaction between *Gardnerella vaginalis* and several anaerobic bacteria. Diagnosis is made by examination of vaginal secretions for "clue cells" and production of a fishy odour (positive whiff test) on adding 10% KOH, and not by culture of *G. vaginalis*.

Human Immunodeficiency Virus (HIV)

Increasingly requests are being made for screening of victims of CSA for HIV. The majority of infections convert within 3 months, and Lacey (1993) recommends testing at 3 and 6 months after the last date of an assault. Serological tests (ELISA) are the most widely used, being highly sensitive and specific. Positive tests should be repeated, and other tests used to confirm if still positive. Passively acquired maternal HIV antibody may persist for over 1 year after birth.

Hepatitis B

Serological tests for hepatitis B surface antigen are indicated if there is supportive epidemiological evidence. The incubation period is up to 3 months.

Syphilis

Children with syphilis acquired through abuse may present with either primary or secondary disease or with positive serology only. Rarely, it is diagnosed by dark ground microscopy from active mucous membrane lesions, but more often antibody screening is employed (e.g. VDRL or TPHA).* Repeat in 3 months. Congenital acquisition from maternal untreated disease can be difficult to diagnose because of transplacental passage of IgG antibodies. Bone changes are present in most children with overt clinical disease.

Forensic Investigations in Sexual Abuse

It is important that when CSA is investigated that correct procedures are carried out for the collection of evidential material and forensic samples (Royal College of Physicians 1991) (Table 11.8). Joint medical examinations will in some cases meet the need, but increasingly paediatricians will become competent at this aspect of the medical examination. Paediatricians should have access to the necessary materials, usually in the form of a "rape kit" provided by the local police child abuse unit.

It is important that a chain of evidence is established so that any exhibit can be clearly demonstrated to have followed the unbroken chain. For example, the doctor who takes a forensic swab should hand it to the police officer who will in turn hand it to the technician at the forensic laboratory. The doctor must seal and label fully the swab, hand it to the next person in the chain and note the date time and person to whom it was handed.

The time limits for detection of spermatozoa are:

- Oral: 12–14 h.
- Vaginal: 6 days.
- Anal: 3 days.
- Seminal fluid: 12–18 h vagina; 3 h in anus.

Dried semen can be identified by green fluorescence under a Wood's lamp.

With a recent assault, e.g. by a stranger, the child is undressed on a spread sheet of clean paper to collect any debris and all stained items and clothes should be separately bagged and labelled, preferably with a police officer present.

Forensic samples fall into two categories:

- Evidential samples.

*TPHA: Treponema Pallidum Haemagglutinin Adsorption
VRDL: Venereal Diseases Reference Laboratory

Table 11.8 Forensic medical samples: guidelines (modified from Royal College of Physicians (1991)

Samples	Examination	Sampling materials, packing/containers	Comments
Clothing and bedding	Damage, stain location, pubic hairs	Paper bags (dry), polythene bags (wet)	More likely to be positive in CSA than swabs
Saliva	Detection of semen	Bottle (no additive)	Child given bottle can be difficult to obtain
Mouth swab	Dection of semen	Plain sterile swabs	Saliva sample better
Skin swabs	Detection of lubricants, blood, semen, saliva	Plain sterile swabs	Moisten with tap water if stain dry
External vaginal swab	Detection of lubricants, blood, semen, saliva	Plain sterile swabs	External taken before internal
Internal vaginal swab	Detection of lubricants, blood, semen, saliva	Plain sterile swabs	In prepubertal only if obvious penetration
Internal and external anal swabs	Detection of blood, semen, saliva, lubricants	Plain sterile swabs	External taken before internal, consider both even if no injury
Penile swab (swabbing from outside of penis)	Detection of semen, saliva, lubricants	Plain sterile swabs	Urethral swab not required
Hairs – matted head/pubic	Detection of semen	Polythene bags	Matted hair is cut out
Loose pubic hairs	Identification of alien	Polythene bags	—

Notes:
For further details contact the Forensic Science Laboratory for your area.
Forensic Science Laboratories will not handle specimens for sexually transmitted disease investigation.

- Control samples (blood and saliva) for comparison purposes.

Taking swabs may be uncomfortable for the victim, and can be dampened with water but not grease.

Perpetrator Identification

A group of tests, including paternity testing, will enable identification of specific offenders. These include blood typing and DNA fingerprinting techniques. For details the reader is referred to standard forensic texts.

PHOTOGRAPHY IN CHILD ABUSE

Photographs are an important aspect of the investigation of suspected child abuse (Ricci 1990, Hobbs et al 1993a). They are a routine part of the documentation of these cases. Consent should be sought from parents and child, where appropriate. Photographs have various uses:

- As a record to supplement drawings and written descriptions.
- Can be used in court to inform the court more precisely of the nature of the findings.
- Should be available for any second medical opinion required to assess the evidence.
- May be used to avoid the need for a further examination of the child.
- Sometimes prove valuable to illustrate concerns to a parent or other, e.g. social worker, who needs to understand clearly the basis for those concerns.

Hospitals may have a department of medical photography working office hours; the police employ their own photographers. Alternatively, the doctor may have the necessary skills, or where using a colposcope routinely photograph all findings.

Procedure

- Ensure a system of clear identification of date and name of child. Data backs are useful here and can be added to the use of frame counter system on the camera.

- Close-up and more distant shots allow full appreciation of the injury, including relationship to other injuries. Include anatomic landmarks. A scale may be incorporated.
- As with all procedures, time taken for explanation and reassurance, and the assistance of someone who understands what is required yields better results.
- Instant processing cameras can be used, but usually a single lens reflex (SLR) 35 mm camera with interchangeable lenses offers the best quality and flexibility. Hotshoe and/or ring flashes are usually required. The most useful lens for medical photography of this kind has a focal length of between 85 and 105 mm.
- Colour film (slide or reversal) is the best film for general use. Accuracy of colour is important and care must be taken if using artificial light. Quality control is best achieved through a department of medical photography who will monitor material processed commercially.

Slides can be stored in separate storage and be used to generate prints for inclusion in medical records. They can also be used in court or for teaching purposes.

REFERENCES

Ablin AS, Greenspan A, Reinhart M, Grix A (1990) Differentiation of child abuse from osteogenesis imperfecta. *Am J Radiol* 154: 1035–1046.

Branch G, Paxton RA (1965) Study of gonococcal infections amongst infants and children. *Public Hlth Rep* 80: 347–352.

Carty H (1991) Differentiation of child abuse from osteogenesis imperfecta. *Am J Radiol* 156: 635.

Chapman S (1993) Recent advances in the radiology of child abuse. In: Hobbs CJ, Wynne JM (eds) *Baillière's Clinical Paediatrics: Child Abuse*, pp. 211–233. Baillière Tindall, London.

Coant PN, Kornberg AE, Brody AS, Edwards-Holmes K (1992) Markers for occult liver injury in cases of physical abuse in children. *Pediatrics* 89: 274–278.

Cooper A (1992) Thoracoabdominal trauma. In: Ludwig S, Kornberg AE (eds) *Child Abuse: A Medical Reference*, 2nd edn, pp. 131–150. New York, Churchill Livingstone.

Frank DA, Zeisel SH (1988) Failure to thrive. *Pediatr Clin N Am* 35: 1187–1206.

Haller JO, Kleinman PK, Merten DF et al (1991) *Diagnostic Imaging of Child Abuse: Pediatrics*, pp. 262–264. American Academy of Pediatrics, Section on Radiology.

Harvey DR, Kovar IZ (1991) *Child Health*. Churchill Livingstone, Edinburgh.

HMSO (1991) *Working Together under the Children Act 1989. A Guide to Arrangements for Inter-agency Co-operation for the Protection of Children from Abuse.* HMSO, London.

Hobbs CJ, Hanks HGI, Wynne JM (1993) Failure to thrive. In: *Child Abuse and Neglect – A Clinician's Handbook*, Chap. 3, pp. 17–45. London, Churchill Livingstone.

Lacey CJN (1993) Sexually transmitted diseases in the prepubertal child. In: Hobbs CJ, Wynne JM (eds) *Baillière's Clinical Paediatrics*, Chap. 9, volume 1, pp. 165–185. Baillière Tindall, London.

Rosenberg DA (1987) Web of deceit: a literature review of Munchausen syndrome by proxy. *Child Abuse Neglect* 11: 547–563.

Royal College of Physicians (1991) *Physical Signs of Sexual Abuse in Children.* A report of the Royal College of Physicians, London.

Samuels MP, McClaughlin W, Jacobson RR, Poets CF, Southall DP (1992) Fourteen cases of imposed upper airway obstruction. *Arch Dis Child* 67: 162–170.

Shaw JCL (1988) Copper deficiency and non-accidental injury. *Arch Dis Child* 63: 448–455.

Taitz LS (1987) Child abuse and osteogenesis imperfecta. *Br Med J* 295: 1082–1083.

12
Infectious Disease

M J Tarlow

INTRODUCTION

Although infectious illnesses are among the commonest reasons for medical consultation and for admission to hospital, most of those that occur in normal children are relatively trivial. In few of these are investigations either desirable or relevant, and when performed with excessive zeal they may cause distress to the child, affecting the doctor–patient and the doctor–parent relationship for no good reason. However, a minority of childhood infections cause serious or even life-threatening disease; in these any information that clarifies the clinical picture aids management, and in these situations as well as those where epidemiological information is important, investigations are essential. This chapter considers the investigation of some of the more serious or unusual infections of childhood. Our ability to investigate infectious disease is rapidly advancing; the advent of monoclonal antibodies and of DNA probes has revolutionized the approach to diagnosis and, although many techniques are still research rather than clinical tools, it is certain that any future editions of this chapter would need to be extensively rewritten as advances are incorporated in clinical practice.

MENINGITIS

Lumbar Puncture

When to do a Lumbar Puncture

Because of the risks of missing the diagnosis, it is important to have a very high index of suspicion that a child may have meningitis and perform a lumbar puncture on the slightest suggestion. It is widely held that if a unit is finding less than 80–90% of its lumbar punctures negative, its index of suspicion is not high enough.

A lumbar puncture is the critical investigation for the diagnosis of meningitis. It should be performed in all patients in whom meningitis is a possibility, although not always immediately (see below). These should include:

- Those with clinical features characteristic of meningitis; i.e. stiff neck, photophobia, or a positive Kernig's sign (inability to straighten the knee joint when the hip is flexed, due to spasm of hamstrings as a result of irritation of spinal nerves) or Brudzinski's sign (spontaneous flexion of the legs when the neck is passively flexed).
- Those with fever and a disturbance in the level of consciousness, even if the specific features listed above are not clearly present.

Although stiff neck and a bulging fontanelle are frequently considered to be the characteristic features of meningitis, vomiting and headache are actually more sensitive indicators, and an alteration in conscious level or state of alertness is probably the most valuable clinical sign.

Lumbar Puncture in Febrile Fits

The routine performance of a lumbar puncture in children who apparently have a "benign" febrile fit is controversial, and practice differs in different countries and between different individuals. Most consider an initial febrile fit in a child without another obvious focus of infection is sufficient reason to exclude the possibility of meningitis unless the child is obviously alert and well. If this is not done, then any delay in recovery or deterioration in status should certainly lead to a lumbar puncture.

Delay and Contraindication of Lumbar Puncture

Lumbar puncture should be *delayed* (but treatment started) if:

- There is a rapidly deteriorating conscious level, or the patient is comatose.
- Focal neurological signs are present (papilloedema is rare in bacterial meningitis and should suggest a superadded problem such as venous sinus thrombosis, subdural effusion, or brain abscess).
- There is marked bradycardia.

It is *contraindicated* in the presence of a severe bleeding disorder, or of local infection at the proposed site of needle insertion.

If delayed, lumbar puncture can usually be performed within a few hours of the onset of clinical management without significant risk.

In situations where lumbar puncture is not performed, blood culture will reveal the organism in 80% of patients with previously untreated meningitis, since bacteraemia is frequently associated.

Interpretation of Lumbar Puncture (Table 12.1)

The following applies to children outside the neonatal period (in the neonate, the normal values for cerebro-spinal fluid differ from those in later childhood).

Appearance

Approximately 500 cells/mm^3 are necessary to produce cloudiness or opalescence in the sample. *Xanthochromia* is yellow discoloration of the cerebrospinal fluid due to bilirubin, either as a consequence of jaundice or derived from red cell lysis in the cerebrospinal fluid following bleeding. In the latter situation, blood must be present in the cerebrospinal fluid for about 12 h before the colour changes from pink to yellow.

Cell Count

This should be performed immediately. Cerebrospinal fluid neutrophils are rapidly lysed, and decrease after only 1 h to two-thirds, and after 2 h to one-half of their original value.

With regard to *white cells*, outside the neonatal period, any polymorphs in the cerebrospinal fluid are abnormal, although occasional lymphocytes may be found in normal cerebrospinal fluid samples (in neonates, up to 30 cells/cm^3 may occur, some of which will be polymorphs; this is normal and should not be taken as evidence of meningitis).

Approximately 5% of patients with meningitis will have no cells in the cerebrospinal fluid at the time of

Table 12.1   Typical cerebrospinal fluid findings in different forms of meningitis

Condition	White cell numbers mm³	White cell types	Protein	Sugar	Microbiology
Acute bacterial meningitis	Usually 500–10,000	Predominantly polymorphs	High >0.4 g/l. Usually <3 g/l	<2 mm/l in most cases	Organism identifiable on stain or culture in >90% of cases
Brain abscess*	Scanty, usually <200	Usually predominantly lymphocytes; sometimes polymorphs	Usually <0.4 g/l	Normal	No organisms present
Tuberculous meningitis	Up to 500. Usually <100	Predominantly lymphocytes (polymorphs may predominate in early infection)	Raised. May be very high (>10 g/l)	Low in most cases	Acid fast organism in cerebrospinal fluid deposit or culture
Viral meningitis	Usually <1000	Predominantly lymphocytes (polymorphs may predominate in early infection)	Mildly elevated	Normal	

*Note that, in this case, lumbar puncture is dangerous and seldom helpful.

lumbar puncture. This is particularly likely in infancy and in the neonate.

Protein

Protein concentrations of $>0.4\,\text{g/l}$ (40 mg/dl) are abnormally high, denoting increased permeability of the blood–cerebrospinal fluid barrier consistent with infection. They do not differentiate between bacterial and viral meningitis, although in tuberculous meningitis the protein concentration in the cerebrospinal fluid is often particularly high.

Glucose

There are multiple causes of the low cerebrospinal fluid sugar associated with bacterial meningitis. Particularly important is a local switch to anaerobic metabolism, associated with ischaemia and hypoxia. When glucose is metabolized anaerobically less energy is produced than by aerobic metabolism, and so more glucose needs to be broken down to provide enough for local tissues. In most cases of bacterial meningitis the cerebrospinal fluid glucose is $<40\%$ of the blood glucose, which should be checked at approximately (but not necessarily exactly) the same time. Normal cerebrospinal fluid glucose is approximately two-thirds of the blood glucose level.

Bacteria

Bacteria should be carefully sought on the spun deposit of cerebrospinal fluid following lumbar puncture. Each of the three common organisms causing meningitis in childhood has a different appearance.

- *Haemophilus influenzae* Gram-negative coccobacilli.
- *Neisseria meningitidis* Gram-negative cocci, usually in pairs.
- *Streptococcus pneumoniae* Gram-positive cocci, usually in pairs.

If the lumbar puncture is done at an early stage in the illness, children can have meningitis without any white cells detectable in the cerebrospinal fluid; all cerebrospinal fluid should therefore be cultured even if it is crystal clear.

Cerebrospinal Fluid in Meningitis Pretreated with Antibiotics

Antibiotics seldom significantly affect the findings in the cerebrospinal fluid in meningitis which has been pretreated for 48 h or less, but reduce the likelihood of a positive Gram stain or cerebrospinal fluid culture to around 50% (in untreated meningitis, an organism is identifiable in over 90% of cases).

Gram-positive organisms may not stain easily and, therefore, can appear Gram-negative in some cerebrospinal fluid samples following pretreatment with antibiotics.

How to Interpret a "Bloody Tap"

The absolute ratio of white cells/red cells in the peripheral blood should be calculated (e.g. a white cell count of $10 \times 10^9\text{/l}$ and a concurrent red cell count of $5 \times 10^{12}\text{/l}$ gives a white cell/red cell ratio of $1:500$. If the ratio in the cerebrospinal fluid is significantly different from this it suggests that white cells were present in the cerebrospinal fluid before traumatic bleeding due to the lumbar puncture occurred.

Mistakes can occur in calculating this ratio, especially in the middle of the night; it is anyway not 100% accurate. It is safest to interpret a bloody tap as though the bleeding had not occurred, i.e. if any polymorphs at all are present in the cerebrospinal fluid the patient should be treated as if he or she had bacterial meningitis, at least until this is ruled out by negative cerebrospinal fluid culture results.

Rapid Diagnostic Techniques

Countercurrent Immunoelectrophoresis

This is a useful technique for the detection of bacterial antigen. It detects capsular polysaccharide antigens by producing an antibody–antigen precipitation line in an agar gel. It can be used for meningitis due to *Haemophilus influenzae*, pneumococcus, and meningococcus of groups A, C and D, and W 135, but group B meningococci (the common type in the UK) cannot be reliably detected.

Antigen can be detected in samples of urine, cerebrospinal fluid, and serum; the test is most sensitive when all are screened together, although positive results can be obtained from urine (which is concentrated before analysis) when cerebrospinal fluid is negative. A result can be obtained within 1 h. The sensitivity of this technique means that even after antibiotic therapy sufficient antigen may still be present to make a diagnosis when no growth is obtained on culture. A negative result, however, does not exclude the diagnosis.

Latex Agglutination

This also detects bacterial antigen, and can be used for all common meningitis producing organisms, although the commercially available kits are relatively insensitive in detecting group B meningococci. The technique overall is more sensitive than countercurrent immunoelectrophoresis. Interpretation of positive latex tests in urine and sera may be difficult, because of non-specific agglutination or of cross-reactions between different organisms.

Positive latex tests in urine can be obtained for 10 days or so after *Haemophilus influenzae* immunization. Both latex agglutination and countercurrent immunoelectrophoresis may be positive after previous antibiotic therapy, when the organism cannot be detected by direct culture.

DNA Hybridization and Polymerase Chain Reaction (PCR)

These techniques, which detect bacterial DNA, are just becoming available to the routine laboratory, and will revolutionize the rapid diagnosis of pathogens in clinical specimens. They are likely to be particularly valuable in diagnosis of viral infections.

Bacterial Cultures from other Sites

These are neither sensitive nor specific, and apart from blood cultures have little part to play in the aetiological diagnosis of bacterial meningitis. In meningococcal meningitis with septicaemia and purpura, Gram stain and culture of fluid obtained by puncture of a purpuric lesion may directly show the organism.

When to do a Computerized Tomography (CT) Scan in Meningitis

If only a few instances is a CT scan helpful in the management of bacterial meningitis. These include:

- Prolonged impairment of conscious level (most patients with meningitis will show significant improvement within 48 h of the initiation of appropriate antibiotic therapy).
- Focal neurological abnormalities.
- Rapid increase in head circumference.
- Relapse or recurrence of illness during or shortly after treatment.

CT scan is the investigation of choice for the confirmation of a suspected cerebral abscess.

UNEXPLAINED FEVER

Fever without Localizing Signs

The term "fever without localizing signs" has been used by many for patients with fever of 7 *days or less* duration with no obvious focus of infection.

Most of these children do not need detailed investigation unless there is other clinical cause for concern.

Occult Bacteraemia

Blood cultures in this group of children will yield positive results in about 5% of cases, even though the children are not particularly ill. *Pneumococcus* is the commonest organism found, and the peak incidence is in the toddler age group. The white blood cell count, sedimentation rate, toxic granulation of the neutrophils or the response to antipyretics are of limited value in predicting bacteraemia in these children. It is, however, important to identify them, since if they are not treated with antibiotics a significant proportion will go on to get meningitis, localized infection, or persisting bacteraemia and fever.

If bacteraemia is thought possible on clinical grounds (i.e. the child looks ill, or has some predisposing factor detected in the history or on physical examination), investigations should include a full blood picture, urine culture, and blood culture. Other investigations need only be performed if clinically indicated.

Any child who has visited a malarial area within the last 6 months should have at least one thick blood film taken for malaria parasites; this should be examined immediately. There are approximately 12 deaths annually in Britain from malaria – all of them potentially preventable.

Pyrexia of Unknown Origin (PUO)

This is defined by fever lasting 8 *days or more* in which initial history, examination and investigations have not revealed the cause.

Most patients with a PUO have common conditions. These will usually be localized infections, expecially upper respiratory or urinary infections, occult abscesses in the pelvis or abdomen (although in the latter cases there will almost always be a clinical clue) or, in younger children, osteomyelitis. Important systemic infections to be considered include infectious mononucleosis, cytomegalovirus, tuberculosis, brucellosis, salmonellosis, and hepatitis (which may be non-icteric). Cat-scratch fever, Q-fever and leptospirosis need only be considered where there is some clinical indication from the history that they might be relevant.

Important non-infectious causes include juvenile chronic arthritis, systemic lupus erythematosus and inflammatory bowel disease; ectodermal dysplasias and diabetes insipidus should be considered where relevant.

Clinical Management

Good history and examination are paramount, and will usually give clues (e.g. mild clubbing, anal skin tags in inflammatory bowel disease). In most series, 20% or more of children with an apparent PUO had strong diagnostic clues evident when history was retaken or the child re-examined. Zoonoses should be considered and contact with pets or wild animals defined carefully.

A significant minority of children have "factitious" fever produced by the child himself or herself or by a parent (Munchausen's syndrome by proxy); in the absence of other physical signs in a child with fever this possibility should be considered carefully before embarking on lengthy and costly hospital investigations.

Pattern of Fever

This is less helpful than the older textbooks suggest.

Intermittent fever, returning to normal at least once daily, occurs in pyogenic infections, tuberculosis, juvenile chronic arthritis and lymphoma.

Sustained fever with little fluctuation is said to be characteristic of typhoid fever.

Relapsing fever is associated with a normal temperature for several days at a time before recurring. Malaria, Weil's disease, Lyme disease, and lymphomas are said characteristically to behave in this fashion. However, it must be reiterated that the diagnostic value of fever pattern is limited, and no disorder should be ruled out because of failure to present with a "textbook" temperature chart.

Investigations

These include: a full blood picture, including platelet count, a blood film for differential count, atypical lymphocytes suggestive of viral infection, the presence of toxic granulation suggests infection, and the presence of abnormal white cells suggestive of leukaemia.

Non-specific indices of inflammation such as the ESR, plasma viscosity, or C-reactive protein are of very limited value, except to follow the progress of the condition; even here clinical observation is generally more helpful.

Blood cultures should be taken routinely; if there are clinical grounds for suspecting an unusual organism (e.g. *Leptospira* in a child who has been exposed to rats or standing water) this should be discussed with the laboratory since unusual media or culture conditions may be necessary.

Urine microscopy and culture are obligatory and comprise one of the most valuable investigations in these children.

Chest X-ray should be performed on all children. If clinically indicated, sinus and mastoid X-rays should be checked.

A Mantoux test (10TU-PPD) should be performed on all patients. If this is negative and there are strong clinical reasons to suspect tuberculosis (TB), higher strength tuberculin should be used.

Bone marrow examination should be performed in relevant patients. This will indicate not only the presence of a leukaemia or other malignancy, but will also allow the detection of a wide variety of infectious organisms including *Mycobacterium tuberculosis*, rickettsia and fungi.

HIV testing should be done if clinical grounds exist for suspicion.

Radio-isotope scans (e.g. gallium or indium labelled leucocytes) can be used to detect the site of an infection. These need only be performed if there are good grounds for suspecting a localized but deep-seated infection. Most clinicians have found them of limited value.

Liver biopsy, lymph node biopsy, etc., need be done only if clinical indications exist.

Trial of Drugs

Aspirin is of value in possible juvenile chronic arthritis. Anti-TB therapy in probable (or even possible) disseminated TB may be life-saving. Otherwise, antibiotic or steroid trials without a diagnosis confuse the clinical picture and delay appropriate therapy. They should not be used except as a last resort in a sick child.

KAWASAKI DISEASE

Diagnosis

There is no diagnostic test for Kawasaki disease. Conventionally, *five* of the following *six* clinical criteria have to be met:

- *Fever* – lasting more than 5 days and not responding to antibiotics.
- *Conjunctivitis* – bilateral and non-purulent.
- *Changes of lips and mouth* – one or more of the following:
   (a) dry, reddened, fissured lips;
   (b) reddened oropharyngeal mucosa;
   (c) strawberry tongue.
- *Changes of peripheral extremities*:
   (a) reddened palms and soles;
   (b) oedema of hands or feet;
   (c) desquamation of hands and/or feet.
- *Rash*.
- *Acute non-purulent cervical lymphadenopathy*.

If coronary aneurysms can be recognized on echo-cardiography or coronary angiography, only *four* of the above criteria need be met.

Atypical Kawasaki Disease

Atypical cases are being recognized with increasing frequency. These patients have the pathognomonic cardiac abnormalities without the four other criteria referred to above.

Laboratory Data

The *platelet count* is almost always raised, especially after the 10th day of illness. In suspicious cases a raised platelet count should be an indication for echocardiography.

Since there is now evidence that immunoglobulin treatment has a beneficial effect, early diagnosis is important, and a case can be made for treating probable or even possible cases who do not fulfil all criteria for diagnosis.

UNUSUAL INFECTIONS

Lyme Disease

This is caused by the spirochaete *Borrelia burgdorferi*. It is a tick-born disease carried especially by ticks of the *Ixodes* genus. It is present in most temperate countries; it is described in Britain especially in the area of the New Forest in Hampshire, being sporadic in many other areas.

A variety of animal hosts exist, particularly mouse and deer.

Transmission

The spirochaete needs to travel from gut to salivary glands of the tick. This takes 24–48 h after attachment; disease is therefore unlikely unless the tick has been attached to the host for many hours.

Clinical Features

Early (up to 1 Month)

This presents with an influenza-like illness with a characteristic erythematous expanding rash (erythema chronicum migrans) and with a migratory arthralgia/myalgia. At this stage, serology or cerebrospinal fluid analysis usually yield normal results, but a skin biopsy may show the organism in up to 50% of patients. The rash and the clinical history considered together are pathognomonic.

Early Disseminated

This presents with neurological symptoms including fatigue, signs of meningism and with cranial nerve palsies, especially Bell's palsy. In addition, cardiac features can occur, including pancarditis and atrioventricular block.

Late Features

Late features of the disease, which may take years to appear, include a characteristic atrophic dermatitis of the extremities, acrodermatitis chronica atrophicans, an intermittent migratory polyarthritis (which can be mistaken for juvenile chronic arthritis), and neurological symptoms which may progress from chronic fatigue to demyelination and dementia.

Diagnosis

Diagnosis is best made on clinical grounds, especially from the characteristic appearance or description of the typical rash of erythema chronicum migrans. Routine laboratory tests are seldom helpful.

Of the *specific investigations*, only serology is sufficiently widely available and accurate enough for routine use.

ELISA detection of specific antibody is currently the most specific technique, but is not likely to be positive less then 1 month after bite.

Blood or tissue culture is difficult and seldom helpful.

Legionnaire's Disease

Legionnaire's disease is very unusual in children except in the immunocompromised and only a handful of cases have been reported. It seldom needs to be considered in the differential diagnosis of severe or unexplained pneumonia in childhood (less than 20 paediatric cases have been reported world-wide). The incidence of seroconversion to the antigen, however, is higher, although still unusual. This suggests that, although infection may occur in normal children, it is almost always asymptomatic.

Investigations

Sputum collection (tracheal aspirate) and culture on selective media is the normal method of diagnosis, although immunofluorescent microscopy of sputum samples is highly specific in experienced hands.

Because of the rarity of Legionnaire's disease in children, serological testing for it is rarely indicated. A single raised titre is not diagnostic and paired acute and convalescent sera are necessary.

Weil's Disease

A wide variety of animals have been described as reservoirs of leptospirosis, but in Britain by far the most likely source of infection is the rat, particularly by contamination of fresh or stagnant water sources with rat urine.

The clinical course is generally of an initial septicaemic phase after an incubation period of 1–2 weeks. This is followed by the so-called "immune" stage, lasting up to a month, and characterized if anicteric by meningitis, uveitis and fever, and if icteric by hepatitis, myocarditis, renal failure and bleeding.

Diagnosis

It is important to have a high degree of suspicion. *Leptospira* are present in the blood and cerebrospinal fluid during the septicaemic stage of the illness, and from the urine in the immune phase. Laboratory cultivation is difficult and special laboratory media need to be used. As blood concentrations of *Leptospira* are often low, multiple cultures should be taken. Cultures may need to be maintained for several weeks at lower temperatures than usual (28–30°C) before growth is detected.

Serology

Slide agglutination tests are used for rapid diagnosis. Killed organisms on a microscope slide are agglutinated by biological fluids (usually serum) containing *Leptospira* antibodies. ELISA assays are available in some laboratories, and a wide variety of other tests are now becoming available. Agglutination titres become positive towards the end of the first week of the illness, and are maximal at about 4 weeks, remaining positive in low titre for years.

Cat-scratch Fever

This is characterized by regional lymph node enlargement following a scratch or bite from a cat. The causative organism has recently been defined – a bacterium known as *Rochalimaea henselae* – although a second organism, *Afipia felis*, may be responsible for some cases. *Rochalimaea* is a small Gram-negative pleomorphic organism detectable in biopsy material from affected lymph nodes. A conjunctival scratch may lead to enlargement of the preauricular lymph node (Parinaud's oculoglandular syndrome) and occasionally cat-scratch disease may be associated with, or even present as, an encephalitis or a hepatitis.

Diagnosis

Diagnosis is generally clinical, depending on three of the following four criteria:

- History of cat scratch or bite approximately 2 weeks earlier.
- No other detectable cause for lymphadenopathy.
- Positive skin test with cat-scratch antigen.
- Characteristic biopsy appearance, preferably with pleomorphic bacteria detectable on silver staining.

Cat-scratch Antigen

This is unstandardized and the reagent (Hanger–Rose skin test antigen) is not readily available. It is injected intradermally into the forearm, and read at 48 h. Induration of 5 mm or more is regarded as positive. Skin testing should not be performed until lymphadenopathy has been present for at least 1 week.

Immunofluorescent antibody tests are available, as are polymerase chain reaction (PCR) detection of *Rochalimaea* rRNA. However, until further progress is made defining the roles of the two putative aetiological agents precisely, neither of these could be considered conclusive.

There appear to be close links between cat-scratch disease, bacillary angiomatosis (a disorder causing multiple nodular skin lesions in AIDS patients), and the skin changes of bartonellosis (a South American infection) and of Kaposi's sarcoma. Trench fever may be related, and all may be caused by similar organisms.

Toxoplasmosis

Toxoplasmosis is due to infection with a protozoon, *Toxoplasma gondii*. The definitive host is the cat, and the disease occurs in children either through congenital infection or by ingesting oocysts from the faeces of infected cats.

Congenital infection only occurs when primary infection of the mother occurs during pregnancy.

Acquired infection is usually the result of contact with cat faeces, but can also occur through eating raw or undercooked meat containing *Toxoplasma* oocysts, or from infected unpasteurized milk (e.g. goat's milk).

Acquired infection is usually asymptomatic. If symptomatic, fever and lymphadenopathy are characteristic, and the illness may present as a glandular-fever-like syndrome.

Ocular toxoplasmosis, usually presenting as visual impairment associated with choroidoretinitis, is usually congenital.

Investigations

Congenital Infection

Serological demonstration of IgM or IgA antibodies in the blood or cerebrospinal fluid in the first 6 months of life is good evidence of congenital infection. In an infant of 12 months or less, IgG antibody may have been derived transplacentally, and therefore cannot be taken as evidence of infection of the infant.

Acquired infection

The presence of IgM antibody to *Toxoplasma* is good evidence of recent infection; if IgG antibody is used for diagnosis, a rising titre over a 3–4 week period needs to be demonstrated to show current rather than old infection.

The Sabin Dye Test

This shows the presence of IgG antibodies to *Toxoplasma* and is the most reliable demonstration of exposure to the organism.

Other Tests

ELISA and immunofluorescence tests for antibodies in blood are also available.

Botulism

This rare toxin-induced disease needs a high index of suspicion for its diagnosis. It should be considered in any patient with (characteristically) a descending symmetrical motor paralysis, without fever or disturbed consciousness. The vast majority of cases are due to improperly preserved foods, either commercially available or home bottled or canned. Serum (30 ml of blood if possible), gastric washings, and faeces should be collected before antitoxin is given. The suspect food should be immediately refrigerated, if possible in its original container and sent to the nearest appropriate laboratory.

Extreme care should be taken in handling potential infected material – even inhalation of minute quantities may be fatal.

The organism and/or the toxin can often be detected in stool or other biological samples relatively late in the course of the illness. The presence of toxin or organism in samples from a symptomatic person is diagnostic.

Wound botulism occurs especially in children with compound fractures.

Infant Botulism

This is due to ingestion of botulinus spores which germinate and colonize the infant colon, leading to a flaccid paralysis because of the local production of botulinus toxin. The organism cannot grow in the colon of older patients except in rare cases after broad-spectrum antibiotic treatment. Honey, which may contain spores of *Clostridium botulinum*, is the only food to date that has been linked with infant botulism. The diagnosis is made by demonstrating *C. botulinum* organism, spores or toxin in a faecal sample from a baby with appropriate clinical signs.

Q-fever

Q-fever is a rickettsial disease due to *Coxiella burnetii*. The disease is contracted from infected livestock, particularly sheep, and it should be considered in any child with a generalized infective illness who has been in contact with farm animals, especially if they have pneumonitis, although hepatitis and carditis are also frequently recognized.

Diagnosis

Diagnosis is serological. No attempts should be made to isolate the organism – this exposes laboratory staff to the risk of infection. A definitive diagnosis is important as Q-fever is treated preferentially with tetracycline, a drug not commonly used otherwise in paediatrics.

Human Herpesvirus-6 (HHV-6)

This has only been recognized in the last few years (since 1986) as the cause of exanthem subitum (roseola) in infants and young children. Diagnostic serological tests are not yet available, although the organism can be cultured from peripheral blood cells in most affected children, the highest incidence being just before the appearance of the rash. Rarely, encephalitis and hepatitis have been described.

Parvovirus B19

This commonly causes "slapped cheek" syndrome (erythema infectiosum), but is also responsible for the aplastic crises which may occur in chronic haemolytic anaemias. Diagnosis is suspected clinically, and confirmed serologically, usually by the demonstration of specific IgM antibody. Viral antigen itself can be detected by gene probes or by the polymerase chain reaction.

PNEUMONIA

Most childhood pneumonias are non-bacterial. In infants, respiratory syncytial virus (RSV), influenza and parainfluenza viruses, Coxsackie, echoviruses, and adenoviruses are important; *Chlamydia* ssp. are recognized pathogens in the neonate and may be much more important than previously recognized in older children. *Mycoplasma pneumoniae* is a significant problem in children over 5 years of age, although it is unusual in younger children.

Viral Pneumonias

Unlike the bacteria which cause pneumonias, the major respiratory viruses are not usually carried asymptomatically in the upper respiratory tract. Isolation of an appropriate pathogenic virus on throat swab is likely to be significant.

Rapid Diagnosis

Most of these common respiratory pathogens can now be diagnosed using rapid techniques such as nucleic acid hybridization or PCR which detect nucleic acid directly, or by rapid immunological techniques (particularly immunofluorescence) that detect viral antigen. Many laboratories can therefore now offer "same-day" diagnosis of serious viral infections.

Serological Techniques

These are of value in the diagnosis of chlamydial and mycoplasma infections where the organisms cannot readily be grown directly.

In infants chlamydial pneumonia IgG antibody is detectable at the onset of the illness.

Diagnosis

Under the age of 5 years sputum cannot easily be collected from children. The following techniques are of value in reaching an aetiological diagnosis in bacterial pneumonias.

Blood Culture

This is positive in about 10% of children with radiological evidence of pneumonia.

Nasopharyngeal Aspiration/Tracheal Aspiration

These samples are often contaminated with upper respiratory tract pathogens and, therefore, results are misleading unless collected through a double-lumen catheter or during direct laryngoscopy.

Pleural Aspiration

This is a particularly valuable technique which should be attempted in all cases of pleural effusion where the aetiological diagnosis is not immediately available.

Aspiration of Pulmonary Exudate

This has been used in sick children in whom an immediate diagnosis is important.

Throat Swabs

In distinction to viral pneumonias, throat swabs are of very little value in the diagnosis of bacterial pneumonia.

Atypical Pneumonia

This term is used to describe a variety of non-bacterial pneumonias in children. The most frequent cause is RSV, followed in younger children (under 5 years) by parainfluenza virus infections. In older children mycoplasmas are the commonest non-bacterial cause of pneumonia.

TUBERCULOSIS

Tuberculosis should be suspected in the following cases:

- *Contact with an adult with active disease* (strongest indicator).
- *Positive Mantoux test*. After intradermal injection of 0.1 ml 1:1000 PPD (10 TU) into the volar aspect of the forearm, the test is read at 48–72 h. The diameter of the induration (*not* the erythema) is measured.

  Previously BCG immunization is associated with a positive Mantoux, but this is usually less than 10 mm in diameter and is transient.

  For skin testing of children who are contacts of known cases, or who are immunocompromised or malnourished, a Mantoux test >5 mm should be regarded as positive, otherwise a 10 mm diameter reaction is needed.
- *Chest X-ray*. Children get primary tuberculosis, which is characterized by hilar lymphadenopathy; only occasionally is the peripheral parenchymal lesion seen, but

lymphadenopathy may lead to lobar collapse or emphysema. Pleural effusions are frequently present if the lung lesion or lymph node has ruptured into the pleural cavity. These are rare under 2 years of age.

Clinical Features

Most children with tuberculosis are asymptomatic, and are diagnosed through contact tracing. When symptoms are present they are often non-specific, with fever, cough, night sweats, and failure to thrive.

Extrapulmonary Tuberculosis

Cervical lymphadenopathy is now usually due to spread from mediastinal lymph nodes, rather than primary tonsillar infection. These should not be biopsied unless absolutely necessary because of the high incidence of sinus formation.

Tuberculosis of the Central Nervous System

This usually develops slowly and insidiously. Involvement of the base of the brain leads to a high incidence of cranial nerve palsies.

Tubercle bacilli are only infrequently cultured from the cerebrospinal fluid, but computerized tomography (CT) scan may be valuable in demonstrating brain-stem meningitis and communicating hydrocephalus.

Diagnostic Tests

Routine chemical or haematological tests are not helpful, but abnormal liver function tests may suggest miliary tuberculosis (liver biopsy is a potentially effective way of diagnosing miliary tuberculosis by detecting granulomas; urine culture is similarly valuable, since organisms are frequently excreted in the urine and can be cultured from it).

Culture for tuberculosis

In most paediatric cases, diagnosis is not dependent on isolation of the organism, but is made on clinical, epidemiological and radiological grounds, together with skin testing. It is important, however, to try to verify the diagnosis in extrapulmonary tuberculosis, and in those cases where no source is evident.

Older children (over 5 years of age) can produce sputum, as can an adult (but remember that most cases of childhood pulmonary tuberculosis will be closed, and the children will not be excreting tubercle bacilli in the sputum). In younger children, early morning gastric washings will detect the organism in about one-third of cases, but should be interpreted with caution, since they can be contaminated with acid-fast bacteria from the mouth.

Cultures normally take about 6 weeks on conventional media. Most authorities would advise treatment of all children with strongly positive Mantoux tests even if they are asymptomatic. Treatment is mandatory for contacts of cases who have positive tests, for those who are immunocompromised or immunodeficient, and for those with chest X-ray abnormalities.

Infants of mothers with tuberculosis in pregnancy should be treated for 3 months or until it is clear that the mother no longer has "open" disease.

Serological Diagnosis

An ELISA assay to detect an antibody to a protein in *Mycobacterium tuberculosis* known as *antigen 5* has recently been introduced. This may be helpful in blood samples of patients with pulmonary tuberculosis, but has only had a poor sensitivity in cerebrospinal fluid samples of patients with meningeal TB.

DNA Probes

Probes for mycobacterial ribosomal RNA have been used in research studies and appear to be very promising diagnostic techniques. They are currently too insensitive to be of clinical value, but PCR methods are under investigation; these should provide a specific, sensitive and speedy way of detecting mycobacterial DNA, and are likely to revolutionize our investigational approach to tuberculosis.

NON-TUBERCULOUS MYCOBACTERIAL INFECTIONS

These have recently become prominent because of the increased incidence of mycobacterial infections, both tuberculous and non-tuberculous in children with AIDS. However, they represent a significant minority of children with mycobacterial infections and deserve attention in their own right. Clinically they usually present with cervical lymphadenopathy or with skin tuberculosis.

The lymphadenopathy is usually painless and is slow-growing, with discoloration of the overlying skin, and later sinus formation. The children are otherwise well.

Investigations

The diagnosis is generally made on epidemiological grounds and clinical features. Acid-fast smears of biopsy material are frequently negative, as only very few organisms may be present. The Mantoux test is generally positive but < 10 mm in diameter.

Confirmation of the clinical diagnosis is difficult and depends on culture and isolation of the organism. In most instances the diagnosis remains a clinical one. Treatment is surgical excision.

BONE AND JOINT INFECTIONS

The diagnosis of bone and joint infections in children may be difficult, particularly since localizing signs are not always present, and bones and joints are difficult to examine directly. Laboratory and other ancillary investigations therefore assume a particularly prominent role (see also Chapter 18).

Radiology

This is very useful in many cases. Oedema of the soft tissues around the site of osteomyelitis or arthritis is a valuable clue to the diagnosis. Evidence of destruction of the bone is a late feature and should not be expected if the history is less than 10–14 days.

Radioisotope Imaging

Technetium scans have a poor sensitivity and specificity except in very experienced hands, and must always be interpreted in conjunction with the clinical data. They are seldom of value in neonates.

Gallium scans should be used sparingly since they involve more radiation than technetium scans, but in osteomyelitis they are more specific and sensitive.

Magnetic Resonance Imaging

This may be a very effective way of differentiating bone from joint or soft tissue infection.

Aspiration of Pus from Bone or Joint

This should be attempted wherever practicable in order to make a bacteriological diagnosis and obtain sensitivities, if the organism cannot be isolated by other means. However, many children with bone or joint infections will have a septicaemia, and the organism can thus be simply confirmed by blood culture.

IMPORTED INFECTIONS

Malaria is by far the most important, and the only one which will be considered here (but see "Gastrointestinal Infections").

Malaria

Malaria is a medical emergency: immediate treatment is essential.

Malaria is usually relatively easy to treat, but if undiagnosed can be fatal. Approximately 12 people die of malaria in Britain each year. Most deaths are due to *Plasmodium falciparum* infections; the other species of plasmodium cause unpleasant fevers but seldom more.

It is most important to have a high index of suspicion for this relatively rare illness.

Clinical Features

The clinical features are non-specific: Fever, malaise, headache, and sweating. The condition is usually misdiagnosed as "influenza". The patient may present with a febrile fit. Other symptoms such as vomiting, diarrhoea, cough or abdominal pain are common, and do not preclude the diagnosis.

Thick Blood Film

All children who have travelled to a malarial area within the last 6 months and present with fever, *or febrile neonates or infants whose mothers travelled in pregnancy*, should have a thick blood film to screen for malaria.

This should be examined *immediately*.

If malaria is diagnosed on the blood film, but the type is unclear, the condition should be treated as falciparum malaria.

Over 90% of patients with falciparum malaria will have been in Africa within the preceding 2 months.

Monitoring

Daily blood films should be examined until asexual parasites have disappeared (should have gone by day 5); gametocytes detectable in red blood cells do not imply treatment failure.

GASTROINTESTINAL INFECTIONS
Acute Gastroenteritis

A distinction should be made between the patient who has profuse watery diarrhoea (a small intestinal infection) usually free of blood or mucus, and the individual who passes blood or mucus in the stool which also contains many polymorphs. This latter dysenteric picture is the clinical hallmark of a large bowel infection.

In Britain the vast majority of infective diarrhoeas are the result of small bowel infection (an enteritis) and the commonest cause is rotavirus, which is particularly prevalent in the winter, and affects children under 5 years.

Enteric Fever (Typhoid Fever)

This is a syndrome of systemic *Salmonella* infection usually caused by *Salmonella typhi*, but which can also be associated with other invasive *Salmonella* infections. It includes typhoid and paratyphoid fevers. Typhoid is now seldom seen in Britain except in those who have recently travelled abroad.

Diagnosis

The blood picture is non-specific, but often shows leucopaenia, and a mild to moderate normochromic anaemia.

Investigations

Stool cultures will be positive in those with diarrhoea. In patients presenting with systemic symptoms, blood cultures should be taken. Several may be necessary as bacteraemia is sometimes intermittent. If blood cultures are negative, e.g. in those children pretreated with antibiotics, bone marrow aspirates should be cultured; these are often positive in the absence of other diagnostic evidence.

Duodenal fluid is said to be as sensitive a source of *Salmonella* isolation as bone marrow.

Serology for *Salmonella typhi*

In general the *Widal test*, which detects antibodies to the O and H surface antigens of *Salmonella typhi*, is of little value, since both false-negative and false-positive results are common.

Latex agglutination and ELISA tests with monoclonal antibodies are both available and in current use; a fluorescent antibody test to *Salmonella typhi* Vi antigen, and molecular probes for the nucleic acid both exist, but are currently research rather than practical procedures.

Dysenteric Infections

In Britain these are usually caused by *Campylobacter* or *Shigella* species, although it must be remembered that both of these can also produce a diarrhoeal illness without blood or mucus.

Diagnosis

In children and infants with bloody diarrhoea, stool culture will usually detect the organism. Rectal swabs are of value when stool is not immediately available. *Shigella* is not viable for long periods outside the body, and stools should therefore be collected and processed without delay. Cultures are more likely to be positive early in the course of the disease when there are large numbers of viable organisms in the stool.

Serological Studies

These are of limited clinical value, since serum antibodies, when present, do not develop until after recovery. However, they are of use in epidemiological studies.

Food Poisoning

"Food poisoning" is the commonly used term for a toxin-induced illness associated with food ingestion. Since the toxin is present in high concentration in the food ingested, the symptoms develop rapidly (within hours) and thus can be distinguished clinically from gastroenteritis or dysentery, which will take days rather than hours to develop. Bacterial food poisoning developing within 6 h of ingestion is usually due to staphylococcal or *Bacillus cereus* toxin, that developing in about 12 h is more commonly clostridial. In all cases attempts should be made to obtain the food incriminated, which should be refrigerated and transported to the laboratory as quickly as possible.

Direct Microscopic Examination of Stool

Indications: Children who have travelled to areas where gut parasites are endemic and who have continuing symptoms for more than 1 week after return.

This will detect leucocytes, and thus separate those infections due to viruses, parasites, or non-invasive (toxin-producing) bacteria from those producing a colitis, usually with dysenteric symptoms.

In addition trophozoites, cysts, and ova will be detected, allowing the diagnosis of *Giardia, Cryptosporidium, Isospora*, and the larvae of *Strongyloides stercoralis*.

Stools should be examined within 1 h of being passed for the greatest likelihood of detecting these parasites. In situations where this is not possible, stools can be collected into a preservative such as 10% formalin.

Some parasites such as *Giardia* and *Cryptosporidium* may not be easily detectable in the stool, although they are present in high concentration in the upper gut. In these children duodenal fluid can be collected by aspiration or by using a commercially available nylon string (Entero-test, Hedeco, Palo Alto, CA) which can be swallowed and withdrawn several hours later; duodenal fluid present on the string can then be examined microscopically. Duodenal biopsy is the most reliable way of diagnosing giardiasis, and biopsies from suspected cases should always be carefully examined histologically; in addition the fluid remaining in the biopsy capsule should be immediately examined microscopically for the presence of trophozoites.

Gastroenteritis – when to culture stools

In most children with mild self-limited diarrhoea, stool culture is not necessary except for epidemiological purposes. All children with colitis should have stools cultured, as should those with severe illness with systemic symptoms, in whom blood cultures should also be taken. In all children with diarrhoea who have returned from areas where gut infections are endemic, both stool cultures and direct microscopy of the stool should be undertaken. If suspicion still exists it is justifiable to collect duodenal fluid or perform a jejunal biopsy to reach a diagnosis.

Serotyping for *Escherichia coli*

Escherichia coli diarrhoeas have been classified according to their pathological mechanism as enterotoxigenic (ETEC), enteropathogenic (EPEC), enteroinvasive (EIEC) and enterohaemorrhagic (EHEC). Serotyping will help identify the EPEC strains and is valuable in tracing outbreaks of infection. It is not necessary for sporadic cases. The EHEC organisms belong mostly to a single serogroup (0157:H7) which produces a shiga-like toxin. These bacteria are associated with haemolytic–uraemic syndrome in some patients and characteristically produce bloody diarrhoea.

Proctoscopy

In children with colitis in whom the condition does not resolve and in whom the diagnosis is obscure, proctoscopy and biopsy may be very valuable. If proctoscopy/sigmoidoscopy is performed biopsy is mandatory when inflammatory bowel disease is a possibility.

FUNGAL AND SKIN INFECTIONS

Most skin infections are diagnosed on clinical grounds if specific diagnosis is considered at all. When an aetiological diagnosis is necessary the following techniques should be used.

- Vesicles should be scraped for cytological study.
- Petechiae should be punctured, petechial fluid obtained, and the fluid stained for meningococci (when appropriate). Apart from Gram-stain of cerebrospinal fluid, this is the only way of immediately confirming a suspected diagnosis of disseminated meningococcal infection.

Fungal skin infections are classified according to their site rather than their aetiology; tinea of the scalp (tinea capitis) is by far the commonest problem in children. Hair is affected and scaling, alopecia and broken hairs are characteristic.

Examination under a Wood's Light

Tinea capitis due to some (but not all) skin fungi exhibits a characteristic green fluorescence under a Wood's light. A positive result is therefore of diagnostic value, while lack of fluorescence does not exclude infection.

When suspected, skin scraping should be performed to obtain material for laboratory examination. The skin is cleaned and then scraped from the centre towards the margin of the lesion. Nail specimens should be taken from the subungual nail bed as far from superficial contamination as possible.

Ringworm (Tinea)

Scalp ringworm can often be confirmed by examination of the hair. The hair follicle itself is the part most likely to be positive; examining a cut hair or hairs will not usually yield any useful results. Hairs can usually be removed by scraping the infected area since they are damaged and loose; otherwise hair bases can be dislodged from the follicles with a pair of forceps.

In addition to culture, all samples obtained for fungal study should be mounted in 20% potassium hydroxide and examined directly. Hyphae are visible more easily if the lighting is turned low, since they may be transparent and therefore invisible in bright light.

Culture is usually on Saboraud's medium which contains both cycloheximide and an antibiotic. Fungi grow slowly, and several weeks may elapse before a positive culture is obtained.

HUMAN IMMUNODEFICIENCY VIRUS (HIV) AND ACQUIRED IMMUNE DEFICIENCY SYNDROME (AIDS)

The demonstration that the HIV virus has been transmitted from an affected mother to her infant is a difficult one. Antibodies to HIV can cross the placenta, and therefore the demonstration that an infant has antibodies is inadequate. It is necessary to show that viral antigen has crossed the placenta, or that the antibodies demonstrated have been produced by the infant rather than the mother and that the infant has therefore been infected with the virus.

The following tests are available, and are used in different centres.

- Direct viral culture in peripheral blood mononuclear cells.
- Detection of HIV p24 (core viral antigen) in peripheral blood.
- Demonstration of infant (IgM or IgA) anti-HIV antibody.
- Detection of part of the viral gene in the infant's peripheral blood cells by the PCR.

Currently, direct viral culture from the baby's blood and PCR are the most sensitive techniques.

By 15 months of age maternal antibody has disappeared from the infants' blood, and standard tests for HIV (ELISA test for serum antibodies to HIV and Western blot to provide confirmation) can be performed as in adults.

The diagnosis is so important that two positive ELISA tests *and* a positive Western blot should be obtained to confirm the diagnosis.

The Diagnosis of AIDS

This is a clinical diagnosis made in HIV-positive children. An inverted CD4/CD8 ratio and hypergammaglobulinaemia are highly suggestive features in an at-risk child.

The diagnosis is confirmed by the development of an opportunistic infection in an at-risk child. Confirmation of the diagnosis and advice on management should be obtained with the assistance of the paediatrician directing the local AIDS service.

THE CHILD WITH RECURRENT INFECTIONS

Who to Investigate for Immunodeficiency

Children get frequent and recurrent mild infections in the absence of any underlying immune defect. Which of these should be investigated further to exclude a possible immunodeficiency? A reasonable clinical rule-of-thumb

is to allow any child one serious infection (e.g. meningitis, pneumonia, septicaemia, etc.) in a 2-year period; any more than that deserves investigation. Remember that most children investigated by these criteria will have normal immune systems.

Two infections of the same site or system should lead to non-immunological causes (including anatomical abnormalities) being ruled out before detailed immunological studies are performed.

Non-immunological Causes of Recurrent Infection

Recurrent meningitis
- Skull fracture, especially involving cribriform plate; cerebrospinal fluid rhinorrhoea or otorrhoea.
- Midline defects, especially sinuses communicating with cerebrospinal fluid.
- Inner-ear abnormalities.
- Chronic middle-ear/temporal bone infection.

Recurrent pneumonia
- Gastro-oesophageal reflux.
- Cystic fibrosis.
- Swallowing disorders.
- Heart disease (especially left-to-right shunt).
- Anatomical or vascular lung abnormalities.

Recurrent urinary tract infections
- Vesicoureteric reflux.
- Anatomical renal problems, particularly those associated with obstruction to urine flow.

Recurrent otitis media
- Defined by the occurrence of more than three infections in 6 months in a child over the age of 5 years.
- Cleft palate (including a submucous cleft).
- Down's syndrome.

History and Examination

This should include a careful family history as well as a personal history. Risk factors for HIV infection should be included. Examination should include a search for lymphoreticular tissue (e.g. tonsils, adenoids, and spleen, and for evidence of albinism (Chediak–Higashi syndrome) eczema, thrombocytopenia and recurrent otitis media (Wiskott–Aldrich syndrome).

Initial investigations should include a full blood count, platelet count, and film, to detect the total and differential white-cell counts.

Screening Tests for Immunodeficiency

These need only be performed in children who meet the above criteria and who have no evidence of any local abnormality that could account for their recurrent infections.

A full blood count and differential should include a platelet count (decreased and/or abnormally small platelets suggest the Wiskott–Aldrich syndrome), and careful examination of a blood film to exclude abnormal white cells or abnormal intracellular granules (Chediak–Higashi syndrome).

Antibody Screening Tests

If two or more serious pyogenic infections (especially of the respiratory or gastrointestinal tract) have been documented, antibody deficiency should be considered.

The following should be performed as screening tests: serum IgG, IgA and IgM, and IgG subclasses. IgG response to immunization should be tested using both a protein antigen (e.g. diphtheria/tetanus vaccine) and a carbohydrate antigen, e.g. pneumococcal vaccine (Pneumovax) and antibody levels measured initially and after 4 weeks. IgM isohaemagglutinins may also be useful. These are natural antibodies that develop to AB blood group substances, probably because of cross-reaction of these with bacterial antigens in the gut. They are not usually present before about 6 months of age, and will only be found to antigens not present in the child's red blood cells. For example, a child who is blood group A should have anti-B isohaemagglutinin present, but not anti-A.

Tests for Cell-mediated Immunity

These should be considered in severe and persistent infections with intracellular pathogens with or without severe pyogenic infections. Screening tests should include:

- Absolute lymphocyte count.
- Delayed hypersensitivity to diphtheria, tetanus or *Candida*. These tests involve intradermal injection of antigen and are read at 48 and 72 h. Induration of 5 mm diameter or greater is regarded as positive.
- HIV testing, where appropriate.
- *In vitro* lymphocyte blastic transformation tests are

usually performed only in patients who appear to have an abnormality on screening, and after discussion with the regional immunology service.

Tests for Complement Deficiencies

These are suggested in children with recurrent pneumococcal or neisserial infections and/or those with collagen-like or vascular diseases.

Screening tests for complement deficiencies should include measurement of total haemolytic complement, and of levels of C3 and C4 complement fractions.

Tests for Phagocyte Defects

These should be considered in children with serious recurrent skin or mucosal infections and/or with chronic mucocutaneous candidiasis. The following tests should be performed:

- Nitro-blue tetrazolium (NBT) dye reduction test for chronic granulomatous disease.
- IgE for hyperimmunoglobulinaemia E (present in Job's syndrome – recurrent severe infections and chronic eczema from infancy inherited as an autosomal dominant).

Any further tests than these should be arranged after discussion with a clinical immunologist, and should only be performed if strong suspicion remains of an immunodeficiency.

REFERENCES

De Rossi A, Mammano F, Pasti M et al (1991) New developments in the diagnosis of pediatric HIV infections. *Antibiot Chemother* 43: 214–226.

Gartner JC Jr (1992) Fever of unknown origin. *Adv Pediatr Infect Dis* 7: 1–24.

Hong R (1989) Assessment of immunity. *Biomed Pharmacother* 43: 545–550.

Lew JF, LeBaron CW, Glass RI et al (1990) Recommendations for the collection of laboratory specimens associated with outbreaks of gastroenteritis. *Morbid Mortal Week Rep* 39: 1–13.

McCracken GH Jr (1992) Current management of bacterial meningitis in infants and children. *Pediatr Infect Dis J* 11: 169–174.

Ostrov BE, Athreya BH (1991) Lyme disease: difficulties in diagnosis and management. *Pediatr Clin N Am* 38: 535–554.

Starke JR (1988) Modern approach to the diagnosis and treatment of tuberculosis in children. *Pediatr Clin N Am* 35: 441–464.

13

Respiratory Disease

R Dinwiddie

INTRODUCTION

Respiratory disease is the commonest cause of illness in childhood. It accounts for 15 million deaths in children under 5 years old annually throughout the developed and developing world (Editorial 1988). The investigation and effective treatment of these conditions therefore provides one of the important keys to improving child health throughout the world. There is also a very considerable morbidity associated with respiratory disease and this too can be alleviated with proper investigation which leads to the correct diagnosis and specific treatment, if this is available.

BASIC INVESTIGATION TECHNIQUES

The major measures of respiratory function are the basic lung volumes and also nowadays sleep studies. These examine oxygen levels during sleep and more complex parameters such as rate and depth of breathing, along with evidence of apnoea and abnormal breathing patterns. The basic lung function tests which are applicable in children over the age of 5 or 6 years are illustrated in Figures 13.1 and 13.2. The most commonly performed examination is a flow–volume curve which gives information on vital capacity, forced expiratory flow in one second, peak expiratory flow rate and the flow during expiration (forced expiratory flow at 25% vital capacity (FEF25%)). Normal values for children are shown in Table 13.1 (Dinwiddie 1990a).

Sleep studies can be performed quite simply by the use of an oxygen saturation monitor and half-hourly observations during overnight sleep. If there are any desaturation episodes these can also be carefully documented. This simple analysis will give a view of the baseline oxygen saturation at rest and also while asleep. Much more sophisticated equipment in specialist centres can measure a considerable range of physiological parameters

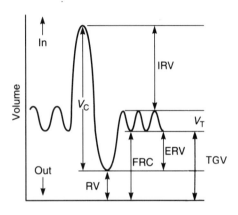

Figure 13.1 ERV, expiratory reserve volume; FRC, Functional residual capacity; IRV, inspiratory reserve volume; RV, residual volume; TGV, thoracic gas volume; VC, vital capacity; VT, tidal volume.

including continuous oxygen saturation level, rate and depth of breathing, movement of chest and abdomen (synchronous in normal breathing but asynchronous during obstructed breathing), presence or absence of central apnoea, heart rate variation during respiration, end-tidal carbon dioxide levels, and eye movements during active and quiet sleep. Other parameters such as EEG, oesophageal pH or continuous video surveillance can also be added, but only under research conditions.

The principal radiological investigations are listed in Table 13.2 and these can be applied at any level dependent on the underlying abnormality. Plain X-rays can be extremely helpful in delineating the anatomy of the airway, indicating evidence of narrowing in particular. Barium swallow gives a dynamic picture of the swallowing mechanisms particularly inco-ordination and aspiration into the lung. It can also be used to evaluate gastro-oesophageal reflux and hiatus hernia. Opportunity should also be taken to examine the airway calibre on screening, since if there is tracheomalacia or broncho-

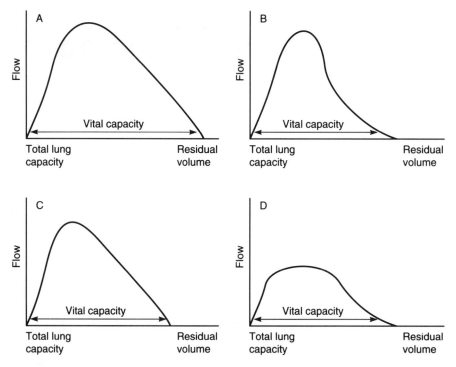

Figure 13.2 Expiratory flow–volume curves. (A) Normal. (B) Obstructed, e.g. asthma or cystic fibrosis. (C) Restrictive, e.g. pulmonary fibrosis. (D) Large airway obstruction, e.g. tracheal stenosis.

malacia the airways may disappear, particularly during expiration. Tracheo-oesophageal fistula is rare except in the presence of oesophageal atresia. It is best searched for by a tube oesophagram, which is a contrast study in which a pressure injection is given directly into the oesophagus via a nasogastric tube.

Ventilation/perfusion lung scans are performed in specialist units and utilize radio-isotopes, such as krypton-81 (^{81}Kr; half-life 13 s) to evaluate lung ventilation and technecium-99 (^{99}Tc; half-life 6 h) given by injection to evaluate pulmonary perfusion (Gordon et al, 1987).

A thoracic computerized tomography (CT) scan is particularly helpful for assessment of bronchial wall

Table 13.1 Lung function tests

Mean value and lower limit (−2sd) in brackets

Height (cm)	Forced vital capacity (FVC) litres				Forced expiratory volume in 1 s (FEVI) litres/sec				Peak expiratory flow rate (PEFR) (l/min)	Functional residual capacity (FRCml)			
	Boys		Girls		Boys		Girls		Boys and girls	Boys		Girls	
100	.98	(.75)	.98	(.75)	.84	(.63)	.84	(.63)	120 (75)	—		—	
110	1.20	(.89)	1.16	(.87)	1.09	(.82)	1.06	(.80)	160 (105)	.69	(.53)	.73	(.61)
120	1.52	(1.14)	1.45	(1.09)	1.36	(1.02)	1.33	(1.00)	210 (140)	.89	(.67)	.91	(.76)
130	1.88	(1.40)	1.78	(1.34)	1.66	(1.25)	1.61	(1.21)	250 (170)	1.11	(.84)	1.11	(.93)
140	2.30	(1.73)	2.18	(1.63)	2.03	(1.52)	1.98	(1.49)	300 (210)	1.37	(1.04)	1.34	(1.13)
150	2.80	(2.12)	2.66	(2.00)	2.44	(1.83)	2.39	(1.79)	350 (250)	1.67	(1.27)	1.60	(1.34)
160	3.44	(2.60)	3.25	(2.44)	2.96	(2.22)	2.89	(2.17)	400 (285)	2.00	(1.52)	1.89	(1.59)
170	4.18	(3.16)	3.92	(2.94)	3.57	(2.67)	3.47	(2.60)	470 (350)	2.38	(1.81)	2.20	(1.85)

Summary values – adapted from Dinwiddie (1990) with permission.

Table 13.2 Respiratory system imaging

Plain films
Chest – PA, AP, lateral
Postnasal space
Filter view of large airways
Sinuses
Lateral neck

Dynamic imaging
Airway screening
Ultrasound
Barium swallow
Tube oesophagram

Special imaging
Ventilation/perfusion lung scan
Magnetic resonance imaging
Pulmonary angiography
Thoracic CT scan
Digital vascular imaging
Bronchography

AP, anteroposterior; CT, computerized tomography; PA, postero-anterior.

thickening, areas of collapse consolidation and evidence of bronchiectasis. Magnetic resonance imaging (MRI) is under evaluation at present.

pH studies for those who may have gastro-oesophageal reflux are becoming increasingly used both in district general hospitals and in specialized units to evaluate this type of functional abnormality as it relates to respiratory disease.

Modern microbiological techniques can elucidate underlying disease particularly the use of immunofluorescence for viruses such as RSV, influenza A and B, adenovirus and measles. Routine bacterial culture should also be taken and serology for viral antibodies can be helpful for those with prolonged symptoms.

Immunological investigation including immunoglobulins and IgG subclasses, which may need to be sent to a regional centre, along with routine blood count and differential and IgE analysis can be helpful in evaluating children with recurrent infections or underlying atopic disease. Immunoglobulin subclass deficiencies are being increasingly recognized as a cause of chronic lung disease in children (Morgan and Levinsky 1988).

COUGH

Persistent cough in a child is one of the most common problems seen in clinical practice. The need for investigation will be determined by a careful review of the history and full physical examination. The majority of children with persistent cough have had recent respiratory tract infection leading to an altered cough threshold which persists for days and sometimes weeks after the acute infection is past. Many will not require detailed investigation at all but rather a clear explanation to the parents of the natural history of such an illness in the young child.

Other significant triggers for persistent cough include inhaled atmospheric pollutants and allergens which cause a recurrent reaction in the upper airway or higher portions of the lower airway. These can be difficult to elucidate at times and this is why it is so important to take a careful history.

Some infants and children also exhibit the phenomenon of bronchial hyper-reactivity (Silverman and Wilson 1985), particularly if they have had previous insults or stress to the lungs. Examples of such prior insults include infection with influenza or adenovirus and bronchopulmonary dysplasia. Infection with pertussis is the best-known example of an infection which leads to persistent cough. This has been described as the "100-day cough" and, although it is now uncommon in the UK due to the high immunization rates, it is still prevalent elsewhere where preventive measures are not practiced at the same level.

The development of the immune system is also an important component of the child's ability to deal with infection. Initially, even in the immune-competent patient resistance is built up by acquisition of "experience" by exposure to recurrent infections. Each will present in the normal way but may be prolonged since the antibody response to each antigen has to be developed. A number of infants and young children, who are otherwise perfectly healthy, have relatively minor immune deficiency, for example IgA or IgG2 subclass deficiency (Morgan and Levinsky 1988). They are much more likely to develop chronic symptoms, especially if the deficiency is permanent. Some children who have these problems show late maturation of the immune system, with complete catch-up within 2–3 years.

Major immune deficiency such as severe combined immune deficiency (SCID) or AIDS will usually present with more generalized features, although persistent respiratory infection is often the first manifestation of significant disease (Marolda et al 1991).

The role of gastro-oesophageal reflux as a cause of persistent symptoms including recurrent cough, wheeze and lower respiratory tract infection is increasingly recognized. This can occur in children who are basically healthy, but is more frequent in those with other problems such as bulbar palsy or an anatomical defect, for example a cleft larynx. Nowadays sophisticated investigation techniques including oesophageal pH studies can supplement basic tests such as barium swallow in elucidating the frequency and severity of this problem. There are still no reliable techniques for demonstrating the subtle aspiration of secretions directly into the lungs unless this is severe enough to cause changes on the chest X-ray.

Asthma is very common in childhood, as has already been mentioned. One type is called "cough variant asthma" which presents only with cough, particularly at night, and not with wheeze (Hollinger 1986). The diagnosis is made by exclusion of other possibilities (see Table 13.3). It can be treated successfully by allergen avoidance or the use of long-acting bronchodilators. Prophylaxis with sodium cromoglycate or inhaled steroids may be necessary for those with persistent symptoms. Although many children are reacting to inhaled allergens, the possibility of certain foods causing these symptoms should also be kept in mind.

Foreign body inhalation, especially in the toddler group, is another important precipitant of persistent cough, especially if it is of sudden onset with or without an obvious episode of choking or aspiration. If this diagnosis is seriously considered then bronchoscopy is vital

Table 13.3 Causes of persistent cough

Chronic or recurrent upper or lower respiratory tract infections

Viral/bacterial, including tuberculosis or pertussis

Bronchial hyper-reactivity

Asthma

Allergic reaction

Gastro-oesophageal reflux ± aspiration

Cardiac failure

Foreign body inhalation

Drugs, e.g. nifedipine

Psychogenic

Cystic fibrosis

Bronchiectasis

Immune deficiency

Immotile cilia syndrome

Tracheo-oesophageal fistula

Extrinsic tracheal compression

Cleft larynx

Bulbar palsy

Smoking

since lung damage in the longer term is directly proportional to the length of time the foreign body is in the lung before being removed.

Cystic fibrosis may present in the infant with persistent or recurrent cough. The history should always aim to elucidate other associated features such as significant lower respiratory tract infection or the presence of steatorrhoea or failure to thrive. The sweat test still remains the simplest and one of the most reliable investigations for this condition (Littlewood 1986).

One of the commonest causes for a truly persistent cough in childhood is that it is psychogenic in origin. The younger child may continue to cough as an attention seeking device. This is usually quite easy to understand from the history, examination and review of the child's behaviour. Indeed, in this situation, many parents are aware of this and only present for confirmation of the diagnosis.

The older child and adolescent, however, often present with a much more complex picture and although the cough is the major feature the underlying triggers, which are usually psycho-social and stress related, can be much more difficult to unravel.

The best approach to investigation is to pursue full organic testing, including bronchoscopy if necessary, while reviewing the psychological factors in detail, from the beginning. The patient and family are much more likely to accept this thorough and comprehensive approach rather than introducing the psychological aspects much later when other investigations have failed to show any underlying organic cause for the symptoms. This method of investigation also facilitates the task of the psychiatrist or psychologist who is likely to become the principal therapist in due course.

A number of rare causes of persistent cough should always be borne in mind, the history and examination will again be important in detecting these. Examples would include a structural defect such as recurrent tracheo-oesophageal fistula after previous surgery for oesophageal atresia or immotile cilia syndrome with or without situs inversus. A drug history is also essential since drugs too, e.g. nifedipine, can result in recurrent cough.

The possible investigations for persistent cough are shown in Table 13.4. The extent to which these are used will of course depend on the circumstances of each individual case.

CHRONIC OR RECURRENT RESPIRATORY DISEASE

Infants and children with chronic or recurrent respiratory disease may require considerable investigation to exclude

Table 13.4 Investigation of persistent cough

Frequent
Throat/nose swabs
Sputum culture
Chest X-ray
X-ray of sinuses/postnasal space
Full blood count
Immunoglobulin ± IgE
Lung function tests
Sweat test
Mantoux test
Skin tests
Respiratory viral antibodies

Infrequent
Full immunology
Barium swallow
Oesophageal pH
Ventilation/perfusion lung scan
Thoracic CT scan

Rare
Laryngotracheobronchoscopy
Oesophagoscopy
Magnetic resonance imaging
Cilia function

CT, computerized tomography.

Table 13.5 Causes of recurrent respiratory disease and wheeze

Cause	Investigation
Acute viral bronchiolitis	Viral immunofluoresence
Asthma	Elevated IgE (not always)
Recurrent aspiration	Barium swallow, pH study
Cystic fibrosis	Sweat test or genotype
Immune deficiency	Immune function, especially immunoglobulins and subclasses
HIV/AIDS	Low CD4 T-cell count, elevated immunoglobulins
Obliterative bronchiolitis	Positive antibodies to viruses, especially adenovirus
Bronchopulmonary dysplasia	Infant lung function
Vascular ring	Barium swallow, ultrasound
Foreign body	Bronchoscopy
Enlarged paratracheal glands	CT scan
Mediastinal cysts or tumours	CT scan
Tracheomalacia	Chest screening, bronchoscopy
Tracheal or bronchial stenosis	CT scan, bronchoscopy, bronchography
Congenital lobar emphysema	Ventilation-perfusion scan, CT scan
Left ventricular failure	ECG, ECHO

CT, computed tomography; ECG, electrocardiogram; ECHO, echocardiogram.

the most common causes of this problem. These are shown in Table 13.5 along with the appropriate investigations. The important aim of these is to elucidate any underlying major disorder such as cystic fibrosis, immune deficiency, gastro-oesophageal reflux, or a congenital abnormality leading to the chronic disease. Examples of these abnormalities would include congenital lung cysts, lobar emphysema or pulmonary sequestration. Chronic damage may have been caused to the lungs by incidental illness in the past such as severe infection with viruses, for example, adenovirus, or bacteria including *staphylococci, Klebsiella*, or *Pseudomonas*. These can lead to persistent damage particularly in the growing and developing lung eventually resulting in bronchiectasis. Inhalation of a foreign body with delayed recognition and subsequent removal can cause similar problems.

Early assessment of chronic respiratory disease is very important since intensive treatment may lead to its reversal. The elimination of recurrent aspiration into the lungs from gastro-oesophageal reflux may be dramatic in its effects, treatment of immunoglobulin deficiency with prophylactic antibiotics such as co-trimoxazole or regular intravenous immunoglobulin therapy can be extremely helpful for those with chronic upper or lower respiratory tract infection secondary to this type of impaired immune

function (Morgan and Levinsky 1988). Sometimes it may be necessary to undertake limited surgical removal of a severely damaged area of lung in order to prevent the spread of infection elsewhere.

There are two types of patient who are seen with this problem. Firstly the basically healthy, well-nourished child without underlying disease who has had a particularly severe infection with limited damage. These children respond well to intensive treatment, and surgery if necessary. The second category of child is either severely malnourished or has a major underlying disorder such as cystic fibrosis or immune deficiency. These children require much more intensive long-term support and care, and have a more limited prognosis. Despite this their general condition and quality of life can be greatly enhanced by appropriate investigation and treatment. Sometimes patients suffer from more than one problem such as, for example, asthma or recurrent reflux in association with cystic fibrosis or immunoglobulin deficiency, particularly of IgG subclass 2, in association with asthma.

THE WHEEZY INFANT

It has often been said that "all that wheezes is not asthma and all that's asthma does not wheeze", this particularly applies to the infant. Wheezing can occur for a variety of reasons which are shown in Table 13.5. The corresponding positive investigations are also shown in this table and these should be applied as appropriate to the investigation of those with persistent symptoms. Nowadays basic tests such as immunofluorescence for respiratory syncytial virus (RSV), sweat test for cystic fibrosis, barium swallow for recurrent reflux and aspiration, immunoglobulins and subclasses should be available to most hospitals. Those with persistent symptoms should be referred to a specialist unit for further investigation which may include more detailed immune work-up, pH studies and possibly bronchoscopy.

It is very important to take into account the family history for those with recurrent wheeze, particularly the prevalence of atopy in the family such as eczema, hayfever, allergic conjunctivitis or food allergy, and evidence of other markers for atopic disease such as eosinophilia in the blood count and elevated IgE level.

ASTHMA

Asthma is extremely common in children with a prevalence of 10–15%. It may manifest itself in a number of different ways and with a large variety of precipitating factors. Important features to take into account in the history include the role of exercise, changes in atmospheric humidity and temperature, effect of respiratory tract infections, extrinsic allergic factors including inhaled allergens but also foods, particularly acidic drinks such as Coca-Cola, fruit juices with or without additives and preservatives and cold drinks or ice-cream. Emotional factors and those due to excitement are also important especially if there is underlying family stress.

Basic investigations, which should be applied judiciously depending on the frequency and severity of the asthma, are listed in Table 13.6 (Dinwiddie 1990b).

Table 13.6   Investigation of asthma

Simple	Complex
Peak flow rate	Functional residual
Spirometry	capacity
Chest X-ray	Thoracic gas volume
Full blood count –	Skin tests
eosinophilia	Total IgE
Immunoglobulins	Immunoglobulin
Sweat test	subclasses
Respiratory viral	Exercise test
antibodies	Specific IgE antibodies
	(RASTs)
	Oesophageal pH study

RASTs, radioallergosorbent test.

The routine investigation of the asthmatic child should include lung function tests. Children of 4 years of age or more can often perform peak flow rates. By the age of 5 or 6 years they can undertake spirometry and flow–volume curves (Figure 13.1) which are probably the most helpful tests for monitoring regular progress. It is always useful to perform flow–volume curves before and after a bronchodilator such as salbutamol, terbutaline or atrovent in order to assess response. Specialist units are able to carry out more complex tests such as the measurement of functional residual capacity (FRC) and thoracic gas volume (TGV).

Reactions to specific allergens using skin tests or measuring individual IgE antibodies in the blood via radioallergosorbent (RAST) tests are also best undertaken in specialist units.

CONGENITAL ABNORMALITIES OF THE RESPIRATORY SYSTEM

A number of congenital defects of the respiratory system occur in infants and children. The simplest way of analysing these from the point of view of investigation is to consider them anatomically. They may be simple defects or they may be seen in conjunction with other abnormalities elsewhere (Falconer et al 1990), such as hemivertebrae or oesophageal atresia, which should alert one to the increased risk of associated respiratory tract anomalies.

The common types are shown in Table 13.7 with the appropriate investigations also outlined. Treatment is complex, and, although in some cases surgery is clearly indicated, in others such as congenital lobar emphysema this may not always be the case and careful follow-up with investigations such as ventilation/perfusion lung scan

Table 13.7 Congenital anomalies of the lung

Site	Investigations
Trachea/bronchi	
Stenosis	CT scan, bronchoscopy
Tracheomalacia	Screening, bronchoscopy
Bronchomalacia	Screening, bronchoscopy
Tracheo-oesophageal fistula	Tube oesophagram, oesophagobronchoscopy
Extrinsic airway	
Compression	Barium swallow, CT scan
Vascular ring	Barium swallow, echocardiography
Duplication cyst	CT scan, MRI scan
Bronchogenic cyst	CT scan, MRI scan
Intrapulmonary	
Congenital lobar emphysema	V/Q scan, CT scan
Cystic adenomatoid malformation	CT scan
Lung cysts	V/Q scan, CT scan
Lobar sequestration	V/Q scan, angiography
Pulmonary hypoplasia	V/Q scan, CT scan
Pulmonary agenesis	V/Q scan, CT scan
Arterio-venous (A-V) fistula	Angiography
Diaphragmatic hernia	Barium swallow, ultrasound
Extrapulmonary	
Rib-cage defects	Chest X-ray
Neuromuscular disease	EMG

CT, computerized tomography; EMG, nerve conduction studies electromyogram; MRI, magnetic resonance imaging; V/Q, radio-isotope ventilation perfusion lung scan.

will indicate the progress and control of the disease with time (Kennedy et al 1991).

The outlook for most congenital malformations of the chest is remarkably good considering the major effect they can have on the baby in the neonatal period. Lung growth and development is particularly rapid in the first 2–3 years of life. It has been shown that intrauterine abnormalities will inhibit alveolar development and numbers in both lungs, even though the defect may be unilateral. However, long-term follow-up in many cases indicated that the lungs are able to adapt to removal of significant areas involved in congenital anomaly with good long-term functional results. The earlier the abnormality can be detected and dealt with the better is the outlook for growth and development. Routine lung function tests including radio-isotope lung scans are a useful way of following these patients over several years.

ACUTE LIFE-THREATENING EVENTS

Recent data have shown that the incidence of sudden infant death syndrome (SIDS) has decreased significantly (Busuttil and Brutchell 1992). Nevertheless, a significant number of infants, about 1:1000 will still suffer from acute life-threatening events (ALTE) and will be referred to paediatric units for further investigation and treatment. The appropriate investigations are shown in Table 13.8 and the degree to which these are pursued will depend on the frequency and severity of the attacks. Another important feature is the level of anxiety in individual cases both as displayed by the parents and family but also by the clinicians who are involved in day-to-day management of the patient.

The possibility of parental interference with the child's breathing must always be borne in mind as this can be very subtle and even intermittent (Samuels et al 1992). It may involve direct occlusion of the airway or the subtle administration of respiratory depressant medication. The investigation and treatment of these patients is one of the most difficult and time-consuming challenges to the paediatrician. Fortunately, most children will outgrow this tendency and the condition is unusual after the first year of life.

CYSTIC FIBROSIS

Cystic fibrosis is the commonest cause of bronchiectasis in children. The incidence of the disease is about 1:2500 of

Table 13.8 Investigation of acute life threatening events

Simple	Complex
Full blood count	Full sleep study
Urea and electrolytes	pH monitoring of oesophagus
Liver function tests	
Arterial blood gases	Metabolic screen
Chest X-ray	Respiratory function tests
ECG	Video surveillance
EEG	
Barium swallow	
Viral antibodies	
Immunoglobulins	

ECG, electrocardiogram; EEG, electroencephalogram.

newborn infants. Recently there have been major advances in our knowledge and understanding of the underlying gene disorder and its genetic expression in the respiratory tract through a disabled transmembrane regulator protein (CFTR) (Dodge et al 1993). The possibility of gene therapy for this disease has been successfully demonstrated in animals and trials in humans have now begun.

The diagnosis of cystic fibrosis can be made in a variety of ways, although the sweat test remains the simplest and most reliable test if carried out properly in a centre performing it on a regular basis (Littlewood 1986). The levels required for the diagnosis have been reviewed and they do vary at different ages and with different volumes of sweat (Hjelm et al 1986).

Analysis of the genotype is even more precise than the sweat test but, unfortunately, a very large number of alleles (over 400) have now been recognized and testing for the commonest four or five will only confirm the diagnosis in about 80% of cases. Other methods such as the measurement of transnasal potential difference are either less reliable or much more complex to perform. Cases where there is particular diagnostic difficulty should be referred to a specialist centre for detailed evaluation.

Neonatal screening for cystic fibrosis can be satisfactorily performed utilizing immunoreactive trypsin. Levels of this enzyme in the blood are elevated particularly during the first 3 months of life in the affected infant. There are, however, a small but significant number of false-positive results, although the recent addition of screening for the common gene types on the same sample has reduced these (Dodge et al 1993).

Although neonatal screening is practiced in a number of countries and within certain regions in the UK, the overall advantages have so far not been sufficient to make the Government introduce it nationally in this country.

The routine care and management of the cystic fibrosis patient in the long term is best carried out by a system of joint care between the district general hospital and the specialist cystic fibrosis centre. This enables the patient to be seen locally but also to receive specialist advice regularly and to have early access to the many new treatments which are now becoming available. Regular monitoring of the cystic fibrosis patient is illustrated in Table 13.9. A number of cystic fibrosis centres carry out an "annual review" where more intensive investigation is carried out on an annual basis. Others perform more continuous assessment, but still generally covering the same tests on a regular basis.

Specific lung pathogens in cystic fibrosis such as *Pseudomonas cepacia* and *Aspergillus fumigatus* require special microbiological culture techniques, skin tests and

Table 13.9 Regular monitoring of cystic fibrosis patients

Test	Frequency
Throat swab	Every visit
Lung function – spirometry	Every visit
Oxygen saturation	Every visit
Full lung function including TGV	6 monthly
Chest X-ray, frontal and lateral	6–12 monthly
Full blood count	Annually
Liver function tests and clotting studies	Annually
Immunoglobulins	Annually
Special tests, e.g. *Aspergillus* antibodies, vitamin levels, liver scan	As indicated clinically

TGV, thoracic gas volume.

serological assays for their detection and to assess response to treatment. The microbiological investigations are routine in laboratories servicing large clinics. The serology may need to be sent to a regional reference laboratory.

Assessment for heart–lung transplantation in cystic fibrosis is very much confined to the few centres designated for this very specialized form of treatment (Higgenbottom and Whitehead 1991). Although a proportion of patients do well, there are still many who will die before organs become available and others who will suffer from chronic rejection of the donated organs. Further research is being undertaken to improve the outcome of these patients in the future.

HIV/AIDS AND THE LUNG (see also Chapter 12)

Infants and children who are HIV antigen positive and who are developing AIDS are particularly prone to opportunistic infection of the lungs. As many as 80% of affected patients suffer from pulmonary complications (Marolda et al 1991). In a significant proportion of cases lung infection, especially with *Pneumocystis carinii*, may be the first manifestation of the acute illness. Bacterial infections with common organisms such as *Streptococci*, *Staphylococci*, *Haemophilus*, *Pseudomonas*, and *Klebsiella* are frequently seen. Fungi, especially *Candida albicans* and *Aspergillus fumigatus*, are not infrequent pathogens. Viruses such as cytomegalovirus and herpes simplex are also important in this group.

The common respiratory viruses such as respiratory syncytial virus (RSV), influenza, parainfluenza, and adenovirus are also seen but appear to cause less severe problems than one might otherwise expect in this situation. Measles is a major pulmonary pathogen among

AIDS patients in developing countries where immunization rates are low.

Other important opportunistic organisms in these children are *Mycobacterium tuberculosis*, *Mycobacterium avium* intracellulare (MAI), toxoplasmosis, histoplasmosis and *Cryptococcus* (Marolda et al 1991).

Another lung pathology seen in AIDS patients is lymphoid interstitial pneumonia (LIP) (Pitt 1991), also known as pulmonary lymphoid hyperplasia (PLH). This is an infiltrative disease due to interstitial thickening caused by lymphocytes. Although it has a typical chest X-ray appearance, diagnosis can only be confirmed by lung biopsy.

Since a large number of potential pathogens exist in these patients special diagnostic techniques are necessary. The most important of these are direct bronchoalveolar lavage (BAL) (Alpert et al 1992) and transbronchoscopic or open lung biopsy. BAL is increasingly used in order to obtain sufficient lung secretions so that full diagnostic techniques can be applied in the search for common and uncommon pathogens.

UNUSUAL LUNG DISEASE

A few children will be seen who are suffering from a number of uncommon diseases of the lung (Dinwiddie 1990c). The individual experience of these is rare and so it is important that they should be seen in a specialist centre where appropriate investigation can be carried out and where a knowledge and understanding of the pathophysiology and treatment can be built up. Examples of these conditions are shown in Table 13.10.

Those which involve infiltration of the interstitium of the lung such as fibrosing alveolitis, autoimmune lung disease, and Langerhans' cell histiocytosis will lead to oxygen desaturation which can readily be detected by a saturation monitor. The decreased oxygen passage across the alveolar surface "transfer factor" can be detected by measuring impairment of the carbon monoxide transfer

Table 13.10 Unusual lung disease

Fibrosing alveolitis
Autoimmune lung disease
Langerhans' cell histiocytosis
Pulmonary haemosiderosis
Sarcoidosis
Swachman's syndrome
Alveolar proteinosis
Central hypoventilation syndrome
Pulmonary lymphangiectasia
Asphyxiating thoracic dystrophy

factor in specialist laboratories. Most of these conditions however require an open lung biopsy for complete diagnosis.

Specialized investigation and treatment is also required for children exhibiting central hypoventilation syndrome. This would include sophisticated sleep studies which show rate and depth of breathing and relative movements of chest and diaphragm during different phases of sleep.

The treatment of these rare disorders often requires the use of agents with significant risk of side-effects including steroids, hydroxychloroquine, azothiaprine or cyclophosphamide. Close and careful monitoring is therefore required.

REFERENCES

Alpert BE, O'Sullivan BP, Panitch HB (1992) Non-bronchoscopic approach to bronchoalveolar lavage in children with artifical airways. *Pediatr Pulmonol* 13: 38–41.

Busuttil A, Brutchell A (eds) (1992) Symposium on sudden infant death syndrome. *J Clin Pathol* 45 (Suppl 11): 1–48.

Dinwiddie R (ed) (1990a) Physiology of breathing. In: *Diagnosis and Management of Paediatric Respiratory Disease*, pp. 9–19. Churchill Livingstone, Edinburgh.

Dinwiddie R (ed) (1990b) Asthma. In: *Diagnosis and Management of Paediatric Respiratory Disease*, pp. 147–175. Churchill Livingstone, Edinburgh.

Dinwiddie R (ed) (1990c) Rare diseases of the lung. In: *The Diagnosis and Management of Paediatric Respiratory Disease*, pp. 247–254. Churchill Livingstone, Edinburgh.

Dodge JA, Brock DJH, Widdicombe JH (eds) (1993) *Cystic Fibrosis. Current Topics*, pp. 1–347. Wiley, Chichester.

Editorial (1988) Acute respiratory infections in under fives: 15 million deaths a year. *Lancet* ii: 699–701.

Falconer AR, Brown RA, Helms PJ, Gordon I (1990) Pulmonary sequelae in survivors of congenital diaphragmatic hernia. *Thorax* 45: 126–129.

Gordon I, Matthew DJ, Dinwiddie R (1987) Respiratory system. In: Gordon I (ed) *Diagnostic Imaging in Paediatrics*, pp. 27–57. Chapman & Hall, London.

Higgenbottam TW, Whitehead B (1991) Heart–lung transplantation for cystic fibrosis. *J R Soc Med* 84 (Suppl 18): 18–21.

Hjelm M, Brown P, Briddon A (1986) Sweat sodium related to amount of sweat after sweat test in children with and without cystic fibrosis. *Acta Paediatr Scand* 75: 652–656.

Hollinger LD (1986) Chronic cough in infants and children. *Laryngoscope* 96: 316–322.

Kenndey CD, Habibi P, Matthew DJ, Gordon I (1991) Lobar emphysema: long term imaging follow up. *Radiology* 180: 189–193.

Littlewood J (1986) The sweat test. *Arch Dis Child* 61: 1043–1045.

Marolda J, Pace B, Bonforte RJ et al (1991) Pulmonary manifestations of HIV infection in children. *Paediatr Pulmonol* 10: 231–235.

Morgan G, Levinsky R (1988) Clinical significance of IgG subclass deficiency. *Arch Dis Child* 63: 771–773.

Pitt J (1991) Lymphocytic interstitial pneumonia. *Pediatr Clin N Am* 38: 89–95.

Samuels MP, McLaughlin W, Jacobson RR, Poets CF, Southall DP

(1992) Fourteen cases of imposed upper airway obstruction. *Arch Dis Child* 67: 162–170.

Silverman M, Wilson N (1985) Bronchial responsiveness in children: a clinical review. In: Milner AD, Martin RJ (eds) *Neonatal and Pediatric Respiratory Medicine*, pp. 161–189. Butterworths, London.

14
Allergy

T J David

INTRODUCTION

Tests for allergy are overvalued and overused. That they are used at all reflects the highly unscientific nature of current allergy practice, and the fact that simple or reliable tests are not available. The lack of useful conventional tests is a major factor in the current widespread use of unorthodox and often bizarre diagnostic approaches.

The whole area is beset by frequent misuse of terminology, so it is essential to define a few terms.

Allergy. An allergic response is a reproducible adverse reaction to a substance mediated by an immunological response, irrespective of the precise mechanism. The substance provoking the reaction may have been ingested, injected, inhaled or merely have come into contact with the skin or mucous membranes.

Antigen. An antigen is a substance which is capable of provoking an immune response.

Antibody. An antibody is an immunoglobulin which is capable of combining specifically with certain antigens.

Allergen. An allergen is a substance which provokes a harmful (allergic) immune response.

Food intolerance. Food intolerance is a reproducible adverse reaction to a specific food or food ingredient, and it is not psychologically based. Food intolerance occurs even when the subject cannot identify the type of food which has been given.

In practice, in relation to allergy diagnosis and identification, the doctor is faced with three types of question:

- Are the symptoms caused by allergen exposure?
- Which allergen (if any) was responsible for a specific exacerbation or adverse event?
- Will the condition improve if specific allergens are avoided?

This chapter will examine the tools which are available to help doctors answer these questions.

TAKING A HISTORY

Standard textbooks on allergy make little or no mention of tests, except to say that allergy tests can only be interpreted in the light of the history. Given that allergy tests are of little value, information obtained in the history assumes central importance. Here are two illustrations.

Penicillin allergy

A 14-year-old was reported to be penicillin allergic by his mother, penicillin was carefully avoided, and he was referred by a paediatrician for allergy testing. Enquiry as to the basis of the penicillin allergy revealed that at the age of 15 months, the boy developed loose stools 24 h after starting antibiotics for otitis media.

Comment. It is idle to write the word "allergy" in a patient's notes without any description of the evidence for the diagnosis. All sorts of untoward events are wrongly labelled as allergies. There are several reasons why penicillin administration may be followed by an adverse event, but few justify a diagnosis of penicillin allergy. A rash during antibiotic therapy may be caused by an underlying infection, or by a colouring agent or preservative included in a liquid preparation of the antibiotic. Loose stools are likely to be due to an underlying viral infection or a disturbance of the gut flora, but it is common to find this described by parents as an allergy to the antibiotic. It is common for parents to report penicillin allergy when enquiries reveal that the adverse event occurred during treatment with a completely different antibiotic. The incorrect and careless labelling of a child as having penicillin allergy may rob the patient of penicillin treatment for life.

Allergy to "Baked Beans"

A 5-month-old infant was referred for an allergy consultation because minutes after eating "baked beans", while in the care of his grandmother, he developed generalized urticaria, florid angioedema of the face, wheezing, coughing, and a stridor, which resulted in emergency admission to hospital. He had previously eaten "baked beans" without difficulty. The parents insisted that no other food could have been given immediately prior to this reaction. It was pointed out that, although in theory such a reaction could be attributable to intolerance to beans or tomato, in practice the history was much more typical of a reaction to egg. The parents denied that this was possible, and insisted that the baby had never received egg, but when the grandmother was confronted she admitted that it was boiled egg and not baked beans which had been given.

Comment. Parental reports of reactions, especially to food, can be unreliable. There are three main reasons. Firstly, because eating food is a common activity, occurring upwards of three times a day, it is quite likely that any adverse event will commence within a few hours of ingesting food. Secondly, parents find it difficult to be objective, and once a reaction is suspected facts are easily "tailored" to the belief. Thirdly, the parents may have been misled by others, or may be hoping to find an allergic and "external" explanation for a problem (such as behaviour difficulty) rather than contemplating a problem within the child or the family.

How to Take a History

The history should include questions about:

- When symptoms occur.
- Where symptoms occur.
- When or where is the patient free of symptoms.
- The presence of other allergic symptoms.
- Family history of allergy or atopic disease.

In general, the quicker the onset of the allergic reaction, the more reliable is the history. A history of an allergic reaction is more reliable if exposure to an item has been followed by the same symptoms on more than one occasion. Other clues from the history are listed in Table 14.1. The possible sources of confusion with symptoms which occur after exposure to pet animals are explained in Table 14.2. A major source of confusion is that parents equate allergy with immediate reactions, and are unaware

that constant exposure to pet antigen in the home tends to cause chronic rather than acute symptoms.

The interpretation of the observation that exposure to a single item (e.g. a cat) is followed within minutes by an obvious adverse event (e.g. sneezing and orbital oedema) should be quite simple, but there are pitfalls. The history is more reliable if it is based on the parents' unprompted original observations. The parents' observations may, however, be unreliable, especially in the following situations:

- If there is a strong emotional underlay, e.g. strong attachment to a family pet, underdiagnosis of allergy may occur because the family do not want to part with the animal.
- In the case of food intolerance, double-blind studies have repeatedly shown parental histories to be particularly unreliable (David 1993).
- In the case of behavioural symptoms, there is a widespread but incorrect belief in the importance of adverse reactions to foods or food additives (David 1993).
- In the context of Munchausen's syndrome by proxy, child abuse, or psychiatrically disturbed parents, a parent's report of alleged allergic reactions may have been fabricated (Warner and Hathaway 1984).

SKIN AND BLOOD TESTS

Skin Prick Tests

The principle of skin prick tests is that the skin weal and flare reaction to an allergen demonstrates the presence of mast-cell-fixed antibody. This is mainly IgE antibody, although in theory it could also be IgG4 antibody (Bernstein 1988). IgE is produced in plasma cells distributed primarily in lymphoid tissue in the respiratory and gastrointestinal tract, and is distributed in the circulation to all parts of the body, so that sensitization is generalized and therefore can be demonstrated by skin testing.

Effect of Drugs

Drugs with H1 receptor antagonist properties (e.g. antihistamines and tricyclic antidepressants) suppress the histamine-induced weal and flare response of a skin prick test. The suppressive effect may last up to a week or more, and in the case of the long-acting astemizole for 5 months or more. H2 receptor antagonists (e.g. ranitidine) partially suppress skin test reactivity. Systemic steroids do not reduce the response to skin prick tests, but local applications of potent topical steroids markedly suppress the skin test response.

Table 14.1 Clues from the history

Clue from the history	Comments
The symptoms are worse at night	Circadian rhythms which control airway calibre, bronchial reactivity and cortisol secretion account for some of the increase in symptoms at night in asthma. In eczema, heat, tiredness and low cortisol secretion may contribute to nocturnal symptoms. Contrary to popular belief, nocturnal symptoms do not point to house dust mite allergy
The symptoms are worse at certain times of the year	A convincing history (e.g. sneezing and conjunctivitis each June and July) will support the usual inference that the symptoms are attributable to a seasonal allergen. Often, the history is not so easy to interpret. For example, a worsening of asthma in September could be due to allergy to inhaled moulds, an increase in the number of house dust mites in the autumn, changes in the weather, or catching viral respiratory infections when returning to school after the summer holidays
The symptoms are worse in certain weather conditions	Possible reasons for attacks of asthma after thunderstorms or heavy rain are allergy to inhaled fungal spores, a fall in the barometric pressure or a sudden fall in air temperature
The symptoms improve when the patient is away from home (e.g. on holiday)	This is commonly noted in atopic eczema, but it is unknown whether it is due to the absence of pet or dust mite antigen, exposure to ultraviolet light, sea bathing, relaxation, or some other factor. The improvement or complete disappearance of asthma at alpine resorts is generally attributed to the absence of mite and pet antigens, but this is unproven
Multiplicity of symptoms	Especially where food intolerance is concerned, single symptoms are less likely to have an allergic aetiology than are multiple symptoms. The infant with wheezing as an isolated symptom is far less likely to have food intolerance than the infant with wheezing, rhinitis, eczema and loose stools
Unilateral symptoms	Unilateral symptoms, whether nasal, ocular or respiratory, suggest the presence of a non-allergic condition
The presence or absence of a family history of atopic disease	Atopic disease is so common in the normal population that a positive family history is a rather non-specific finding. In an apparently atopic child, the *absence* of a positive family history is more important, and should make one re-consider a diagnosis of atopic disease

Control Solutions

Because of the variability of cutaneous reactivity, it is necessary to include positive and negative controls whenever performing skin tests. The negative control solution consists of the diluent used to preserve the allergen extracts. The positive control solution usually contains histamine 1–10 mg/ml (or 0.1 mg/ml for intradermal tests), and is mainly used to detect suppression of reactivity, for example caused by H1 receptor antagonists.

Scratch Testing

A drop of allergen solution is placed on the skin which is then scratched so as to penetrate the skin superficially. As well as providing non-specific weal reactions which are the result of trauma, the scratch test introduces a variable amount of allergen through the skin. The test is therefore poorly standardized and produces results which are too variable for routine clinical use.

Prick Testing

A drop of allergen solution is placed on the skin which is then pricked with an hypodermic needle. Prick tests can also produce variable results, but the introduction of standardized precision needles for prick testing has made the method potentially more reproducible. However, the delegation of skin testing to untrained staff, and the continued use of unstandardized hypodermic needles leads to frequent errors and poor reproducibility.

Table 14.2   Possible sources of confusion with symptoms which occur after exposure to pet animals

Observation and incorrect conclusion	Comments
A child is noted to have an immediate allergic reaction when stroking or being licked by, for example, a dog, but is otherwise apparently able to live in the same house as the animal without obvious immediate allergic reactions. It is concluded that the dog has nothing to do with the child's asthma	Delayed reactions or enhanced bronchial reactivity may have been overlooked. The animal may be an important contributory cause of the asthma
It is reported that a child experiences an immediate allergic reaction to certain cats but not others. It is concluded that cats are not a cause of the asthma	As above, delayed reactions or enhanced bronchial reactivity may be overlooked
The onset of a boy's asthma, in early infancy, predates the acquisition of a dog when he was 3 years old. The boy is now aged 12 years, and it is concluded that the dog cannot have anything to do with the child's symptoms	In infancy the main trigger is likely to have been viral respiratory infections. However, children with atopic disease often become allergic to their pet, and now that the child is older, the animal could be an important contributing cause of the asthma
The child's symptoms did not improve when the pet was sent to live elsewhere for a few weeks	Sufficient pet antigen to provoke disease is likely to remain in the household for months or years, unless exceptionally rigorous steps are taken to remove such antigen (e.g. by replacing carpets and upholstered furniture, and by washing the walls)

Method of Skin Prick Testing

A small drop of each test extract and control solution is placed on the volar aspect of the forearm (or occasionally on the back). The implication of a recent study showing that positive reactions affect the reactivity of adjacent skin (Terho et al 1989) is that drops must be placed more than 4 cm apart. The needle is pressed through the drop of allergen extract into the skin at an angle of $90°$ to the skin, to a standard depth of 1 mm. Some devices are passed through the drop, penetrating the skin at a $45°$ angle, and the skin is then gently lifted to create a small break in the epidermis.

Result: Timing

The skin prick test induces a response that reaches a peak in 8–9 min for histamine, 10–12 min for compound 48/80 (a histamine-releasing agent), and 12–15 min for allergens. The standard advice is to read the histamine control result at 10 min (Bernstein 1988) and the remaining skin test sites at 15 min, and to reinspect at 25–30 min as in some patients reactions take a little longer to develop (Dreborg 1989). Late reactions can also occur, but are not usually sought as their significance is unclear; they are discussed briefly below.

Result: Size

The size of the reaction, which is often oval or irregular in shape, is measured with a ruler. The largest diameter (D) and the diameter at right angles to this (d) is measured, and the reaction is expressed as $(D + d)/2$.

Result: Weal or Flare?

Most authorities recommend measurement of the size of the weal alone, but others suggest that the size of the flare should also be measured.

Criteria of Positivity

There is a lack of agreed definition about what constitutes a positive reaction. Most definitions of a positive reaction are based on the absolute diameter of the weal, with arbitrary cut-off points for positivity at 1, 2 or 3 mm (Bousquet 1988). A major difficulty is that the size of the weal depends to some extent on the potency of the extract.

Problems with Interpretation

It is far easier to perform the test than to interpret the results. Skin tests tell you what is going on in the skin. Trying to extrapolate from skin test results, which is the whole purpose of the exercise, is fraught with difficulties. The numerous problems are listed in Table 14.3. The current doctrine is that a positive skin prick test is an indication of clinical sensitivity, past, present or future, and that prick tests are worth doing to provide confirmatory evidence. From a carefully taken history, one might

Table 14.3 Problems with interpretation of skin prick tests

False-positive tests
Asymptomatic or subclinical hypersensitivity; positive tests in those with no symptoms of allergy. A few such subjects develop symptoms later, but the test cannot identify this subset
Persistent positivity, in subjects who have grown out of their allergy

False-negative tests
Negative tests in those with genuine IgE-mediated allergy
Negative tests in those in whom the mechanism is not IgE-mediated
Due to drugs (e.g. H1 receptor antagonists)

Problems in infancy
False-negative reactions in infants and toddlers
Lack of age-related guidelines as to what constitutes a positive reaction

Poor correlation with provocation tests

Varying potency of skin testing allergen extracts

Effect of IgE level
There is a correlation between the total serum IgE concentration and the degree of positivity of skin prick test results, leading to false-positive reactions in those with very high IgE concentrations

Poor reproducibility
Due to the poor reproducibility of the histamine-induced weal

Variation in skin reactivity depending upon the skin site chosen

Placing the histamine control site too near an adjacent site (4 cm or less)
May induce a non-specific weal reaction, and it is probable that a similar problem may occur between two adjacent allergens

Circadian variation in skin test reactivity

suspect a particular allergen, and the finding of a positive prick test would increase the likelihood that the allergen was causing symptoms. Few people, however, would be prepared to ignore a strong history of allergy in the face of a negative prick test, yet it is illogical to regard the prick test as significant only when it confirms the history and to disregard it when it fails to do so.

Intradermal Testing

Intradermal testing comprises the intradermal injection of 0.01–0.05 ml of an allergen extract. It can cause fatal anaphylaxis, and is only performed if a preliminary skin prick test is negative. Intradermal tests are more sensitive than skin prick testing (Dreborg 1989), and hence also produce even more false-positive reactions. The difficulty in the interpretation of the results, the pain of intradermal injections, and the risk of anaphylaxis mean that intradermal testing has no place in the routine investigation of IgE-mediated allergic reactions or food intolerance in childhood.

Late-phase Reactions

In an IgE-dependent skin test reaction, the weal and flare at 10–20 min can be followed by a late-phase reaction comprising induration and inflammation that begins, peaks and terminates within 1–2 days. The clinical significance of these late-phase reactions is at present unclear.

Conclusion

The enthusiasts for skin prick testing are mainly "allergists", for whom there may be a need to demonstrate "allergy expertise" or where the performance of tests is associated with a fee for service. Although skin prick testing has a place in research studies, it is difficult to see a place for skin testing in the general diagnosis or management of suspected allergy. The contentious issues in clinical practice are whether a child with atopic disease or symptoms suggestive of allergy will benefit from allergen avoidance measures, but there is no evidence that skin prick test results are of any value at all as predictors of response to such measures.

Patch Testing

In contact dermatitis, sensitization affects the whole body. The principle of patch testing is that if an allergen is applied to a small area of normal skin and enough is absorbed, inflammation develops at the site of application. The allergen is usually applied as a patch test. A positive reaction may confirm that a subject has allergic contact sensitivity to the substance tested, but does not necessarily mean that the substance is the cause of the patient's dermatitis.

Allergens are usually applied to the skin on the back, on 1 cm diameter patches of filter paper, which are either placed on an impermeable sheet or in a cup, which holds a test substance closely applied to the skin. The patches or cups are left on for 48 h. The distinction between irritant and allergic reactions may be difficult. The features of irritant reactions are sharp delineation corresponding to the margins of the test patch, no infiltration, lack of itching, and redness with a brown hue. Positive reactions of an allergic nature are red and infiltrated with minute papules or vesicles (which in severe reactions coalesce into bullae), diffuse, and extend beyond the margins of the patch.

Tests for Circulating IgE Antibodies

The radioallergosorbent test (RAST) is the best known of a number of laboratory procedures for the detection and measurement of circulating IgE antibody. This type of test avoids possible confounding variables in skin testing, namely IgE affinity for mast cells, their tendency for degranulation, and skin reactivity to released mediators. Thus, in theory, the in vitro test should be more reliable than skin testing. In practice, since the test is detecting IgE antibodies, the test suffers from very similar drawbacks to those for skin prick testing, outlined in Table 13.3. Additional difficulties are:

- The high cost.
- The fact that a very high level of total circulating IgE (e.g. in children with severe atopic eczema) may cause a false-positive result.
- The fact that a very high level of IgG antibody with the same allergen specificity as the IgE antibody can cause a false-negative result.
- The fact that, for each allergen, the test differs in the degree to which it is influenced by the total serum IgE concentration.
- *In vitro* IgE assays are slightly less sensitive than skin testing.
- The IgE antibody concentration in the plasma varies with allergen exposure. A few patients with allergic rhinitis are RAST negative before the pollen season, but become positive after the pollen season.

In vitro tests for IgE antibody are preferable to skin testing:

- Where the child has had a very severe reaction to the allergen in question (because of the small risk of anaphylaxis with skin testing).
- Where the child has widespread skin disease (e.g. atopic eczema).
- Where the skin shows dermographism.
- When H1 antihistamines cannot be discontinued.

The degree of correlation between RAST results and skin prick test results depends on the criteria used for positivity, and thus there is endless scope for manipulation of data. However, in general there is a good correlation between the two tests.

ANTIGEN PROVOCATION CHALLENGE

With the exception of food challenges in patients with suspected food intolerance (see later), provocation tests have little place in routine clinical practice but have been helpful in the study of the pathophysiology and pharmacology of atopic disease. In clinical practice, the results suffer from the same major limitation as the results of skin or IgE antibody testing, which is that a positive result from an allergen challenge does not prove that the allergen is contributing to the patient's disease.

Bronchial Challenge Tests

There are two categories of test:

- Tests of specific airway responsiveness to an individual allergen. Increasing concentrations of allergen are inhaled until a 20% fall in FEV_1 occurs.
- Tests of non-specific airway responsiveness. Increasing concentrations of pharmacological agents with airway smooth muscle contractile effects, such as histamine or methacholine, are inhaled. The most common variable used to express non-specific responsiveness is the concentration of drug causing a 20% fall in FEV_1, as determined by interpolation between points on the dose–response curve.

Nasal Challenge Tests

The use of semi-quantitative objective parameters (counting sneezes, weighing tissues after the nose has been blown), and the introduction of the measurement of nasal airflow (rhinomanometry), have facilitated studies using nasal challenges. Interpretation of the results is complicated by factors which may affect the response to nasal challenge such as seasonal variation of nasal reactivity, mucociliary clearance, and the migration of basophils, mast cells and eosinophils into the nasal submucosa.

Conjunctival Testing

A small quantity of dry pollen or diluted allergen extract is dropped into the lower conjunctival sac, and the patient is observed for lacrimation, sneezing, or injection of the conjunctivae or sclerae.

Food Challenges

Food challenges are helpful either: to confirm a history; to confirm the diagnosis, for example of cow's milk protein intolerance in infancy, where the diagnostic criteria include improvement on elimination diet and relapse on reintroduction; to see if a child has grown out of a food intolerance; or as a research procedure. The food challenge should replicate normal food consumption in terms of dose, route and state of food. It should also be performed in such a way that the history can be verified. Thus, for example, it is no good solely looking for an immediate reaction if the parents' report a delayed reaction.

Open Food Challenges

Open food challenges are the simplest approach. The parents, doctor and the patient know what food is being given. An advantage is that the challenge can be made directly with the freshly prepared foodstuff concerned, rather than a freeze-dried or dehydrated preparation. Open food challenges run the risk of bias influencing the parents' (or doctor's) observations. Often this is unimportant. But in some cases parental belief in food intolerance may be disproportionate, and where this is suspected there is no substitute for a double-blind placebo-controlled challenge. An open challenge may be an open invitation to the overdiagnosis of food intolerance. For example, in the UK parents widely believe that there is an association between food additives and bad behaviour, but in one series, double-blind challenges with tartrazine and benzoic acid were negative in all 24 children with a clear parental description of adverse reaction (David 1987).

Double-blind Placebo-controlled Food Challenge

The test comprises the administration of a challenge substance, which is either the item under investigation or an indistinguishable inactive (placebo) substance. Neither the child, the parents nor the observers know the identity of the administered material at the time of the challenge. The procedure is as follows.

Step 1 Obtain a Detailed History

Which food or foods are suspected? What symptoms are produced? How long after ingestion do the symptoms occur? What is the smallest quantity of food which will produce the symptoms? How frequently does the reaction occur? How reproducible is the reaction? In other words, does it always happen when a food is ingested, or only on

certain occasions? Does the reaction only occur in the presence of some additional factor? For example, does the reaction only occur if ingestion of the food is followed by exercise?

Step 2 Elimination Diet

Suspect foods need to be avoided for approximately 2 weeks prior to challenge, on the grounds that regular administration of a food trigger could obscure a reaction to a single dose. The regular administration of salicylates to patients with salicylate intolerance quickly leads to a state of tolerance to salicylate. It is possible, although unproven, that a similar phenomenon can occur with foods and food additives.

Step 3 Recording Results

The results should be recorded systematically, with details of the time given, the times of observation, the dose of food material given, and the nature of the symptoms observed.

Step 4 Preparation of Foods

Dehydrated or dried powdered food is either administered in opaque white (tinted with titanium oxide) gelatin capsules containing up to 500 mg test material, or disguised in a carrier food such as milk, apple or vegetable purée, or lentil soup (Bock et al 1988, Bock 1991).

Step 5 Placebos

Where capsules are used, the simplest placebos are dextrose or lactose powder. Liquid vehicles, without the addition of anything else, can be used as a placebo.

Step 6 Medication Avoidance

Drugs which may need to be avoided before food challenge are H1 histamine antagonists, and where bronchoconstriction is an end-point, any bronchodilator drugs. A potential drawback to withdrawing treatment is that this alone may precipitate symptoms, which may happen to coincide with either active or placebo challenge. This problem can only be avoided (a) by not stopping the medication, or (b) by performing multiple challenges.

Step 7 Food Administration

Food administration should start with a small quantity, less than that estimated by the parents to produce symptoms. The dose is then doubled at intervals specified by the history, so that if the reaction is said to occur after 30 min then the dose could be doubled every 45–60 min. The doubling dose is continued until the patient has obvious symptoms, or until about 10 g of dried or 100 g of untreated food have been given. In some cases, particularly those with delayed reactions, larger quantities of food may be needed (e.g. 200 ml of cows' milk per day).

Risk of Anaphylactic Shock

There are certain situations that carry a risk of anaphylactic shock occurring during a food challenge. These are:

- Where there is a previous history of anaphylactic shock great caution is required. Is the challenge really needed? There may be a case for directly applying the food to the skin, prior to food challenge. A negative reaction is no guarantee of safety, but a strongly positive reaction should make one reconsider whether the challenge is really necessary.
- Certain foods (cows' milk, fish, nuts, egg) carry a greater risk of anaphylactic shock than others.
- Food challenges in patients with atopic eczema who have been on elemental diets may constitute a special risk for anaphylactic shock (David 1989).

Repeat Challenges

A high proportion of children with food intolerance "grow out" of the intolerance, the exception being intolerance to peanuts which is usually life-long (Bock and Atkins 1989). This means that where a child has a positive food challenge, it may be worth repeating the challenge at 6–12 monthly intervals to detect the development of tolerance.

Limitations of Double-blind Food Challenges

The technique is subject to a number of potential limitations:

- In some cases of food intolerance, minute quantities of food (e.g. traces of cows' milk protein) are sufficient to provoke florid and immediate symptoms. In other cases, much larger quantities of food are required to provoke a response. For example, Hill et al (1988) demonstrated that, whereas 8–10 g of cow's milk powder (corresponding to 60–70 ml of milk) was adequate to provoke an adverse reaction in some patients with cows' milk protein allergy, others (with late onset symptoms and particularly atopic eczema) required up to 10 times this volume of milk daily for more than 48 h before symptoms developed.
- It is often unclear from the history what dosage of different foods is required to exclude food intolerance.

- Standard capsules which contain up to 500 mg of food are suitable for validation of immediate reactions to tiny quantities of food, but concealing much larger quantities of certain foods (especially those with a strong smell, flavour or colour) can be very difficult. If capsules are not used then performing challenges which are truly double blind (i.e. the parents do not know whether active substance or placebo is being given) at home becomes much more difficult.
- Reactions to food occurring within the mouth (Amlot et al 1985) are likely to be missed if the challenge bypasses the oral route, for example by administration of foods in a capsule or via a nasogastric tube.
- Capsules are unsuitable for use in small children, and this is a major limitation as most cases of suspected food intolerance are in infants and toddlers. Nasogastric tubes are too invasive for routine clinical use. This means trying to disguise one food in another carrier food. It is unsatisfactory to allow patients (or parents) to break open capsules and swallow (or administer) the contents mixed into food or drink, as the colour (e.g. tartrazine) or smell (e.g. fish) will be difficult or impossible to conceal and the challenge will no longer be blind.
- Difficulties arise if a cooked food is used for testing and the patient is only sensitive to a raw food, or vice versa.
- There is a danger of producing anaphylactic shock, even if anaphylactic shock had not occurred on previous exposure to the food. For example, in Goldman's classic study of cows' milk protein intolerance, anaphylactic shock had been noted prior to cows' milk challenge in 5 children, but another 3 out of 89 children developed anaphylactic shock as a new symptom after cow's milk challenge (Goldman et al 1963). In a study of 80 children with atopic eczema treated with elimination diets, anaphylactic shock occurred in 4 out of 1862 food challenges (David 1984). The risk appears to be greatest for those who have received elemental diets (David 1989).
- A food challenge performed during a quiescent phase of the disease may fail to provoke an adverse reaction. In chronic urticaria, intolerance to salicylates is confined to patients with active disease. The same phenomenon is commonly observed in atopic eczema, and is particularly noticeable when the skin lesions improve during a holiday in the sun (Turner et al 1991), during which parents may note that the child can tolerate foods which are not tolerated at home.
- Although some patients react repeatedly to challenges with single foods, it is possible (but unproven) that some patients only react adversely when multiple allergens are given together. The additive effect of

allergens has been best validated in patch testing (McLelland and Shuster 1990).

- Where food intolerance exists in children with atopic eczema, it is common for the patient to be intolerant to several foods. The removal of only one offending item may fail to help the patient. For the same reason it is possible that when this item is reintroduced into the diet in the form of a food challenge, the food may not provoke any detectable worsening of the dermatitis.

- In some situations, factors other than a food are necessary for positive challenges to occur. For example, in a subgroup of patients with exercise-induced anaphylaxis, symptoms only occur if exercise follows the ingestion of a particular food. Exercise or the food alone fail to provoke symptoms. In some cases, the nature of the "other factor" is obscure. For example, tartrazine challenges in children with asthma who are intolerant to tartrazine may fail to provoke any significant change in lung function, although histamine challenge testing may reveal enhanced bronchial reactivity (Hariparsad et al 1984). It is not known what additional factors are required to produce symptoms in such patients. The point here is that a conventional double-blind challenge, using as an endpoint, for example, a 20% fall in FEV_1, would fail to confirm genuine tartrazine intolerance.

Clinical Usefulness

Double-blind placebo-controlled food challenges are clearly the best available tool to confirm food intolerance. However, it is evident that single food challenges fail to take into account any possible additive effect of allergens. They also may fail to provoke a reaction if an underlying disease (e.g. urticaria or atopic eczema) is inactive, and unless performed with great care may fail to replicate natural exposure in which some other factor such as exercise is required to produce a positive reaction.

REFERENCES

Amlot PL, Urbank R, Youlten LJF et al (1985) Type I allergy to egg and milk proteins: comparison of skin prick tests with nasal, buccal and gastric provocation tests. Int Arch Allergy Appl Immunol 77: 171–173.

Bernstein IL (ed) (1988) Proceedings of the task force on guidelines for standardizing old and new technologies used for the diagnosis and treatment of allergic diseases. J Allergy Clin Immunol 82: 487–526.

Bock SA (1991) Oral challenge procedures. In: Metcalfe DD, Sampson HA, Simon RA (eds) Food Allergy. Adverse Reactions to Foods and Food Additivies, Chap 6, pp. 83–112. Blackwell, Oxford.

Bock SA, Atkins FM (1989) The natural history of peanut allergy. J Allergy Clin Immunol 83: 900–904.

Bock SA, Sampson HA, Atkins FM et al (1988) Double-blind, placebo-controlled food challenge (DBPCFC) as an office procedure: a manual. J Allergy Clin Immunol 82: 986–997.

Bousquet J (1988) In vivo methods for study of allergy: skin tests, techniques, and interpretation. In: Middleton E, Reed CE, Ellis EF, Adkinson NF, Yunginger JW (eds) Allergy. Principles and Practice, 3rd edn, Vol. 1, Chap. 19, pp. 419–436. Mosby, St Louis.

David TJ (1984) Anaphylactic shock during elimination diets for severe atopic eczema. Arch Dis Child 59: 983–986.

David TJ (1987) Reactions to dietary tartrazine. Arch Dis Child 62: 119–122.

David TJ (1989) Hazards of challenge tests in atopic dermatitis. Allergy (Suppl 9): 101–107.

David TJ (1993) Food and Food Additive Intolerance in Childhood. Blackwell, Oxford.

Dreborg S (ed) (1989) Skin tests used in type I allergy testing. Position paper. Prepared by the sub-committee on skin tests of the European Academy of Allergology and Clinical Immunology. Allergy 44 (Suppl 10): 1–59.

Goldman AS, Anderson DW, Sellers WA et al (1963) Milk allergy. I. Oral challenge with milk and isolated milk proteins in allergic children. Pediatrics 32: 425–443.

Hariparsad D, Wilson N, Dixon C, Silverman M (1984) Oral tartrazine challenge in childhood asthma: effect on bronchial reactivity. Clin Allergy 14: 81–85.

Hill DJ, Ball G, Hosking CS (1988) Clinical manifestations of cow's milk allergy in childhood. I. Associations with in-vitro cellular immune responses. Clin Allergy 18: 469–479.

McLelland J, Shuster S (1990) Contact dermatitis with negative patch tests: the additive effect of allergens in combination. Br J Dermatol 122: 623–630.

Terho EO, Husman K, Kivekas J, Riihimaki H (1989) Histamine control affects the weal produced by the adjacent diluent control in skin prick tests. Allergy 44: 30–32.

Turner MA, Devlin J, David TJ (1991) Holidays and atopic eczema. Arch Dis Child 66: 212–215.

Warner JO, Hathaway MJ (1984) Allergic form of Meadow's syndrome (Munchausen by proxy). Arch Dis Child 59: 151–156.

15

Heart Disease

M L Rigby

INTRODUCTION

The paediatrician will be alerted to the presence of congenital or acquired heart disease by a heart murmur, tachypnoea, cyanosis, failure to thrive, recurrent chest infection, or heart failure in infancy and by effort intolerance, syncope, palpitations or cyanosis in the older child.

In many instances a short history, competent physical examination, chest X-ray and electrocardiogram will be sufficient to allow an accurate diagnosis. As a general rule, innocent murmurs, small ventricular septal defects and mild aortic or pulmonary stenosis do not require referral of the patient to a cardiologist. However, the presence of symptoms or of an abnormal chest radiograph or electrocardiogram warrant a specialist's opinion.

In many cases an echocardiogram will be advised, but this must be performed and interpreted by an expert. Any additional investigations, such as magnetic resonance imaging (MRI), computerized tomography (CT) or cardiac catheterization and angiography will also be performed in a specialized referral centre.

THE ELECTROCARDIOGRAM

Routine Reporting

It is good practice to have a routine for reporting every electrocardiogram (ECG). The following list forms a satisfactory basis in most infants and children. (See later text for details.)

- Heart rate (describe atrial and ventricular rates if they are different).
- Rhythm (P wave axis differentiates sinus from non-sinus).
- QRS mean frontal axis.
- T wave mean frontal axis.
- PR interval, QRS duration, QT interval.
- QRS amplitude, R/S ratios and Q waves.
- T wave and S–T segments.

Heart Rate

The usual paper speed for recording an electrocardiogram is 25 mm/s. As a consequence 1 mm is equivalent to 0.04 s and 5 mm equal to 0.20 s. Heart rate can therefore be calculated by one of the following methods:

- 60 ÷ RR interval.
- Number of RR intervals in six large squares × 50 (for tachycardia).
- 300/number of large squares between two R waves (for bradycardia).

Normal heart rates for age are listed in Table 15.1.

PR Interval

The PR interval (Table 15.2) is measured from the onset of the P wave to the beginning of the QRS complex. Prolongation occasionally occurs without any obvious cause. Otherwise, it is found in association with the following conditions:

- Atrioventricular septal defects (primum ASD or complete AV canal).

Table 15.1 Normal heart rates for age

Age	Heart rate (beats/min)				
	Min.	5%	Mean	95%	Max.
0–24 hours	85	94	119	145	145
1–7 days	100	100	133	175	175
8–30 days	115	115	163	190	190
1–3 months	115	124	154	190	205
3–6 months	115	111	140	179	205
6–12 months	115	112	140	177	185
1–3 years	100	98	126	190	190
3–5 years	55	65	98	132	145
5–8 years	70	70	96	115	145
8–12 years	55	55	79	107	115
12–16 years	55	55	75	102	115

Table 15.2   Normal PR intervals for age

Age	PR interval (s)				
	Min.	5%	Mean	95%	Max.
0–24 hours	0.07	0.07	0.10	0.12	0.13
1–7 days	0.05	0.07	0.09	0.12	0.13
8–30 days	0.07	0.07	0.09	0.11	0.13
1–3 months	0.07	0.07	0.10	0.13	0.17
3–6 months	0.07	0.07	0.10	0.13	0.13
6–12 months	0.07	0.08	0.10	0.13	0.15
1–3 years	0.07	0.08	0.11	0.15	0.17
3–5 years	0.09	0.09	0.12	0.15	0.17
5–8 years	0.09	0.10	0.13	0.16	0.19
8–12 years	0.09	0.10	0.14	0.17	0.27
12–16 years	0.09	0.11	0.14	0.16	0.21

- Rheumatic or viral myocarditis.
- Hyperkalaemia.
- Digitalis toxicity.
- Myocardial ischaemia or profound hypoxia.
- Atrioventricular discordance (congenitally corrected transposition).

A short PR interval is most likely to be found in one of the following:

- Wolff–Parkinson–White syndrome.
- Lown–Ganong–Levine syndrome.
- Pompe's disease.

QRS Duration

The QRS duration (Table 15.3) is measured from the onset of the QRS complex to the termination of the S wave. Factitious prolongation occurs when the QRS complex is large.

Table 15.3   Normal QRS duration for age

Age	QRS duration (s)				
	Min.	5%	Mean	95%	Max.
0–24 hours	0.05	0.05	0.065	0.084	0.09
1–7 days	0.04	0.04	0.056	0.079	0.08
8–30 days	0.04	0.04	0.057	0.073	0.08
1–3 months	0.05	0.05	0.062	0.080	0.08
3–6 months	0.06	0.06	0.068	0.080	0.08
6–12 months	0.05	0.05	0.065	0.080	0.08
1–3 years	0.05	0.05	0.064	0.080	0.08
3–5 years	0.06	0.06	0.072	0.084	0.09
5–8 years	0.05	0.05	0.067	0.080	0.08
8–12 years	0.05	0.05	0.073	0.084	0.09
12–16 years	0.04	0.04	0.068	0.080	0.10

An abnormally wide QRS duration may occur in the following circumstances:

- Right or left bundle branch block.
- Ventricular pre-excitation.
- Interventricular block.
- Ventricular ectopic beat.
- Ventricular tachycardia.
- Hyperkalaemia
- Toxicity due to certain anti-arrythmic drugs such as flecainide or procainamide.

Mean Frontal QRS Axis

The mean frontal QRS axis is most conveniently calculated by measuring the R and S waves in leads V1 and AVF as shown in Figure 15.1. The normal values are listed in Table 15.4, showing that extreme right axis is a common finding in the neonatal period. The presence of a superior axis at any age is unusual and is of considerable diagnostic importance. The cyanosed neonate or infant

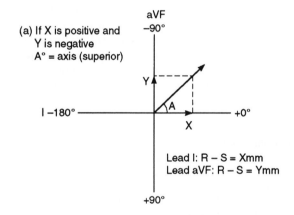

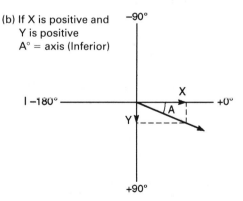

Figure 15.1   Diagram illustrating a method of determining the mean frontal QRS axis which can also be applied to the P-wave axis and T-wave axis.

Table 15.4 Normal mean frontal QRS axis values for age

Age	QRS axis (frontal plane)				
	Min.	5%	Mean	95%	Max.
0–24 hours	60	60	135	180	180
1–7 days	60	80	125	160	180
8–30 days	0	60	110	160	180
1–3 months	20	40	80	120	120
3–6 months	40	20	65	80	100
6–12 months	20	0	65	100	120
1–3 years	0	20	55	100	100
3–5 years	0	40	60	80	80
5–8 years	−20	40	65	100	100
8–12 years	−20	20	65	80	120
12–16 years	−20	20	65	80	100

with a superior axis is likely to have classical tricuspid atresia or, less commonly, double inlet ventricle. The acyanotic infant with a superior axis and heart failure will almost certainly have an atrioventricular septal defect with common valve orifice. A superior axis is also found in about one-tenth of infants with ventricular septal defects presenting with heart failure. The child with a superior axis with signs of an atrial septal defect is likely to have an atrioventricular septal defect with separate valve orifices – the so-called "primum" defect. Physical signs of pulmonary stenosis associated with superior axis are a feature of Noonan's syndrome. Tetralogy of Fallot coexisting with an atrioventricular septal defect can be anticipated in the child or infant with the combination of Down's syndrome, cyanosis and a superior axis. A superior axis may also indicate left anterior hemiblock associated with transient myocardial ischaemia of the newborn, or may follow surgery for ventricular septal defects or tetralogy of Fallot. Thus a superior axis may occur in the following circumstances:

- Absent right atrioventricular connexion (tricuspid atresia).
- Double inlet ventricle (< 10%).
- Atrioventricular septal defect (> 90%).
- Atrioventricular septal defect with tetralogy of Fallot (> 90%).
- Large perimembranous ventricular septal defect (< 10%).
- Left anterior hemiblock.
- Ebstein's anomaly of the tricuspid valve.
- Noonan's syndrome.
- Following surgical closure of ventricular septal defect.

The term "left axis deviation" includes the group with a superior axis but more specifically is present when the axis is below the lower limit of normal for age and may occur in the presence of:

- Left ventricular hypertrophy.
- Left bundle branch block.
- Left anterior hemiblock.

Right-axis deviation is present when the QRS axis is greater than the upper limit of normal for age. It may occur in:

- Right ventricular hypertrophy.
- Right bundle branch block.

QT Interval

The QT interval is measured from the onset of the Q wave to the end of the T wave in leads with visible Q waves. It varies with heart rate but not with age, except in infancy. According to Bazett's formula, the corrected QT interval is equal to QT divided by the square root of the RR interval. It should not exceed 0.425 s. However, a value of up to 0.49 s may be normal in the first 6 months of life.

A prolonged QT interval may be seen in:

- Hypercalcaemia.
- Rheumatic or viral myocarditis.
- Long QT syndrome.
- Head injury or cerebrovascular accidents.
- Congestive cardiomyopathy.
- Following the administration of certain drugs including Procainamide and Quinidine.

A short QT interval may be seen in:

- Hypocalcaemia.
- Digoxin toxicity.

Determination of Amplitude

The amplitude of any positive deflexion is measured from the upper margin of the baseline to the very top of the deflexion. Similarly, the amplitude of any negative deflexion is measured from the lower margin of the baseline to the lowest point of the wave.

T-wave Amplitude

Tall peaked T waves may be seen in:

- Hyperkalaemia.
- Left ventricular hypertrophy.

Flat or low T waves may be seen in:

- Normal newborn infants.
- Hypokalaemia.
- Carditis.
- Myocardial ischaemia.
- Digoxin toxicity.

Normal RS Progression Pattern in Precordial Leads

In symptomatic infants with congenital heart disease it is more useful to consider the RS progression pattern in the precordial leads (Figure 15.2) than the presence or absence of ventricular hypertrophy. The majority of children over the age of 2 years have a characteristic RS progression pattern in these leads. Thus, in leads V4R and V1 there is a dominant S wave while there is dominant R wave in lead V6. This is the so-called "adult pattern" of left ventricular dominance. The characteristic RS progression pattern at birth includes a dominant R wave in leads V4R and V1 and a dominant S wave in lead V6. This "neonatal pattern" of right ventricular dominance persists for up to 1 month. The majority of children between the ages of 1 month and 2 years have a dominant R wave in V6. This is the so-called "infant pattern" of balanced ventricular forces. The infant pattern may be present soon after birth and may persist up to the age of 3 years. In the normal child the RS voltages will be normal.

RS Progression Patterns Associated with Cardiac Malformations

The Neonatal RS Progression Pattern

When a symptomatic neonate demonstrates the normal neonatal RS progression pattern there is a variety of diagnostic possibilities, but it may be assumed either that there are two normal ventricles or that the left ventricle is small. Thus, in the neonate with central cyanosis, the most likely diagnoses are:

With normal left ventricle:
- Complete transposition.
- Persistent foetal circulation.
- Obstructed total anomalous pulmonary venous connection.
- Critical pulmonary valve stenosis.
- Tetralogy of Fallot with severe infundibular stenosis.
- Pulmonary atresia with ventricular septal defect.

With small left ventricle:
- Univentricular connection to right ventricle.
- Hypoplastic left heart syndrome.

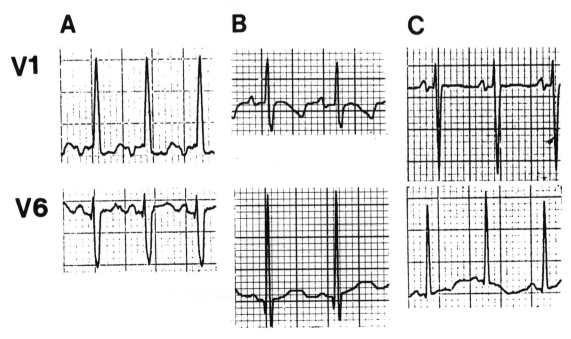

Figure 15.2   (A) Neonatal precordial RS progression pattern. (B) Infant precordial RS progression pattern. (C) Adult precordial RS progression pattern.

In the presence of two normal ventricles there is also likely to be evidence of right ventricular hypertrophy (see below).

The symptomatic neonate without desaturation but with the normal neonatal pattern will almost certainly have the coarctation syndrome.

When the neonatal pattern persists after the age of 1 month, it indicates right ventricular hypertrophy with either a normal or a rudimentary left ventricle. Complete transposition, hypoplastic left heart syndrome and coarctation syndrome are unlikely to present outside the neonatal period, so that in early infancy the major diagnostic groups are:

- Severe obstruction to pulmonary blood flow (usually pulmonary valve stenosis).
- Pulmonary atresia with ventricular septal defect (and pulmonary blood flow via major systemic-pulmonary collaterals).
- Total anomalous pulmonary venous connection.
- Univentricular connection to right ventricle.

In later infancy, or after the age of 1 year, persistence of the neonatal precordial RS progression pattern again indicates right ventricular hypertrophy as in tetralogy of Fallot or ventricular septal defect with infundibular stenosis or pulmonary stenosis. The pulmonary vascular resistance occasionally does not fall after birth in the presence of a ventricular septal defect, persistent patency of the arterial duct or atrial septal defects. Under these circumstances, the resultant right ventricular hypertrophy leads to persistence of the neonatal pattern.

The Infant RS Progression Pattern

The symptomatic infant with a dominant R wave in both leads V1 and V6 will usually present outside the neonatal period because of one of the following:

- Large ventricular septal defect.
- Multiple ventricular septal defects.
- Large arterial duct.
- Complete transposition with ventricular septal defect.
- Double outlet right ventricle.
- Atrioventricular septal defect with common orifice.
- Common arterial trunk.
- Aortopulmonary window.
- Double inlet left ventricle.
- Critical aortic stenosis.

In practice, some of these conditions may present during the neonatal period. Irrespective of the time of presentation there is often not only an infant RS progression pattern but also evidence of biventricular hypertrophy (see below).

The Adult RS Progression Pattern

An adult RS progression pattern (left ventricular dominance) in the symptomatic neonate or infant almost always signifies the presence of a rudimentary or hypoplastic right ventricle such as might be found in hearts with:

- Classical tricuspid atresia.
- Double inlet left ventricle.
- Pulmonary atresia with intact ventricular septum.
- Ebstein's malformation of the tricuspid valve.

Less frequently, an adult RS progression pattern in the neonate or infant may indicate left ventricular hypertrophy in the presence of a normal right ventricle as a consequence of volume overload because of an arterial duct or pressure overload in critical aortic stenosis.

Right ventricular hypertrophy (Figure 15.3(B)) The following are important features of ventricular hypertrophy:

- A pure R wave of more than 10 mm in lead V1.
- An R wave in V1 of more than 20 mm.
- Upright T waves in lead V1 after the age of 3 days and before puberty.
- A neonatal RS progression pattern after the age of 1 month.
- An infant RS progression pattern after the age of 18 months.
- Right axis deviation for age.
- A Q wave in lead V1 (also found in 50% of hearts with atrioventricular discordance).

Left ventricular hypertrophy (Figure 15.3(A)) The following features suggest the presence of left ventricular hypertrophy:

- An R wave in lead V6 of more than 25 mm.
- An S wave in lead V1 of more than 20 mm.
- A Q wave in lead V5 or V6 of more than 4 mm.
- T-wave inversion in leads V5 and V6 (so-called left ventricular strain).
- An adult RS progression pattern before the age of 18 months.
- An infant progression pattern during the first month of life.

Biventricular hypertrophy Biventricular hypertrophy is characterized by voltage evidence of both left and right ventricular hypertrophy. It is likely that the sum of the R

A   **B**

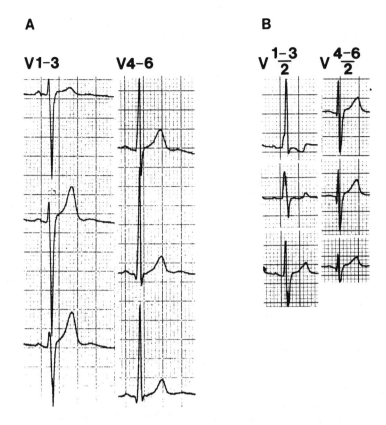

Figure 15.3   (A) Precordial leads in left ventricular hypertrophy with tall R waves in leads V5 and V6 and deep S waves in leads V1 and V2. (B) Precordial leads in right ventricular hypertrophy with tall R wave in lead V1 and prominent S waves in leads V5 and V6.

and S waves in leads V3 and V4 will be greater than 60 mm.

Tachycardia

Sinus Tachycardia

Sinus rhythm originates in the sinoatrial node and has two important characteristics:

- A P wave precedes each QRS complex with a regular PR interval.
- The mean frontal P-wave axis (calculated in the same way as the QRS axis) is in the range 0–90 so that an upright P in lead II and an inverted P in a VR are almost always present.

When there is sinus tachycardia the usual characteristics of sinus rhythm are present, but the heart rate is

above the upper limit of normal for age although rarely above 200/min. Important causes include:

- Anxiety.
- Fever.
- Hypovolaemia.
- Shock.
- Heart failure.

Supraventricular Tachycardia (SVT)

Classification

Junctional tachycardia:
- Atrioventricular re-entry tachycardia (AVRT).
- Atrioventricular nodal re-entry tachycardia (AVNRT).
- Long RP tachycardia.

Atrial tachycardia:
- Atrial re-entry tachycardia.
- Ectopic atrial tachycardia.
- Atrial flutter.
- Atrial fibrillation.

Clinical Presentation

- Unexplained fetal hydrops.
- Neonatal cardiogenic shock.
- Tachypnoea, poor feeding, pallor in neonate or infant.
- Palpitations in older children.
- Syncope.
- Cardiomegaly on routine chest radiograph.
- Unexplained rapid pulse.

Mechanisms

The most common type of SVT results from a re-entry circuit between atria and ventricles which involves the atrioventricular node as the antegrade limb and an accessory connection between ventricle and atrium as the retrograde pathway (AVRT). During sinus rhythm only antegrade conduction through the accessory pathway gives rise to the characteristic features of pre excitation. These are a short PR interval and a delta wave at the onset of the QRS complex. Although junctional tachycardias can be associated with structural heart disease (Ebstein's anomaly of the tricuspid valve, congenitally corrected transposition, double inlet left ventricle) atrial tachycardias are much more likely to occur with coexisting heart disease.

General Characteristics of Junctional Tachycardias (Figure 15.4)

- Heart rate 180/min or above.
- Extremely regular narrow QRS complexes (occasionally aberrancy causes wide QRS).
- One to one relationship of P wave and QRS.
- P wave follows QRS (AVRT).
- P wave within QRS and often hidden (AVNRT).
- P wave before QRS (Long RP tachycardia).
- Abnormal P wave axis.
- Associated heart disease uncommon.

Characteristics of Re-entry or Ectopic Atrial Tachycardia (Figure 15.4(A))

- Heart rate 180/min or above.
- Extemely regular narrow QRS complexes (occasionally aberrancy causes wide QRS).
- Atrioventricular block is frequent.

- P wave may be hidden in T wave.
- Abnormal P-wave axis.
- Associated heart disease common.

Atrial Flutter (Figure 15.4(B))

- Atrial rate about 300/min with "saw-tooth" configuration.
- Atrioventricular block (2 : 1, 3 : 1 or 4 : 1) is frequently present so that the ventricular rate is usually 150/min or less.
- QRS duration is normal.
- Associated heart disease common.

Atrial Fibrillation

- Extremely fast atrial rate.
- Irregularly irregular ventricular response and pulse.
- Normal QRS complexes.
- Associated heart disease common.

Ventricular Tachycardia (Figure 15.4(C))

This is characterized by:

- A heart rate of 120–180/min.
- Wide QRS complexes (so-called "ventricular fusion complex").
- No visible "P" waves.
- Underlying ventricular dysfunction (often after cardiac surgery).

Ventricular Fibrillation

This is characterized by:

- Bizarre ventricular QRS patterns of varying size and configuration.
- Rapid and irregular rate.
- Extremely low cardiac output.

Bradycardia

A heart rate of less than 80/min in the neonate or infant and less than 60/min in older children can be considered a bradycardia. The important types of slow heart rate are:

- Sinus bradycardia.
- Junctional (nodal) rhythm.
- Sinoatrial dysfunction (sick sinus syndrome).
- Second-degree heart block.
- Complete heart block.

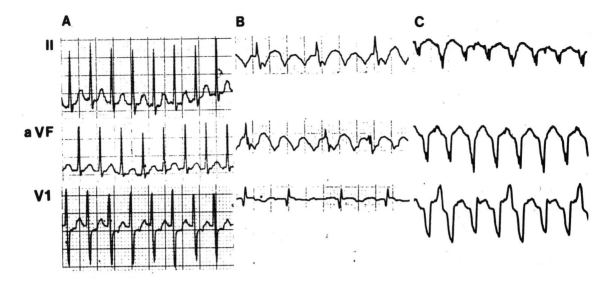

Figure 15.4 (A) AV re-entry tachycardia. (B) Atrial flutter. (C) Ventricular tachycardia.

Sinus Bradycardia

All rhythms that orginate in the sinoatrial node (sinus rhythm) have two important characteristics:

- The "P" wave precedes the QRS complex with a constant PR interval.
- The "P"-wave axis is between 0° and 90° so that there are upright T waves in lead II and inverted P waves in AVR.

The causes of sinus bradycardia include:

- Vagal stimulation.
- Increased intracranial pressure.
- Hypothyroidism.
- Hypothermia.
- Hypoxia.
- Hyperkalaemia.
- Digoxin.
- Beta-blocking agents.

In most instances, however, sinus bradycardia is of little significance.

Junctional (Nodal) Rhythm

Heart rhythms which originate from the atrioventricular node are characterized by:

- An absent P wave or an inverted P wave following the QRS complex.

- A QRS complex which is almost always normal in duration and configuration.

If there is a persistent failure of the sinoatrial node, the atrioventricular node will become the main pacemaker of the heart. As a consequence there is a relatively slow heart rate. Nodal rhythm is characterized by:

- Absence of P waves (hidden in the QRS complex).
- An inverted P wave or P wave with abnormal morphology following the QRS complex.
- QRS rate of 40–60/min.
- Normal QRS duration and configuration.

A junctional rhythm often occurs during sleep, but may follow some types of cardiac surgery, pharyngeal stimulation and digoxin toxicity.

Sick Sinus Syndrome (Sinoatrial Dysfunction)

Because the sinoatrial node fails to function as the dominant pacemaker a variety of dysrhythmias result. They include sinus bradycardia, sinoatrial block, sinus arrest with junctional escape beats and ectopic atrial tachycardia. The causes of sinoatrial dysfunction include:

- Cardiac surgery involving the atria, e.g. surgical repair of atrial septal defect, or Mustard operation.
- Myocarditis.
- Unknown cause.

Second-degree Heart Block

In first-degree heart block there is a prolongation of the PR interval beyond the upper limits of normal for the patient's age. This can occur in acute rheumatic fever, cardiomyopathies, atrioventricular septal defects, following cardiac surgery or with digoxin toxicity. It is also found in healthy individuals. In contrast, second-degree heart block is diagnosed when some but not all of the P waves are followed by a QRS complex. The causes include those found with first-degree heart block.

Complete Heart Block

The characteristics of complete heart block are the following:

* The P waves are regular and there is a regular PP interval.
* The QRS complexes are also regular so that the RR interval is constant but the rate is slower than the P-wave rate.
* The duration of the QRS complex is normal in congenital complete heart block and in these circumstances the ventricular rate may be greater than 60/min.
* In surgically induced or acquired complete heart block the QRS duration is frequently prolonged and the ventricular rate is less than 50/min.

The causes of congenital complete heart block include:

* An isolated anomaly of unknown cause associated with a structurally normal heart.
* Maternal connective tissue disorders.
* Structural heart disease of which the most common is congenitally corrected transposition of the great arteries.

In children the most important causes of acquired heart block include:

* Cardiac surgery.
* Myocarditis.

THE CHEST RADIOGRAPH

The chest radiograph is an essential part of the clinical evaluation of the cardiovascular system. The X-ray should be exposed in full inspiration. For the most part a posteroanterior projection is sufficient, although initial evaluation is often accompanied by a lateral view as well.

A systematic approach to the reporting of an X-ray film should include the following:

* Determination of bronchial situs with location of the liver and stomach bubble.
* Cardiac position.
* Heart size and cardiothoracic ratio.
* Cardiac silhouette.
* Evaluation of cardiac chambers and great arteries.
* Pulmonary vascular markings.
* General features of the skeleton and lung.

Determination of Bronchial Situs

There are four types of atrial arrangement (situs) and usually there is concordancy between atrial and bronchial situs so that determination of the latter from a posteroanterior chest X-ray (or filtered films of the bronchi) allows atrial arrangement to be inferred.

* *Usual atrial arrangement (situs solitus).* This is characterized by a short right main bronchus, long left main bronchus, right sided liver and left-sided stomach.
* *Mirror-image atrial arrangement (situs inversus).* This is associated with a long right-sided bronchus, short left-sided bronchus, left-sided liver, right sided stomach and usually dextrocardia.
* *Right atrial isomerism (asplenia syndrome).* Characterized by bilaterally short bronchi, right isomerism is associated with variable position of the stomach (right, left or midline), a rather centrally located liver and any position of the heart.
* *Left atrial isomerism (polysplenia syndrome).* When there is polysplenia bilaterally long bronchi are present, a centrally positioned liver is frequently found and in the majority of cases there is a left sided stomach.

In general terms, the cardiac apex should be on the same side as the stomach or opposite to the liver. When the cardiac apex and stomach are at opposite sides or the liver is a midline (central) structure, the likelihood of a major congenital heart defect is considerable.

Cardiac Position

When describing the position of the heart, it is neither desirable nor necessary to infer situs or the mechanism for any abnormality. Thus terms such as dextroversion or dextrorotation should be avoided. In fact there are only three possibilities:

* Laevocardia (left-sided heart).

- Dextrocardia (right-sided heart).
- Mesocardia (central or midline heart).

Dextrocardia is most frequently encountered in the following:

- Congenitally corrected transposition with usual atrial arrangement.
- Left or right atrial isomerism.
- Scimitar syndrome.
- A few cases of tricuspid atresia with usual atrial arrangement.
- Most cases of mirror image arrangement of the atria (situs inversus) with or without associated congenital cardiac malformations.

Heart Size and Cardiothoracic Ratio

The simplest measurement of heart size is the cardiothoracic ratio. This is obtained by relating the largest transverse diameter of the heart to the widest internal diameter of the chest (usually at the level of the costophrenic angles). A cardiothoracic ratio of >0.5 is considered to indicate cardiac enlargement, although the cardiothoracic ratio cannot be used with any accuracy when there is not a good inspiratory chest film which is frequently the case in small infants. When there is a narrow anteroposterior diameter of the chest a posteroanterior film may erroneously show cardiomegaly. It is noteworthy that cardiac enlargement on a chest X-ray more reliably reflects volume overload than pressure overload and is therefore particularly characteristic of lesions with a high pulmonary blood flow or valve regurgitation. Cardiac enlargement is also characteristic of a dilated cardiomyopathy, whatever the cause.

Cardiac Silhouette

In the posteroanterior projection of a chest X-ray, the right cardiac border is formed by the superior caval vein superiorly and by the right atrium inferiorly. The left heart border is formed from top to bottom by the aortic arch, the pulmonary trunk and the left ventricle. The left atrial appendage is located between the pulmonary trunk and left ventricle and is not prominent in the normal heart. The right ventricle forms no part of the cardiac border. When there is a lateral projection the cardiac silhouette is formed anteriorly by the right ventricle and posteriorly by the left atrium above and left ventricle below.

In newborn infants the presence of a large thymus means that the typical cardiac silhouette is often absent. The thymus is situated at the superoanterior mediastinum so that the base of the heart will be widened on a posteroanterior view and the retrosternal space will be obliterated on the lateral view.

The overall shape of the heart, however, is rarely of any value in diagnosing cardiac defects although the following are frequently described:

- *Egg-shaped heart*. This is characteristic of simple transposition of the great arteries of the neonate and is characterized by a narrow pedicle.
- *Boot-shaped heart*. This is said to be typical of tetralogy of Fallot but may be found with tricuspid atresia.
- *Snowman sign*. This is said to be characteristic of infants with supracardiac total anomalous pulmonary venous connection. The head of the snowman is made up by the vertical vein on the left, the left innominate vein superiorly and the dilated superior caval vein on the right.

Evaluation of Cardiac Chambers and Great Arteries

Right Atrial Enlargement

This is characterized by increased prominence of the right lower cardiac silhouette in posteroanterior projection.

Right Ventricular Enlargement

This is rarely obvious on a posteroanterior projection and frequently there is a normal cardiothoracic ratio. The right ventricular enlargement is best seen in the lateral view, when there is filling of the retrosternal space anteriorly.

Left Atrial Enlargement

In the lateral projection there is a posterior protrusion of the left atrial border. In the posteroanterior view there is frequently a double density seen towards the right, the left atrial appendage becomes prominent on the left cardiac border and the left main bronchus is elevated.

Left Ventricular Enlargement

In the posteroanterior view the cardiac apex is displaced to the left and downwards. In the lateral projection, the lower posterior cardiac border is displaced posteriorly.

Enlargement of the Pulmonary Trunk

This can be seen in posteroanterior projection on the

upper left heart border. It is likely to be due to one of the following:

- Post-stenotic dilatation in pulmonary value stenosis.
- Increased pulmonary blood flow through the pulmonary artery (atrial septal defect, ventricular septal defect, etc.).
- Pulmonary hypertension.

Hypoplasia of the Pulmonary Arteries

This is characterized by a concave segment of the upper left heart border. It is characteristic of the following:

- Tetralogy of Fallot.
- Tetralogy of Fallot with pulmonary atresia.
- Classical tricuspid atresia with severe pulmonary stenosis or pulmonary atresia.
- Other conditions with pulmonary hypoplasia.

Dilatation of the Aorta

An enlarged ascending aorta in the posteroanterior projection is seen as a rightward bulge of the right mediastinum. It is characteristic of the following:

- Aortic stenosis.
- Tetralogy of Fallot.
- Long-standing aortic coarctation.
- Systemic hypertension.

The Aortic Arch

When the descending aorta is seen along the left margin of the spine this usually indicates a left aortic arch while a right aortic arch is associated with a descending aorta along the right margin of the spine. Alternatively, the position of the trachea may help locate the descending aorta. The left aortic arch is usually associated with a trachea located slightly to the right of the midline. When there is a right aortic arch, the trachea is shifted to the left. A right aortic arch is important because it may be associated with tetralogy of Fallot or common arterial trunk. In long-standing coarctation of the aorta the so-called pre-coarctation and post-coarctation dilatation may be seen as a "figure-of-three" at the upper left heart border.

Pulmonary Vascular Markings

Increased Pulmonary Blood Flow (Pulmonary Plethora)

The characteristics of increased pulmonary vascularity include:

- Enlargement of the pulmonary arteries.
- Extension of the pulmonary arteries into the lateral third of the lung fields.
- Increased vascularity to the lung apices.
- A right pulmonary artery diameter greater than the internal diameter of the trachea.

Increased pulmonary blood flow without cyanosis is characteristic of an atrial septal defect, ventricular septal defect, arterial duct or atrioventricular septal defect. When cyanosis is associated with an increased pulmonary blood flow the possibilities include: (a) total anomalous pulmonary venous connection; (b) common arterial trunks; (c) hearts with univentricular atrioventricular connection (e.g. tricuspid atresia or double inlet ventricle) without pulmonary stenosis; (d) complete transposition of the great arteries; and (e) transposition with ventricular septal defect.

Decreased Pulmonary Blood Flow (Pulmonary Oligaemia)

The characteristics of diminished pulmonary blood flow include:

- Small hilar blood vessels.
- "Black" lung fields.
- Small and thin pulmonary vessels.

Pulmonary oligaemia is characteristic of cyanotic heart disease with diminished pulmonary blood flow. Typically it's found in: (a) tetralogy of Fallot; (b) tetralogy of Fallot with pulmonary atresia; (c) tricuspid and pulmonary atresia; and (d) congenital cardiac lesion associated with severe pulmonary stenosis.

Pulmonary Venous Congestion

The characteristics of pulmonary venous congestion include the following:

- Hazy and indistinct pulmonary vascular markings.
- Upper lobe blood diversion.
- Kerley B lines.
- Pulmonary oedema.

Pulmonary venous congestion is found in conditions with left ventricular failure (e.g. large ventricular septal defect, dilated cardiomyopathy) or obstruction to pulmonary venous drainage (congenital mitral stenosis, obstructed total anomalous pulmonary venous connection, cortriatriartum, hypoplastic left heart syndrome).

Normal Pulmonary Vascularity

Normal pulmonary vascular markings can readily be encountered with major or severe congenital heart disease. For example, severe obstructive lesions such as aortic stenosis or aortic coarctation and even pulmonary stenosis are associated with normal pulmonary vascularity. Similarly complex lesions such as tricuspid atresia or double inlet left ventricle can be associated with normal pulmonary vascularity when there is moderate pulmonary stenosis (and balanced systemic and pulmonary blood flow).

General Features of the Skeleton and Lung

Pectus excavatum may flatten the heart in the anteroposterior dimension giving rise to a compensatory increase in its transverse diameter. Vertebral abnormalities and thoracic scoliosis are frequent findings in patients with congenital heart disease. Rib notching of the 4th to 8th ribs is a feature of older children with coarctation of the aorta.

In many infants the thymus is large giving rise to a false impression of cardiomegaly. In the lateral view, the thymus occupies the superoantero mediastinum obscuring the upper retrosternal space. When there is severe cyanosis the thymus may be very small. This is particularly evident in complete transposition. When the thymus cannot be seen Di George syndrome has to be considered particularly in the presence of aortic interruption or common arterial trunk.

A long-standing density at the right lower lung field is found with bronchopulmonary sequestration in which a segment of the lung is supplied directly by an anomalous artery arising from the descending aorta below the diaphragm. A vertical vascular shadow along the right lower cardiac border due to partial anomalous pulmonary venous return from the lower lobe is characteristic of the scimitar syndrome which is usually associated with bronchopulmonary sequestration.

OTHER METHODS OF INVESTIGATION

Echocardiography

Transthoracic Echocardiography

Transthoracic echocardiography is the most important investigative technique available to the paediatric cardiologist. It is used to obtain morphological information and to make quantitative measurements of ventricular function. It should not, however, be considered as an alternative to careful clinical examination and accurate evaluation of an ECG and chest X-ray. Echocardiography should be performed by an individual who is expert in the technique. Unreliable information is probably more dangerous than none at all. Many infants and children with a heart murmur do not require investigation by echocardiography. The important indications are listed below:

- Any neonate or infant with tachypnoea, cyanosis or heart failure which is not thought to be caused primarily by a lung abnormality.
- A heart murmur accompanied by an abnormality on the ECG or chest X-ray.
- Any infant or child with cyanosis or heart failure.
- A loud heart murmur.
- A diastolic or continuous murmur.
- Absent femoral pulses.
- Fixed splitting of the second heart sound.
- A single second heart sound.
- A loud pulmonary component to the second heart sound.
- Any patient with a precordial or cervical thrill.

Doppler Echocardiography

Doppler echocardiography is used to measure peak instantaneous gradients across discrete sites of obstruction. It can be used, therefore, to estimate the severity of aortic or pulmonary stenosis and mitral or tricuspid stenosis. Similarly it will estimate the systolic pressure drop across a VSD or across a mildly regurgitant tricuspid valve allowing measurement of the RV systolic pressure. Other uses include measurement of the diastolic aortic or pulmonary arterial pressures and measurement of cardiac output.

Colour-flow Doppler

Colour-flow doppler is a non-quantitative technique which allows the rapid recognition of regurgitant or stenotic valves, intracardiac shunts or an arterial duct.

Transoesophageal Echocardiography

Transoesophageal echocardiography in infants and children is performed under sedation or general anaesthesia. The major indications are an inadequate transthoracic window (usually in older children with complex cyanotic heart disease) and some types of interventional cardiac catheterization (umbrella closure of an interatrial communication or ventricular septal defect).

Magnetic Resonance Imaging

On the whole, resonance scanning is inferior to echo-cardiography in its ability to demonstrate cardiac morphology and make quantitative physiological measurements. It is, however, becoming a useful alternative to cardiac catheterization and angiography, when imaging of the aortic arch and the pulmonary arteries is required.

Computerized Tomography

Computerized tomography (CT) is rarely used for the investigation of heart disease in infants and children. It probably has a role in the diagnosis of a vascular ring. So called "ultrafast CT" can be used to display the pulmonary arteries and aorta as an alternative to conventional angiography.

Cardiac Catheterization and Angiography

Cardiac catheterization and angiography is still practised widely by paediatric cardiologists, although only about 50% of patients undergoing cardiac surgery will have been subjected to this investigation. The major indications for cardiac catheterization include:

- The measurement of pulmonary vascular resistance (when it is thought to be elevated on clinical grounds).
- Angiographic demonstration of the great arteries and coronary arteries.
- Interventional cardiac catheterization.

THE INVESTIGATION OF SPECIAL PROBLEMS

Cardiomyopathy

There are essentially two major groups of cardiomyopathy. The first has predominantly dilated ventricles (most commonly the left in isolation) and the second has predominantly thick walled ventricles. The former is characterized by obvious cardiac enlargement on the chest X-ray, while a normal heart size or mild cardiomegaly is characteristic of the latter.

Dilated Cardiomyopathy

In most cases no cause will be identified and generalized T-wave abnormalities will be seen on the ECG. The following should be excluded.

- Aortic coarctation (absent/delayed femoral pulses).
- Anomalous origin of left coronary artery from the pulmonary trunk (infarct pattern on the ECG).
- Refractory and persistent supraventricular tachycardia (ECG).
- Kawasaki disease (myocardial ischaemia on ECG).
- Transient perinatal myocardial ischaemia (myocardial ischaemia on ECG).
- Myocarditis (viral titres, immune complexes, ESR).
- Autoimmune disorders.

Rare causes of dilated cardiomyopathy include:

- Type-IV glycogen storage disease (see Chapter 4).
- Mucopolysaccharidosis.
- Gangliosidosis.
- Refsum's disease.
- Fabry's disease.
- Haemochromatosis.
- β-Oxidation defects (e.g. cartinine deficiency).
- Disorders of pyruvate metabolism.
- Respiratory chain defects.

Useful investigations include:

- Plasma carnitine.
- Plasma amino acids.
- Urine amino acids.
- Serum lactate and pyruvate.

Hypertrophic Cardiomyopathy

In most cases no cause will be found and the ECG will demonstrate generalized T-wave changes and left or right ventricular hypertrophy. Possible causes and association include:

- Classical hypertrophic cardiomyopathy.
- Maternal diabetes.
- Severe neonatal distress (e.g. septicaemia).
- Noonan's syndrome.
- Friedreich's ataxia.
- Leopard syndrome.
- Neurofibromatosis.
- Lipodystrophy.
- Glycogen storage disease.
- Mucopolysaccharidosis.

Infective Endocarditis

The most common infective organisms are:

- *Streptococcus veridans*.

- *Streptococcus faecalis*.
- *Staphylococcus aureus*.

Less commonly encountered organisms include:

- *Pneumococcus*.
- *Haemophillus influenzae*.
- *Pseudomonas*.
- *Escherichia coli*.
- *Candida albicans*.

Characteristic clinical features include fever of several days duration in a patient with an underlying cardiac abnormality. There is usually an insidious onset of fever, fatigue, anorexia and pallor. On physical examination there is usually a heart murmur, fluctuating fever and splenomegaly. Skin manifestations such as petechiae, Osler's nodes and splinter haemorrhages are frequently encountered. Pulmonary and systemic emboli may occur together with haematuria and even renal failure. Four to six blood cultures should be performed over a period of 24–48 h before commencing antibiotic treatment. Anaemia is common together with a leukocytosis with a shift to the left, increased sedimentation rate, microscopic haematuria and sometimes vegetations demonstrated on the cross-sectional echocardiogram.

Isolation of the infecting organism is mandatory for adequate antibiotic therapy. In patients referred to hospital already receiving antibiotic treatment it may be necessary to discontinue antibiotics for up to 48 h in order to obtain positive blood cultures. Therapy is dictated by the antibiotic sensitivities of the organisms isolated. Bactericidal drugs, such as penicillins, cephalosporins and aminoglycosides, must be used rather than bacteriostatic agents.

Rheumatic Fever

The diagnosis of acute rheumatic fever is made by the use of revised Jones criteria which consist of three groups of important clinical and laboratory findings.

Five major criteria:
- Polyarthritis.
- Carditis.
- Chorea.
- Erythema marginatum.
- Subcutaneous nodules.

Five minor criteria:
- Fever.
- Arthralgia.
- Previous history of rheumatic fever or rheumatic heart disease.
- Raised ESR and positive C-reactive protein.
- Prolonged PR interval.

Supporting evidence of preceding streptococcal infection includes:
- Increased ASO titre.
- Positive throat culture for group A *Streptococcus*.
- Recent scarlet fever.

The diagnosis of acute rheumatic fever is probable when two major criteria or one major criterion with two minor criteria are present. With the exception of chorea the absence of evidence of preceding streptococcal infection is a warning sign against acute rheumatic fever.

REFERENCES

Burnard ED, James LS (1961) The cardiac silhouette in newborn infants: a cinematographic study of the normal range. *Pediatrics* 27: 713–717.
Datey KK, Bharucha PE (1990) Electrocardiographic changes in the first week of life. *Br Heart J* 22: 175–180.
Hastreiter AR, Abella JB (1971) The electrocardiogram in the new-born period I. The normal infant. *J Pediatr* 78: 146–151.
Jones RS, Baumer H, Joseph MC, Shinebourne EA (1976) Arterial oxygen tension and the response to oxygen breathing in the differential diagnosis of congenital heart disease in infancy. *Arch Dis Child* 51: 667–672.
Talner NS, Sanyal SK, Halloran KH, Gardner TH, Ordway NK (1965) Congestive heart failure in infancy. I. Anomalies in blood gases and acid-base equilibrium. *Paediatrics* 35: 20–24.

16

Ear, Nose and Throat

K Pearman and D W Morgan

THE ASSESSMENT OF HEARING

Most audiological tests in childhood are directed at determining the quietest sounds which can stimulate the auditory system (the auditory threshold). The auditory threshold of a normal ear varies between individuals and with frequency. The range of intensity which can be perceived is vast so that absolute measures of sound pressure (in pascals (Pa)) are not helpful in clinical audiology and the intensity (loudness) of sound stimuli is more conveniently measured in decibels (dB). Decibels are comparatiave logarithmic units based on the threshold of hearing of normal ears. Thus the threshold of hearing of a normal ear at a given frequency is 0 dB and the quietest sound an ear with a 30 dB loss can perceive is 1000 times more intense.

The human ear can perceive a frequency range of approximately 20–20 000 Hz. Within this range, the speech frequencies have the most practical importance and clinical audiometry spans the range 250–8000 Hz, with most elements of human speech lying between 500 and 4000 Hz.

A child's auditory ability is mainly determined by how well his or her auditory system can interpret speech signals. Different elements of speech are produced not only with different frequencies but also with different intensities with the vowels tending to be lower pitched (voiced) and, therefore, of greater intensity than the consonants which are mostly produced by subtle tongue and lip movements. Clarity of perception may therefore be significantly hampered by a relatively modest hearing loss.

In terms of disability, a child with a 30 dB loss perceives a conversational voice with about the same intensity as a normally hearing child perceives a whisper, making it hard work to keep up with conversations of no immediate interest. This is about the level at which a hearing aid may be beneficial in a permanent loss. With a 60 dB loss a shout is perceived as a whisper and this is about the level at which the unaided child may fail to develop speech.

It is important to remember that hearing tests require interpretation in the context of the child as a whole. The handicap produced by a particular hearing impairment is subject to wide variation between individuals and is also affected by factors such as personality and social background. Age is a major factor; a 10-year old with good language development and social skills will be much better able to overcome auditory disability than a 2-year old with an identical hearing loss.

HEARING TESTS

Hearing tests can be broadly classified into behavioural tests which are age-appropriate, and electrophysiological tests which are more age independent. Not all childhood ear tests are strictly tests of hearing, e.g. the impedance test. The tests most commonly used in British clinical practice are described below.

Behavioural Testing

Age 0–6 Months

Newborns are able to distinguish their mothers' voices from a very early age and an experienced mother's assessment of whether or not her baby can hear may be very useful clinically. Startle responses, blink reflexes and stilling can often be elicited by sound stimuli, but it is not possible to obtain repeatable behavioural responses to quiet test sounds close to threshold level and no simple clinical test exists for this age group. So far devices for screening hearing using physiological responses (e.g. auditory response cradle), have not gained widespread clinical acceptance.

Distraction Testing: Age 6–18 Months

Distraction testing is most commonly used in testing the hearing of infants, both for screening and diagnostic purposes. If properly performed under reasonable conditions, the test is both reliable and repeatable. The principle of the test it to induce the child to turn his or her head to locate the source of a sound presented outside the range of vision.

The test is performed by two testers in a quiet room. The child sits on a parent's knee facing the first tester across a low table. The child's visual attention is lightly occupied by a bright object held by the first tester on the table top. The object is then covered and while the child continues to look in its direction, the second tester presents the test sound from about 1 m away and 30° behind the coronal plane so as to avoid a visual stimulus. The first tester observes the child's response and the test is repeated on either side and with different stimulus intensities and frequencies to establish minimum response levels. The stimuli used are usually appropriately calibrated warble tones, although voice, high frequency rattles and everyday noises such as rustling paper can be used.

The main pitfalls of the test are response to non-test stimuli such as parental nudging, shadows, perfume or incidental noise and patient noncompliance. The test requires an appropriate level of physical, mental and visual ability and this must be borne in mind when testing the developmentally delayed.

The results of distraction testing should not be regarded as being equivalent to those of a pure tone audiogram. It is unrealistic to expect to measure precise thresholds in this age group and a "pass" level (typically about 30 dB) is often quoted according to local circumstances.

Visual Reinforcement Audiometry: Age 6 Months to 3 Years

Visual reinforcement audiometry (VRA) is an increasingly used technique in UK clinical practice. The equipment required is somewhat bulky and the technique is therefore more suited for use in audiology centres than for community screening programmes.

The principle of VRA is to give the child a visual reward for responding to a sound stimulus (usually by head turning). The reward, particularly if complex and interesting maintains the child's interest and improves response rates compared with distraction so that frequency specific and threshold information can be obtained.

The test is most conveniently performed in a sound treated room, ideally with an adjacent observation room which contains the audiometric equipment and from which one tester can observe the child through one way glass. The child sits with a parent facing a low table on which there are objects of interest. At 45° on either side are loudspeakers with adjacent visual reinforcers, for example an animated toy which becomes visible only when the tester turns it on. The test stimuli are usually warble tones at 0.5, 1.2 and 4 kHz played through the loudspeakers.

At first a loud tone is presented for a few seconds simultaneously with the visual reward in order to attract the child's interest. After the child turns away, the stimulus is repeated and when the head-turn response is established, the tone is presented alone and the reward only given for an adequate head-turn. The stimulus intensity is adjusted until the threshold at that frequency is established. The complexity of the test can be varied according to the needs of the individual patient. A single loudspeaker may be adequate for screening purposes but both sides and more tones can be tested where appropriate. The test setup is flexible and can be modified in various ways and used for assessment of sound localization, responsiveness to speech and for free field testing of hearing aid wearers in appropriate cases.

As with distraction testing, VRA is subject to the constraints of patient interest, cooperation and developmental status. As the test is usually performed in a free field, using loudspeakers it is possible to underestimate unilateral hearing losses, although this is not usually of great practical significance. Overall VRA is reliable, repeatable and requires fewer retests than most behavioural tests in this age group.

Results are typically expressed in decibels, with pass levels of about 30 dB, depending upon the local set-up.

Play Audiometry: Age 18 Months to 5 Years

Behavioural testing in this age group has its difficulties but requires simple equipment and is therefore appropriate to community screening as well as having a continuing role in diagnostic work. Testing is play based. In the earlier part of the age range it relies mainly on testing discrimination of speech by gauging responses to simple instructions (co-operative testing). As maturity increases, testing is based on conditioning the child to perform a simple task in response to an auditory stimulus (performance testing).

In co-operation testing, familiar objects such as toys are used in structured play with the object of finding the quietest level at which the child can successfully distinguish between them when asked. The names of the objects are often similar sounding, e.g. "tree and key"' There are various modifications of the technique which can be increased in complexity by the use of pictures, puzzle boards, etc., depending on the maturity of child.

In performance testing, the task is a simple one such as putting a wooden peg in a board. The auditory stimulus may be verbal such as saying "go" but is usually provided by a free field audiometer which can produce tones at various volumes and frequencies so that thresholds can be established. An older child may be able to wear earphones so that performance testing merges into pure tone audiometry.

Shyness, difficulties in maintaining interest and differences in maturity make the younger end of this age range the most difficult of all to test audiologically. There are also potential pitfalls with standardization of testers' voices and the giving of non-verbal clues. It may be particularly difficult to assess developmentally delayed children or those with behavioural problems since the test is not purely auditory. This is not necessarily a drawback since hearing testing in its wider sense is part of the assessment of communication ability and this type of testing may be helpful in building up an overall picture in difficult cases. Co-operative testing does not give frequency specific information but is sufficiently sensitive to pick up mild hearing losses. The test is completed by the child achieving 80% correct responses. Normals typically pass at 40 dB. The presentation of performance test results may vary according to the complexity of the test procedure and is usually on audiogram charts.

Pure Tone Audiometry: Age 4 Years Upwards

Pure tone audiometry is the most commonly used hearing test in clinical practice for both diagnostic and screening purposes. It is relatively simple to perform and presents a graphical illustration of auditory function which is easy to interpret. Pure tone audiometry can be administered to all but the most mentally retarded.

The principle of pure tone audiometry is to determine the minimum intensity at which each of a number of frequencies can be perceived in each ear separately.

The stimuli used are pure tones generated by an audiometer and presented by earphones (air conducted sound) or by a bone conductor on the mastoid process. Thresholds are usually established by presenting an easily heard tone and working down in 10-dB steps until the tone is no longer heard. Intensity is then increased again in 5-dB steps until the tone is just heard. The process is then repeated until a threshold is established.

The usual frequencies tested are 0.25, 0.5, 1.0, 2.0, 4.0 and 8.0 kHz. Patient response is usually signified by pressing a button which illuminates a light on the audiometer. Age-appropriate modifications of the tech-

nique include presentation of the stimuli by hand-held earphones, reduction in the number of frequencies tested, less stringency in precise threshold determination and use of more interesting and playful methods of indicating response.

The audiogram chart shows decibels of hearing loss at various frequencies, so that a normal test should be a straight line at the 0-dB level for both air- and bone-conducted sound. In practice this is seldom achieved and air-conduction thresholds of 20 dB or better through the speech frequencies (0.5–4.0 kHz) would be unlikely to be associated with disability and can be regarded as normal in childhood. Bone conduction can be regarded as a test of cochlear function, while air conduction is an indicator of hearing ability. Thus the test can be used to distinguish between conductive, sensorineural and mixed loses.

An experienced tester can usually detect inattention and boredom in a test subject. Difficulties can arise, however, when there is a significant difference in air-conduction threshold between the two ears since it can be difficult to be certain which cochlea is being stimulated. This is particularly true of bone-conducted stimuli which are transmitted across the skull with little attenuation. This can be overcome by masking the non-test ear with white noise presented through an earphone. Masking needs to be quite loud, and can prove confusing and frightening to small children so that audiometric differentiation between conductive and sensorineural losses may proved difficult under the age of 7 years.

Electrophysiological Tests

Electric Response Audiometry: All Ages

Electric or evoked response audiometry (ERA) can be used in a variety of situations where behavioural audiometry is unreliable or impossible, such as in the very young, the handicapped and individuals with non-organic hearing loss. Although some portable screening machines are available, their usefulness is limited. As ERA requires expensive equipment and technical expertise, its use is mainly confined to audiology units.

The principle of ERA is the detection of electrical activity in the auditory pathway. As with other evoked responses, the potentials generated are extremely small and multiple stimuli and computer averaging of signals is required to cancel out random electrical activity in the brain and neck muscles so that the potential under investigation can be detected. Responses can be obtained from various points on the auditory pathway, although the precise point of generation is not known in every case. (See Table 16.1.)

Table 16.1   Electrophysiological tests

Potential	Latency (ms)	Origin
Electrocochleography (ECochG)	0–10	Cochlea/VIII nerve
Brain-stem audiometry evoked potentials (BSER or AER)	0–10	VIII nerve/brain stem
Post-auricular myogenic response (PAM)	10–24	Auricular muscles
Middle latency responses (MLR)	10–60	Thalamus/cortex
Cortical-evoked responses (CERA)	60–5000	Cortex

Electrocochleography

Electrocochleography (ECochG) records activity in the cochlea and eighth nerve and gives good auditory threshold information at any age, as well as some information about inner ear pathology. The auditory stimulus comes from an earphone and recordings are taken from the middle ear using a needle electrode passed through the tympanic membrane. This usually necessitates general anaesthesia in childhood, making the test expensive and time consuming.

Brain-stem Auditory-evoked Potentials

The brain-stem auditory-evoked potential (BSER) is the most commonly used auditory-evoked potential (AEP) in clinical practice. It can be performed at any age and gives robust threshold information to within 10 dB of behavioural thresholds. Athough the test can be performed without sedation in co-operative subjects, it is affected by excessive muscular activity and may take up to an hour to perform so that it is usually performed under sedation. Stimuli are presented by earphone and recordings are made via vertical and mastoid electrodes. The recording obtained is a series of peaks corresponding to the various relay stations on the brain-stem auditory pathway. When a response is obtained, the test is successively repeated at lower intensities until no response is detected.

Middle and Late Latency Responses

Middle and late latency responses (MLAs) and cortical-evoked responses (CERA) are not suitable for clinical use in childhood because they are both dependent on subject maturation, conscious level and other factors. CERA is the most useful AEP for giving frequency-specific information, but this is seldom of practical value in paediatric clinical practice.

Post-auricular Myogenic Potentials

This test is based on the recording of potentials arising in the muscles which "prick up" the ears. It can be used as a screening test, but is not sufficiently sensitive to obtain accurate threshold information and is rarely used clinically.

Interpretation of Results

BSER and ECochG should be regarded as a supplement to behavioural audiometry, rather than a replacement for it. For a variety of reasons no evoked response test has yet been developed which can give information equivalent to that obtained by pure tone audiometry. Modern ERA equipment is very reliable but its use requires a high level of technical expertise and its output requires skilled interpretation which can be subjective. A good recording requires a synchronous burst of electrical activity in the auditory pathway, this can be hampered by conductive losses which may give disproportionately bad recordings.

Bone-conducted BSER can be performed but tends to give unreliable results. It is difficult to obtain information about low tone hearing by these techniques and the click stimuli usually used in clinical practice test mainly 2.0 kHz and above. This is not usually important but occasionally leads to underassessment of impairment in low tone losses and overassessment in high-tone losses. Behavioural audiometry goes some way towards assessing, however crudely, the brain's ability to respond to auditory stimuli and ERA cannot do this. Despite these drawbacks BSERA and, to a lesser extent, ECochG are now regarded as essential clinical tools.

Otoacoustic Emissions: All Ages

Otoacoustic emission testing (OAE) or cochlear echo is a new test which is just coming into routine practice. In essence it is a test of cochlear function. Its use is largely restricted to audiology units at present, but it shows promise for screening populations difficult to test by behavioural audiometry such as neonates, the handicapped and patients with non-organic loss. It is simpler and quicker to perform than ERA, which can be reserved for those cases failing the test.

OAE is based on the discovery that normal ears emit sound when stimulated acoustically. Mechanical activity, probably generated in the outer hair cells, which are actively contractile takes place in the cochlea in response to sound. This generates vibrations which are transmitted back through the sound conducting mechanism and can be detected in the ear canal by a sensitive microphone.

The test, which does not usually require sedation, can be performed at any age. It is performed by the insertion of a probe containing a speaker and microphone into the ear canal. Repeated click stimuli are used and the output is computer averaged in a similar manner to ERA.

OAE's can only be obtained from normal, or near-normal ears. The results come in the form of a print-out, which shows the response of the individual ear and gives some frequency-specific information. The test is highly sensitive, but since it is essentially a pass/fail test, it does not give threshold information in cases of hearing impairment and the presence of temporary middle ear problems may cause a child with normal cochlear function to fail the test. The need for sound-attenuated test conditions may limit the use of this test to audiology units.

Tympanometry

Tympanometry, also known as impedance audiometry, is strictly speaking a test of middle ear function rather than a direct test of auditory function. Since middle-ear disease accounts for the vast majority of childhood hearing problems, however, it is a useful adjunct to auditory testing and its use is widespread for both screening and diagnostic purposes. Tympanometry is principally used to measure middle ear pressure but can also be used in the asessment of inner ear and facial nerve function.

Sound transmission through the middle-ear mechanism is dependent upon a number of factors, including the resistance, stiffness and inertia of the system. Changes in air pressure in the ear canal or middle ear will affect the stiffness of the tympanic membrane and therefore the ability of the system to transmit sound, most sound being transmitted when there is no air pressure difference between the external and middle ears. Sound not transmitted through the middle ear mechanism is reflected from the drum surface and measurement of the variation of reflected sound energy against ear canal air pressure is the basis of tympanometry.

Clinical tympanometry can be performed at any age and requires only passive co-operation on the part of the patient. It is quite quick to perform taking only a minute or two per ear. The tympanometer has a probe which is inserted into and seals the ear canal. Within the probe are three channels one each for a miniature microphone, a loud-speaker and one connected to a pressure pump. The loud-speaker emits a continuous hum and variations in the ear canal sound pressure against air pressure are detected by the microphone. The apparatus can also be used to detect changes in the stiffness of the system due to contraction of the stapedius muscle which can be induced by sudden loud sound introduced into either ear. Most tympanometers produce a print out giving a graphical representation of middle ear compliance (measured in millilitres of equivalent air volume, which for practical purposes can be regarded as the amount of sound absorbed by the middle ear), against air pressure (in deca-pascals (daPa)).

A normal tracing is a peak showing maximum compliance when there is little or no air pressure difference between the middle and external ears. There is a normal range and negative middle ear pressure peaks going down to −100 daPa are regarded as normal in childhood. Pressure peaks lower than −100 daPA are indicative of eustachian dysfunction and flat traces usually signify the presence of middle ear effusions. The height of the peak may be an indicator of problems with the drum or ossicular chain, but there is too great a normal range for this to be of much practical value.

Other information which may be gained from tympanometry includes ear canal volume and stapedius reflex thresholds. The latter are not particularly valuable in paediatric practice but can give information on cochlear function and are occasionally useful in localizing a lesion of the facial nerve which supplies stapedius.

Although tympanometry gives a rapid "at a glance" method of assessing glue ear, it is subject to misinterpretation. Flat traces may be caused by very narrow ear canals, wax occlusion or the presence of functioning grommets or perforations, since all these conditions prevent the drum being stressed by changes in canal air pressure. This is usually apparent when reference is made to the canal volume which is recorded on the printout and which is small in cases of blockage and apparently unusually large in perforations. Normal canal volumes are usually 0.5 ml, but there is wide normal variation and comparison of the suspect ear with the other side may be helpful in avoiding errors of interpretation.

NON-ACOUSTIC INVESTIGATIONS RELEVANT TO HEARING LOSS

Infection

Intra-uterine infections such as rubella, cytomegalovirus and syphilis and acquired infections, including otitis media, meningitis and all childhood fevers may be associated with hearing loss. Serological or microbiological testing may therefore be appropriate in individual cases. In practice, however, many of these conditions have other sequelae and audiological testing comes after the primary diagnosis has been made.

Genetics

Genetic investigation and counselling is valuable in some cases of syndromal and non-syndromal hearing loss. Cytogenetic tests are becoming available for some conditions associated with hearing loss, e.g. fragile X syndrome, and this aspect of investigation may assume greater clinical relevance in the future.

Imaging

In most cases of congenital sensorineural deafness, the defect is not detectable radiologically and imaging is not part of routine work up in UK clinical practice. High-resolution computerized tomography (CT) scanning of the temporal bone has increased knowledge of anatomical defects in some cases associated with hearing loss and may be particularly useful clinically when surgery is under consideration. This includes some cases of congenital atresia, some trauma cases and cases of inner ear deformity associated with meningitis. In deafness acquired through trauma or infection, and increasingly in congenital cases, CT is necessary to assess cochlear patency when cochlear implantation is under consideration.

Magnetic resonance imaging (MRI) is less useful than CT in imaging anatomical defects of the temporal bone, but superior in demonstrating posterior fossa tumours which are an extremely rare cause of deafness in childhood.

Congenital Deformities of the Outer Ear

Congenital malformations of the ear are usually clinically obvious. They may or may not be associated with deformities of the ear canal, middle ear and cochlea and may be unilateral or bilateral. Many cases (e.g. Treacher Collins syndrome) are syndromal and require general and possibly genetic assessment.

Otologically, the focus of investigation is the assessment of hearing which can be abnormal even in an apparently normal contralateral ear and may not be profound even in cases of bilateral atresia since cochlear function is not necessarily abnormal. The demonstration of hearing thresholds can be extremely difficult audiologically in bilateral cases because newborns cannot be tested behaviourally and the inbuilt conductive loss

makes the interpretation of AEPs difficult. Bone-conducted AEPs can be performed in some centres but do not give an absolutely reliable assessment of cochlear function. Careful follow-up, repeated testing and a trial of a bone-conducted hearing aid may therefore be needed before an accurate assessment of disability is achieved. High-resolution CT scanning is the only imaging technique which gives information of value in these cases. In the newborn it may be of prognostic value in demonstrating the presence or absence of inner ear structures. Anatomical information about middle and inner ear structures and the position of the facial nerve is essential to the planning of any reconstructive surgery, although this is not generally considered for several years.

INFLAMMATIONS OF THE EAR

The management of common childhood ear infection such as acute suppurative otitis media is usually based on clinical findings, and specific investigations may not be needed in every case. Resistant, recurrent or complicated cases may require investigation to determine appropriate management.

Microbiology

If an ear is discharging, a swab sent for bacterial culture and sensitivity will be helpful in determining appropriate antibiotic therapy. The swab must be small enough to enter the child's ear and fine nasopharyngeal swabs are preferable to throat swabs for this purpose. Occasionally, in otitis externa of viral origin with blistering or blood blistering of the ear canal, electron microscopy of blister fluid may yield diagnostic information, but is unlikely to be useful in management. In non-discharging ears, bacteriological information may be obtainable from nasopharyngeal swabs or blood culture in appropriate cases. Paracentesis of the middle ear is practiced in some countries, but is not routinely used in the UK.

Imaging

Mastoid X-rays may show gross pathology such as opacification of the air–cell system or other gross pathology. This can be useful, for example in distinguishing otitis meida from a florid otitis externa with a swollen ear canal, but seldom gives information which changes clinical management.

Sinus and nasopharyngeal X-rays may be of value in demonstrating other upper respiratory tract pathology relevant to otitis such as sinusitis or adenoidal hyper-trophy.

CT scanning is of particular value in the investigation of unusual or complicated cases. It is mandatory where intracranial suppuration secondary to otitis is suspected and is helpful in defining anatomical details prior to surgery in congenital lesions, cholesteatomas and facial nerve lesions.

Audiology

The assessment of hearing is seldom needed in the acute management of otitis media. Routine follow-up hearing tests in all cases would be wasteful of resources, but it should be borne in mind that resolution is not complete until auditory function has returned to normal. Clinical follow-up should take account of this and testing arranged if appropriate. Hearing testing forms an essential part of the management and follow-up of all cases of chronic otitis media and glue ear.

Blood tests

Blood culture and full blood count may be appropriate. Immunoglobin estimation may be indicated where immune deficiency is suspected of underlying recurrent or chronic disease.

VERTIGO

Vertigo and imbalance are very unusual childhood symptoms which may be poorly articulated and described. Many cases are of uncertain aetiology and relatively benign, e.g. paroxysmal vertigo of childhood. Others are due to middle ear disease, epilepsy, migraine, demyelination or intracranial tumours. Careful history taking with clinical neurological and otological examination are essential to the choice of appropriate investigations. Auditory and middle ear function should be assessed bilaterally in an age appropriate manner (see above).

Electroencephalography should be performed in all cases where epilepsy is suspected and may also be helpful in suggesting the source of a focal lesion. In addition to giving threshold information, brain-stem evoked potentials may show an increase in latency in some brain-stem disorders, but this does not give specific diagnostic information.

Imaging is essential in most cases of childhood vertigo. If temporal bone pathology is suspected, CT scanning is the method of choice. MRI, if available, is probably superior in the demonstration of intracranial tumours, particularly those in the posterior cranial fossa.

There are no specific blood tests that are appropriate to the investigation of childhood vertigo, but syphilis serology should be performed in appropriate cases.

The principle of vestibular function testing rests on the demonstration of spontaneous or induced nystagmus. Spontaneous nystagmus can sometimes be observed clinically especially if optic fixation is abolished, e.g. by using an infrared viewer in the dark, but eye movements are more conveniently recorded by electronystagmography. There is a difference in electrical potential between the cornea and retina and changes in this electrical field caused by eye movement can be picked up by electrodes placed on the temples; it is therefore possible to record eye movements against time. Recordings can be made of spontaneous nystagmus. Asymmetry of nystagmus induced by caloric stimulation may indicate end organ disease as may some nystagmus induced by head positioning. Asymmetry of optical pursuit of moving targets, pendula, etc., may indicate brain-stem dysfunction. Unfortunately, vestibular function tests only demonstrate relatively gross changes in a subtle and complex mechanism of balance control and normal tests are not proof of a normally functioning vestibular system, neither do they give specific diagnostic information. Full vestibular function testing can be elaborate, unpleasant and frightening and, although occasionally helpful, its use in childhood must be selective and may require modification.

FACIAL PARALYSIS

Lower motor neurone facial paralysis is relatively uncommon in childhood and has many causes. Idiopathic (Bell's) palsy and paralysis associated with acute and chronic otitis media are the commonest childhood facial palsies. In Möbius syndrome there is agenesis of the facial and other cranial nerve nuclei. Melkersson's syndrome, which is familial, is associated with a lobulated tongue and recurrent palsy. Trauma with obstetric forceps may cause congenital facial palsy and head injury with temporal bone fracture may cause nerve disruption or haematoma causing a paralysis of delayed onset. Viral lesions such as herpes zoster and, rarely, viral encephalitides may also cause facial paralysis. Tumours of the brain-stem, cerebellopontine angle, temporal bone or parotid may cause partial or complete facial palsy. In some tumours and in idiopathic cases the paralysis may be recurrent. Investigation will clearly be directed by clinical considerations.

The facial nerve is principally a motor nerve carrying fibres to the muscles of facial expression. Its principal branches are the greater superficial petrosal nerve carrying secretomotor fibres to the lachrymal gland, the nerve to the stapedius muscle and the chorda tympani nerve supplying taste to the anterior two-thirds of the tongue and secretomotor fibres to the submandibular gland. Tests are available for all these functions and, although seldom used in childhood, may have prognostic value as well as helping in localizing lesions.

The motor function of the nerve can be tested by nerve stimulation in which an electrode is placed on the cheek skin and the current required to elicit a twitch is compared on the two sides. This test can have prognostic value in cases of complete Bell's palsy. Prognosis is worse in cases of complete denervation. In such cases the nerve degenerates in the first two to three days and cannot be stimulated. Nerve conduction studies can also be performed as can electromyography by which denervation and reinervation of individual motor units may be detected.

The nerve to the stapedius can be tested by determining acoustic reflex thresholds (see "Tympanometry").

Lacrimation can be assessed by hanging filter paper strips in the conjunctival sac bilaterally and comparing the rate of wetting (Shirmer's Test). The secretomotor function of the submandibular gland can also be measured by measuring its output but is of little use clinically. The taste function of the anterior tongue can be assessed clinically and also by electrogustometry in which the minimum current required to make an electrode taste metallic is compared on the two sides.

Audiometric testing should be performed in all cases in which intracranial or intratemporal pathology is suspected. Imaging should be performed in all progressive or recurrent cases in order to exclude posterior fossa or intratemporal tumours. This will involve CT scanning but MRI may be appropriate in some cases.

NOSE

Nasal disease may occur at any age in the paediatric population and the spectrum of disease may vary from the trivial to acute life-threatening disorders. As in any other disease a diagnosis is greatly helped by meticulous history taking. The time of onset, duration and rate of progression of symptoms are particularly pertinent, as well as any associated symptoms or signs. A full past medical and family history should also be sought.

Nasal Obstruction

Radiology

Radiology rarely adds anything important to a thorough examination. However, it may be useful in specific circumstances.

Plain X-rays

These are of use in assessing the size of adenoid hypertrophy. They do not exclude the presence of a foreign body. An opacified maxillary antrum is associated with an antrochoanal polyp. In juvenile angiofibromas the bowing of the posterior maxillary sinus wall may be visible on the lateral nasal view.

CT Scanning

This is appropriate in selected cases. It is important to discuss the case with the radiologist to decide the correct plane (axial or coronal) and window setting to enable soft tissue or bony detail to be seen in order to obtain worthwhile information. Prior suction and vasoconstriction is essential. It is the investigation of choice in choanal obstruction and will provide detail as to type of atretic plate (bony or membranous) and length.

It is also useful in assessing neoplasms both benign and malignant. In benign lesions such as dermoids and lipomas extension into the cranial fossa may be confirmed. In malignancy the extension into surrounding tissue and degree of bony erosion is essential in staging and planning treatment.

Magnetic Resonance Imaging

As the sophistication of the scanning techniques develop, wider applications will be found. It is of no use in assessing bony detail. However, it is of great use in assessing soft tissue neoplasms such as gliomas and encephalocoeles as communication with the anterior cranial fossa may be assessed (Lund et al 1990). In capillary haemangiomas the STIR (short tau inversion recovery) highlights the vascular tissue while CT scanning is equivocal (Morgan and Evans 1990).

Angiography

This is indicated in juvenile angiofibromas especially if pre-operative embolization is contemplated.

Biopsy

Biopsy should only be undertaken following a complete assessment including radiology. Ideally it should be excisional unless malignancy is suspected. Care should be taken in vascular lesions and when communication with the CSF is suspected. Needle aspiration may be useful.

Sweat Test

Nasal polyps are present in 10% of children with cystic fibrosis, therefore a sweat chloride test may be indicated.

Nasal Discharge

Radiology

Plain X-rays of the sinuses may be useful if a purulent sinusitis is suspected. Coronal CT scanning using bone window settings is essential if CSF rhinorrhea is suspected.

Microbiology

A nasal swab is rarely of any great help in infective rhinitis, as anaerobes are rarely cultured and the commonest organisms are usually predictable (*Haemophilus influenzae*, *Streptococcus pneumonia* and *Branhamella catarrhalis*).

Biochemistry

CSF rhinorrhea may be confirmed by measuring the sugar and protein content. CSF is usually clear with a specific gravity of 1.004–1.008. Unlike pure nasal secretions it contains glucose. A more reliable method is to perform electrophoretic analysis of nasal secretions for the tau protein (asialo transferrin) which is only present in CSF (Porter et al 1992).

Nasal Smear

Cytological evaluation of a nasal smear may suggest an allergic aetiology if there is a raised eosinophil count. However, these parameters are far from reliable (Lund and Scadding (1991)).

Immunology (see Chapter 14)

Skin prick testing has the advantages of being inexpensive, quick and easy to perform. It allows a wide range of allergens to be tested at one go and has little if any risk of anaphylaxis. It is important to stop antihistamine or oral sympathomimetics at least 3 days prior to testing. Systemic corticosteroids have no effect on the result.

The radioallergosorbent test (RAST) is an *in-vitro* quantitative test to detect circulating IgE antibodies. It is usually reserved for patients who are on therapy which will interfere with skin testing or when there is a documented risk of anaphylaxis to the allergen. Raised serum levels of IgE and eosinophilia may suggest allergy, but are unreliable.

Estimation of IgG subgroups may be useful in patients who suffer from repeated infections and an immunodeficiency is suspected.

Cilial Function Testing

These tests are indicated when ciliary dyskinesia is suspected, e.g. Kartagener's syndrome.

Saccharin Testing

This depends on the co-operation from the child for it to be successful. The saccharin is placed 0.5 cm behind the leading edge of the inferior turbinate. The time taken for the child to taste the bitter–sweet of the saccharin is noted. The normal range is within 20 min. If normal, no further investigation is indicated.

Cilial Beat Frequency

A nasal smear is taken from middle third of the nose using a brush or spatula. The sample of cells is then transferred to Ringer's solution prior to the ciliary beat frequency being measured using a photomultiplying technique. The normal beat frequency is 12–15 Hz.

Cilial Biopsy

This is indicated if the clinical beat frequency is abnormal. The biopsy is taken 1 cm behind the inferior turbinate and submitted for electronmicroscopy to exclude microtubular defects of the cilia.

Sinusitis

The ethmoid sinus is slightly more developed than the maxillary sinus at birth. The sphenoid sinus develops shortly after birth, the frontal does not appear until 5 or 6 years of age.

Radiology

Plain sinus X-rays may show complete opacification of the involved sinuses (if developed) or a fluid level. A tipped view confirms the presence of fluid.

CT scanning is essential if secondary complications have developed such as periorbital swelling, proptosis or neurological sequelae. The presence and extent of an associated abscess can be confirmed prior to operative intervention.

In rare cases of chronic sinusitis where surgery is contemplated a coronal CT scan is essential to delineate the extent of disease and associated anatomical abnormalities prior to surgical treatment.

Microbiology

A simple nasal swab rarely helps. Middle meatal swabbing under endoscopic control is more reliable unless antral washings are available. Culture for anaerobic organisms is mandatory, especially in the presence of complications.

Biopsy

Antroscopy and biopsy may be useful in refractory sinusitis to exclude fungal infection, granulomatous disease or malignancy.

Epistaxis

Epistaxis in childhood is common but rarely serious compared with in adulthood as it is usually due to venous bleeding from the plexus of veins in Little's area on the anterior nasal septum. Rarely, the epistaxis may have a more serious cause such as blood dyscrasias or a juvenile nasopharyngeal angiofibroma (JNA) which occurs in the postnasal space of adolescent males.

Haematology

Blood analysis is indicated if clinical anaemia, a clotting disorder, or blood dyscrasia is suspected. Full blood count, platelet count, blood film and clotting factor assessment including bleeding time may be indicated. (See Chapter 1.)

Radiology

Radiology is rarely indicated unless a JNA is suspected. The bowing of the posterior wall of the maxillary sinus by the JNA may be seen on a lateral sinus X-ray. CT and MRI are the investigations of choice to assess tumour size. Angiography may be indicated.

Olfactory Disorders

Olfactometry

Simple qualitative testing may be performed by asking the patient to identify common odours such as peppermint water and cloves. Smelling salts may be used (with care) to exclude malingerers as this stimulates the trigeminal sensory nerve.

Two quantative assessments of olfaction exist but depend on a cooperative patient. The University of Pennsylvania Smell Identification Test (UPSIT; Sensonics Inc, 15 Haddon Ave, Haddonfield, NJ 08033, USA) is a scratch and sniff test. The Olfactometry Test uses serial dilutions (Olfacto-Labs, PO Box 757, El Cerrito, CA 94530, USA).

Radiology

Plain sinus X-rays may exclude an underlying sinusitis. CT and/or MRI should be reserved for the investigation of space-occupying lesions.

Resonance Disorders

Resonance disorders of speech are due to velopharyngeal dysfunction and can be classified into three types:

- *Hypernasality* (rhinolalia aperta) due to velopharyngeal incompetence resulting in nasal excape. Usually associated with cleft-palate disorders or neurological disease.
- *Hyponasality* (rhinolalia clausa) due to nasal obstruction either posterior (adenoidal speech) or anterior (nasal pinching effect). Usually has an organic basis. Rarely needs further investigation.
- *Mixed nasality* (rhinolalia mixta) due to a combination of velopharyngeal incompetence and nasal obstruction.

Speech Therapy Assessment

This is essential for both diagnosis and treatment. The use of specific sentences will differentiate the type of resonance disorder.

Nasendoscopy

In the co-operative child the flexible endoscope will allow a dynamic assessment of the velopharyngeal sphincter to be performed.

Videofluroscopy

Radiological assessment of the postnasal space may be supplemented by this dynamic assessment of the velopharynx during speech and swallowing. The technique determines the nature of the velopharyngeal disorder and the potential for treatment.

Nasal Anometry

This investigates the abnormal airflow, it's instant of occurrence and its peak value during speech (Ellis 1979).

THROAT

Throat disorders may present with some degree of respiratory embarrassment. Where the obstruction is progressive or distressing, transfer of the patient to a high dependency area where skilled airway support can be provided is essential prior to investigating the cause. It is essential to monitor the clinical condition of the patient as well as using oximetry as the oxygen saturation and pCO$_2$ may be normal immediately prior to a catastrophic deterioration.

Airway Obstruction

Radiology

Head extension is essential to get meaningful results. It should only be attempted if the patient has a stable airway. An anteroposterior and lateral neck (high KV) with a posteroanterior and lateral chest X-ray during inspiration and expiration are the minima. They may show airway narrowing or collapse due to tracheomalacia, anomalous blood vessels, retained foreign body, supra-glottic swelling due to infection or papilloma, tracheal shift, and mediastinum displacement may be visible.

Barium swallow may be indicated in tracheo-oesophageal fistulae, oesophageal stenosis, or vascular anomalies are suspected.

CT and/or MRI scanning may be indicated if mass lesions causing airway compression exist. Further investigation such as angiography and including pressure studies may be indicated.

Endoscopy

Microlaryngoscopy, bronchoscopy and oesophagoscopy should be undertaken if the diagnosis is uncertain or respiratory distress persists.

Dysphonia

Endoscopy

Endoscopy, whether flexible under local anaesthesia or rigid under general anaesthesia, must be performed to obtain a diagnosis. A diagnosis should always be obtained in cases of persistent hoarseness.

Radiology

Radiology rarely has a place unless the hoarseness is associated with other symptoms.

Dysphagia and Aspiration

Radiology

Standard chest X-ray views are essential to assess severity of aspiration.

Videofluroscopy will assess the level of obstruction as well as the site and severity of aspiration. Reflux may also be assessed and the presence of vascular compression or achalasia.

Radiolabelled milk scan will assess the severity of reflux with time, as well as the degree of aspiration.

Endoscopy

Laryngoscopy, bronchoscopy and oesophagoscopy should be performed to exclude anatomical abnormalities such as clefts, fistulae and vascular rings.

pH Monitoring

Twenty-four-hour pH monitoring is the most effective way of assessing the severity of gastro-oesophageal reflux. Microscopy of the sputum following suction aspiration after physiotherapy may demostrate fat-laden macrophages.

Snoring and Obstructive Sleep Apnoea

Any condition which restricts the airway in the nose, nasopharynx or oropharynx is liable to produce stertor or snoring. When the restriction during sleep becomes more severe obstructive sleep apnoea may develop leading to oxygen desaturation and a rise in pCO$_2$.

Radiology

A plain lateral X-ray of the postnasal space and upper airway is useful in identifying the adenoidal and tonsillar obstruction as well as showing the position of the lower jaw and tongue base.

Sleep Study

Polysomnography is rarely indicated unless central sleep apnoea, such as Ondine's curse is suspected. Confirmation of obstructive sleep apnoea may be obtained by using overnight pulse oximetry.

Sleep Nasendoscopy

If the site of obstruction is in doubt, sleep nasendoscopy may be performed using a flexible nasendoscope to observe the site of obstruction during sedation or inhalation anaesthesia. Facilities for cardiorespiratory monitoring and intubation must be available.

SALIVARY DISEASE

Salivary disease in childhood is uncommon. The clinical features are much the same as in adult disease. Congenital abnormalities are rare. Inflammatory, either bacterial or viral, is the most common disease. Chronic sialadenitis usually resolves at puberty. Neoplasia is rare and the majority of tumours are benign and occur in the parotid gland.

Haematology and Serology

A full blood count, serological testing and salivary antibody testing may be useful to distinguish infective from inflammatory cause such as Sjögren's syndrome.

Radiology

Plain X-rays are rarely useful unless sialolithiasis is suspected. Sialography is difficult to perform in children, and is of limited use due to artefacts.

Ultrasound scanning is the initial investigation of choice as it is painless and can distinguish between solid and cystic lesions.

CT scanning has been superseded by MRI scanning in the assessment of salivary disease, especially in terms of tumour extension.

Biopsy

Fine-needle aspiration has a limited role to play as even cystic lesions may co-exist with neoplasia and interpretation may be difficult.

Biopsy of a localized mass in the salivary gland should be excisional rather than incisional. However, if a parotid swelling is diffuse, an incisional biopsy via a modified parotidectomy incision is preferable to a superficial parotidectomy.

Microbiology

Tissue from lymph nodes should be sent fresh for microscopy and culture to exclude tuberculosis.

DROOLING

Some drooling is normal in infancy and early childhood. Persistent drooling beyond this age is generally caused by a functional disability, the most common cause being cerebral palsy with weakening of tongue and lip control.

Examination

Nasal obstruction and adenoidal hypertrophy should be assessed.

Dental examination consists of assessment of occlusion and dentition (primary or secondary).

Tongue movement, lip closure and head posture should also be assessed, ideally by a speech therapist.

Radiology

Videofluoroscopy will allow detailed examination of the pharyngeal phase of swallowing to be assessed. Exclusion of oesophageal disease is essential as well as chronic aspiration.

Isotope scanning will also allow a dynamic assessment of salivary function and swallowing to be made.

REFERENCES

Ellis RE (1979) The Exeter nasal anometer system. In: Ellis RE, Flack FC (eds) *Diagnosis and treatment of palatoglossal malfunction*, pp. 31–36. London: The College of Speech Therapists.

Kearns DB, Wickstead M, Choa D et al (1988) Computed tomography in choanal atresia *J Laryngol Otol* 102: 414–418.

Lund VJ, Howard DJ, Lloyd GAS et al (1990) Magnetic resonance imaging of paranasal sinus tumours for craniofacial resection. *Head & Neck* 11: 279–285.

Lund VJ, Scadding G (1991) Immunologic aspects of chronic sinusitis. *J Otolaryngol* 20: 379–381.

Morgan DW, Evans JNG (1990) Developmental nasal anomalies. *J Layrngol Otol* 104: 394–403.

Myging N, Johnson NJ, Thomsen J (1977) Intranasal allergen challenge during corticosteroid treatment. *Clin Allergy* 7: 69–73.

Porter MJ, Brookes GB, Zeman AZJ et al (1992) Use of protein electrophoresis in the diagnosis of cerebrospinal fluid rhinorrhea. *J Laryngol Otol* 106: 504–506.

17

Ophthalmology

A R Fielder

INTRODUCTION

An ophthalmic symptom can be the first manifestation of a serious systemic disorder. As many infants and young children with visual problems present first to paediatricians clearly the responsibility for identification will often lie with them and they need to have an approach to their investigation. This challenge is heightened by the fact that many of the conditions are uncommon and the symptoms of some of the potentially most sinister disorders are easily misinterpreted and the signs are subtle. The aim of this chapter is to help the paediatrician deal with clinical problems some of which are so uncommon that few paediatricians will be familiar with them but not so rare that they do not need to know about them.

This chapter is divided into two sections: the first dealing with methods of investigation and the second being problem-based. The emphasis is on simple clinical examination methods because in practice these are the most valuable tools we have, and often poorly utilized.

METHODS OF ASSESSMENT

Although visual acuity is the most frequently measured visual parameter, there is far more than this to functional vision. Here we will concentrate mainly on acuity, but the visual field, colour and binocularity will also be considered.

Measurement of Visual Acuity

In adult life visual acuity is almost always measured using the Snellen test-type. In childhood the term "acuity" is often applied incorrectly to all tests of vision, and this causes much confusion and misunderstanding.

Tests of seeing usually test either visual acuity or visibility and these two must not be equated. *Visibility* is the term used when the test object is single and contains no detail. *Visual acuity* may be tested in two ways both of which are based on resolution. *Resolution* acuity refers to the ability to distinguish two separate points such as the bars of a grating or squares of a chequer board. *Recognition acuity* is the term used when the test uses letters or pictures and contains an element of *recognition* as well as resolution.

Recognition acuity (e.g. Snellen) is the major clinical measure of visual acuity. Visibility, which is measured by such tests as Stycar balls or the Catford drum must be distinguished from acuity. This is important in assessing either the history or the significance of a test result (Figure 17.1).

Indirect Assessment of Vision

Often vision can only be assessed indirectly by taking a history, or observing the activities of the infant or child. Other features sometimes used as indirect indicators of vision include the presence of a squint, nystagmus, and pupillary reactions. A history frequently reveals more useful information about vision than examination, especially so for the infant and toddler, and the child with severe learning difficulties. Strong patterns (i.e. with edges) are the most powerful visual stimuli. Thus, ask about visual interest, eye-to-eye contact, and following responses. Ensure that other senses, such as noise are not contaminating the response. Smiling to a visual stimulus commences in the 6th week, an important milestone, as delay in its onset may have a visual basis.

Interpretation

Parental Concern About Vision

This is never ill-founded and concern that a baby has poor vision indicates severely reduced vision. Lack of concern

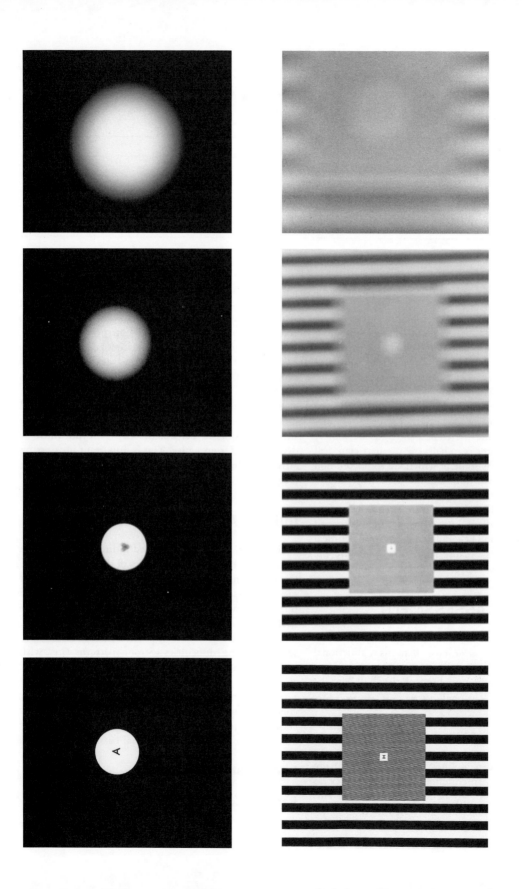

Figure 17.1 Visibility and resolution. Both the white spheres containing the letter A and the gratings are blurred by identical amounts. The sphere is a test of visibility and the A and gratings test resolution. A small blur renders the fine gratings and the letter A indistinct (high acuity is sensitive to blur), but note the A can still be recognized as this letter or an upside down V. Increasing the blur simply increases the size of the sphere which is why low vision children can still see sweets, threads on carpets, etc. Low levels of acuity are difficult to blur, hence the coarse gratings can be seen despite a high degree of defocus.

does not necessarily indicate normal visual development, or even preclude a severe defect. This may be because some parents believe that young babies normally have poor vision or they may be afraid to voice their concerns. Only the most severe visual deficits are readily apparent in infancy, and everyday observations of vision usually involve visibility rather than resolution. Children with learning difficulties may adopt unusual visual strategies which are not easily recognized by the professional, but are known to the parents. Older children may not tell adults about their poor or deteriorating vision, and altered behaviour may be a presenting feature. Although progressive visual loss is uncommon in the older child, doctors need to keep this possibility in mind, since the causes include treatable conditions such as raised intracranial pressure or tumours.

Squint and nystagmus may both point to reduced vision, but the pupillary reflex, on its own, is not useful in this context, as it can be normal in cortical blindness.

Direct Assessment of Vision

Children too Young for Snellen Testing

Up to about 2½ years, and in the older child with learning difficulties, Snellen-based tests cannot be used, so other qualitative and quantitative tests must be used. It is important that the limitations of each test are understood, and only the last two listed in Table 17.1 are quantitative.

When testing each eye in turn always try to assess the better eye first because occluding the better eye may upset the child and make further testing impossible. Use a light or, better, a toy. Look for three features of fixation: central, steady and maintained. With normal foveal fixation, the light reflex lies minimally nasal to the pupil centre, but clinically this is referred to as central fixation. If vision is normal fixation will be central, steady, and maintained on the target. With poor vision fixation may become eccentric, unsteady and is not maintained. This qualitative assessment is frequently used as a test for amblyopia in the very young.

Quantitative Tests of Visual Acuity (Tests of Resolution not Visibility)

Behavioural Tests – Preferential Looking

Preferential looking (PL) is a technique of measuring visual acuity based on the principle that infants prefer to look at a patterned rather than a non-patterned stimulus. PL has increased our understanding of visual development but was not widely used clinically until it was

Table 17.1 Tests of vision for young children

Test	Comment
Fix and follow	Response present after 31 weeks gestation
Orientation	Turning to diffuse light from 32 weeks gestation
Smiling	Onset 6 weeks after full-term birth. Important in history
Reaching for objects	From about 2½ months, disappears, returning again about 4 months. Poor test of vision
Catford drum	Tests visibility – not now recommended
Rolling and mounted balls (Worth and Stycar)	Test visibility – better tests now available
Preferential looking (acuity card procedure and Cardiff cards)	Tests visual acuity (resolution) – quantitative (see text)
Visually evoked potential	See text

simplified as the acuity card procedure (ACP) in the 1980s.

Acuity Card Procedure

Equipment. ACP apparatus consists of a series of grey cards. These contain a square or circular patch of black and white stripes (gratings) pasted onto one surface to either side of a central peep-hole while the other side is either blank or contains a 'balancing' white circle. The card is presented through an aperture in a screen (Figure 17.2). A series of about 18 cards each containing stripes of different width to cover acuities from about 0.18 cycles/degree* (6/1000) to 39 cycles/degree (6/5). The test distance is 38 or 55 cm.

Procedure. The infant will preferentially look at the stripes rather than the blank side, and the tester looking through the peep-hole has to decide to which side the infant is looking (i.e. where the grating is). Increasingly finer gratings are shown until they do not induce a response, and the last consistent response is the visual

---

*Grating acuities are recorded in cycles/degree – the number of pairs of black and white stripes per degree of visual angle. 30 cycles/degree is equivalent to 6/6 Snellen notation, although this conversion is not always directly applicable.

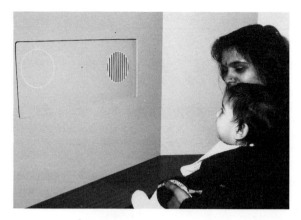

Figure 17.2   Acuity card procedure. An infant prefers to look at the circle containing the grating, if he or she can see it. The observer is looking through the central peep-hole at the child's looking responses.

acuity. For a bed-bound infant or child, cards can be presented without the screen. ACP is adaptable to many clinical situations and takes only a few minutes to perform (about 2–5 min for a binocular test).

ACP can be used from birth with success rates of around 95% for binocular testing and around 65% for monocular testing for children under 2 years of age. PL-based tests have shown that adult acuity levels are not achieved until 3–5 years of age and that the visual development of preterm infants is controlled predominantly by innate rather then environmental influences, i.e. acuity develops according to postmenstrual and not postnatal age. In children with learning difficulties ACP is successful in about 70%. They are not a homogeneous population but some considered clinically inattentive do respond to ACP. PL-based tests, particularly ACP, have provided insight into the natural history of visual pathway disorders. This is of value in assessing and monitoring the functional significance of: ocular malformations, cataract and aphakia, retinal disorders and children with visual impairment.

ACP is an excellent back-up test. Important medical and surgical decisions sometimes depend on a reliable acuity assessment and as ocular signs are often a poor indicator of the level of acuity, using ACP to confirm a Snellen test can be most helpful. Undoubtedly the most important use of ACP is in assessing the infant who may be blind, here it is simple, fast and reliable.

Compared with the "gold standard" Snellen, all PL-based tests overestimate acuity in amblyopia. Thus ACP is not suitable for amblyopia screening although it can be used as an indicator of amblyopia, and to monitor amblyopia therapy.

Cardiff Cards

These have recently been introduced as a toddler test which combines preferential looking with picture cards. It is too early to report on its value, although it has been enthusiastically taken up by orthoptists.

Electrophysiological Methods

The visually evoked potential (VEP) can be used to measure acuity, but requires a far more rigorous protocol than can be adhered to in a routine clinical setting. This is distinct from the frequent qualitative use of the VEP.

Snellen Testing

The Snellen chart is the "gold standard" acuity test against which all other tests are compared. See Table 17.2.

Vision testing is summarized in Table 17.3.

Other Visual Functions

Binocular Single Vision

This is the integration of the images from the two eyes into a single percept. This can only occur when:

● Corresponding points from each retina are coupled,

Table 17.2   Snellen-based tests of visual acuity

Test	Comment
Picture matching (Kay, Beale, etc.)	Useful for some preschool children. Not very accurate. Some cultural difficulties
Single optotype matching (e.g. Sheridan and Gardiner seven-letter test)	Very frequently used but relatively insensitive (crowding effect)
Crowded single-letter optotype (Cambridge crowding cards, Sonksen and Silver test)	Recently introduced letter-matching tests. Surround (crowd) test letter*
Snellen chart	"Gold standard" test. Used from about 3½ to 6 years and above

*Single letters are easier to identify than letters presented in a row, a phenomenon known as "crowding". Single-letter tests therefore tend to overestimate visual acuity. This is a particular problem with amblyopia.

Table 17.3 Summary of vision testing

Differentiate between visibility and resolution/recognition at all times during the assessment – history or examination

In the history, parental concern is very strongly indicative of a serious problem, but lack of concern does not necessarily indicate the reverse – there may still be a severe deficit

Qualitative evaluation must be used for infants (in the absence of ACP), and for monocular testing occlude the defective eye first

ACP is invaluable in evaluating the infant who may be blind

ACP also has some disadvantages, notably in screening for amblyopia

As soon as possible use a Snellen-based test

Picture and single-letter tests may underestimate the degree of amblyopia

Do not use a hand, either yours or the child's, for occlusion during monocular testing. Yours may not be acceptable and the child may have gaps between his or her fingers! Use a card or plastic occluder; these are more child- and user-friendly

Test the worse eye first

ACP, acuity card procedure.

i.e. they point in the same direction and project to the same part of the visual cortex.

- There is fusion. This has sensory and motor components. Sensory fusion is the ability of the cortex to interpret the images from the two eyes as one and is tested by the cover test or Worth's four-dot test. Motor fusion is the ability to maintain this single image when the eyes are diverging or converging, and is tested by prisms.
- There is stereopsis which is the third component of binocular vision and creates a sense of depth. Stereopsis is measured using random dot stereograms, the Titmus test, or Lang's stereotest.

Colour Vision

By about 3 months of age, infants have adult-type colour vision. Testing is another matter and is not usually successful until after 3 years. Rarely are colour defects mentioned voluntarily by the child. Most colour defects in children are congenital. About 8% of boys are red–green colour blind and, as there are career implications, children are screened at school, ideally not before 11 years of age. Colour defects in girls are very rare. Although acquired defects are infrequent, they can occur in retinal or optic nerve disorders. Colour testing should be performed under good natural illumination.

Identifying Coloured Objects

This involves identifying objects such as sweets, toys or articles of clothing. There are pitfalls to this test as a child may know from familiarity that a particular object is red and thus what is being tested is object recognition rather than colour perception. More importantly, certain colours can be differentiated by their brightness rather than hue (sensation of colour).

Ishihara Test

This consists of dots which vary in colour but not brightness. The dots are arranged as numbers which have to be identified or traced. Only red–green defects are detected by this test, but it is ideal for this purpose and is the most frequently used test.

City University Test

The child has to match one of four surrounding colours to the central test dot. It is simple but not very sensitive.

D-15 Test

This consists of a sequence of 15 coloured "targets" which the child has to arrange in the correct sequence, "which colour is closest to?", etc. This is a simplified Farnsworth–Munsell 100 hue test and covers the entire spectrum. This is the most sensitive test for children. It is quite simple to use, but is not as easy to interpret. Its use is usually confined to ophthalmic units.

Electroretinogram (ERG)

Total colour blindness (achromatopsia, or rod monochromatism) is rare. It can be detected electrophysiologically (see p. 244), even in early infancy. The ERG is not used to diagnose other milder colour defects.

Visual Fields

The dimensions of the visual field are: 100° temporal, 75° inferior, 60° superior and medial. This field is studied both around its periphery and across its interior by two types of perimetry:

- *Kinetic perimetry* – the stimulus moves.
- *Static perimetry* – the stimulus is static but its intensity alters. Stimuli are presented at fixed points of the visual field. Computerized automated perimetry is

based on static principles and is being used increasingly. It is applicable around 8–9 years of age.

Abnormalities may help localize and diagnose an ocular or neurological lesion, and knowledge of a field defect can alter management as it may have significant functional effects.

Perimetry Techniques

History. Even large defects can pass unnoticed or, more likely, be falsely attributed to another cause. Thus bumping into objects may be considered to be due to general clumsiness rather than a hemianopia. When taking a history ask about function in such activities as eating, bumping into, or ignoring objects preferentially on one side, etc.

Confrontation. This is crude, but in children often the only method possible. Although scotomas in the central field, but not affecting acuity, are difficult to identify, it is useful for the detection of field constriction, hemianopias and other peripheral defects, which often have important neurological connotations. These are listed below in order of sensitivity.

- *Observer with assistant*. The observer sits, eye-to-eye (on the same level) with the child who is encouraged by using a toy, etc., to keep looking straight ahead. The assistant, standing behind the child, quietly brings a toy slowly in from the periphery towards the centre of the patient's field of vision. The observer notes the point at which the toy causes distraction: the peripheral limit of the field. This is repeated in at least four quadrants. Familiarity, wariness, etc., limit this test, and so the section of the field which might be defective should be tested *first*.
- *Observer without assistant*:
  (a) Observer sits facing child and holds up both hands, asking the child to identify or touch the wiggling fingers.
  (b) As above but this time the tester gradually brings a toy or finger from the periphery. Unfortunately the direction of the tester's arm tells the child where to look.
- *Goldmann perimetry*. This is the "gold standard" kinetic method which permits detailed evaluation of the peripheral and central field. The degree of co-operation required precludes its use before about 8–9 years. Simple kinetic perimeters are used to measure the peripheral field in infants, but are still research tools.
- *Automated computerized perimetry*. This is rapidly gaining popularity in adult work, and adds a new dimension to perimetry. It is applicable after about 8–9 years of age.

Eye Movements

Types of Eye Movement

Eye movements are carefully co-ordinated so that both eyes move synchronously in the same direction as conjugate movements or versions. They are also co-ordinated to move in opposite directions as in convergence: vergence or disjugate movements.

Supranuclear Eye Movements

These include pursuit, saccadic, optokinetic and vestibulo-ocular (VOR), and vergence eye movements. They all share a final common pathway from the ocular motor nuclei, along the cranial nerves to the extraocular muscles. Supranuclear disorders affect the movement of both eyes which cannot move in one direction (e.g. right, or up) but squint is not a feature. Examples include: gaze palsy, and "sunsetting" in hydrocephalus and congenital ocular motor apraxia. These are all quite infrequent. The best known supranuclear disorder is nystagmus (see p. 241).

Nuclear and Infranuclear Pathways

Nuclear and infranuclear disorders affect the movement of one eye only, except when the cranial nerve has either bilateral (3rd) or contralateral representation (3rd and 4th).

Examining Eye Movements

Ocular Excursion

Observe the movement of each eye in all nine positions of gaze and in convergence. This is important because an abnormality may only be apparent in one position of gaze.

Eye Position: The Light Reflex

First assess the position of the eyes in the straight-ahead (primary) position. Normally the corneal light reflex lies centrally, or more correctly, just nasal to centre. The position of this reflex (Hirschberg test) is the simplest method of determining and crudely measuring the angle of a squint.

The Cover Test

This is a "low-tech" test which is often poorly performed. Indeed, for many clinicians the hands and brain seem to discharge randomly producing a flurry of flapping hands in front of the child's eyes, a bemused patient, and a confused clinician. Design a structured examination protocol:

- *Control fixation.* Ensure the child is looking directly at your light or toy. Just because the eyes are stable does not always signify you have the child's attention. I prefer a toy to a light and will move it slightly from side to side to be quite certain that attention is maintained.
- *Use an occluder for the cover test.* Although the tester's hands or thumb are often used, the response is far easier to judge when a card or commercial plastic occluder is employed.
- *Move deliberately.* Try to perform each action only once or twice.
- *Test distance.* Certain squints are present at one distance only. For this reason the cover test must be performed at two distances (at least) while looking (fixing) at:
  (a) a distant object, at least 6 m away,
  (b) a near object, ⅓ m distance.
- *Cover–uncover test.* A test for manifest strabismus (heterotopia).
  (a) Observe very carefully the position of each eye.
  (b) Place the occluder in a definite action over one eye. If the other (non-covered eye) moves in or out, this confirms the presence of a strabismus.
  (c) Take the occluder away from the eyes.
  (d) Reassess eye position.
  (e) Occlude the other eye. A movement on one side only confirms the presence of a unilateral strabismus, but if it occurs on each side in turn, an alternating deviation is present.
- *Alternate cover test.* The test for a latent squint (heterophoria).
  (a) Occlude one eye, as above.
  (b) Pass smoothly and speedily across to occlude the other eye so that neither eye can take up fixation in the interim. This dissociates the two eyes.
  (c) Observe the eye which was first occluded, if it moves in any direction on removing the occluder there is a latent squint assuming a manifest deviation has first been excluded by the cover–uncover test.

Nystagmus

This is one of the more difficult clinical signs to record. Note certain characteristics:

- Direction – by convention this refers to the fast phase.

- Rate – slow, medium or rapid.
- Amplitude – coarse, medium or fine.
- Symmetry between the two eyes.

All four characteristics can be recorded on a simple nine-position chart. The terms "pendular" or "jerky" are not helpful, and both aspects can be present in one patient.

Ophthalmic Assessment

History

Obtain information from any source: helper, teacher, play assistant, etc. Always take a family history.

Determine whether one or both eyes are affected. A homonymous hemianopia may be misinterpreted as a loss of vision in one eye. The time-scale of events is often difficult to determine, especially if the deficit involves only one eye. In children it may be difficult to distinguish between deterioration and failure to progress, the latter causes an apparent falling off in ability relative to the performance of peers.

Family photographs may show signs such as leucocoria (Figure 17.3). A compensatory head posture, ptosis, strabismus, etc., can be most helpful in determining both the time-scale of events and the rate of progress. They can indicate or obviate the need for further investigation.

The complaint *reduced vision* may cover a range of symptoms such as, blur, distortion, a visual field defect, or even diplopia. Blur is the most frequent visual symptom, but may be used to cover all those listed below unless specific questions are asked. *Distortion* may be due to retinal disarrangement, such as in retinal detachment or macular problems. It is rare in paediatric practice. *Photosensitivity* and *poor dark adaptation* can both be clues to serious disorders.

Defects of colour vision are rarely volunteered. Thus concern by the patient about colour vision is most likely to be well founded, but the converse may well not hold true.

Field defects are rarely complained of, but the child may be noted by parents to be clumsy, bump into objects on one side, more than another, etc.

Ocular pain is the hallmark of problems at the front of the eye, raised intraocular pressure, and inflammatory conditions of the eye and orbit. Pain can also be referred from intracranial structures.

Diplopia is characteristic of a cranial nerve palsy, and rarely in other, non-paralytic, types of squint. It is rarely complained of during childhood for a number of reasons:

- Children, unlike adults, have the ability to suppress the second image very rapidly, often within a few days.

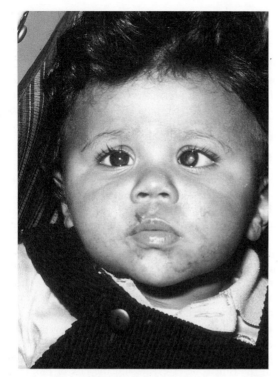

Figure 17.3   Leucocoria. A 1-year-old who presented with leucocoria due to retinoblastoma. The mother said she could "see through" her child's left eye. The ultrasound scans of this child (Figure 17.11) show that both eyes are involved and there is a suspicion of an altered reflex in the lower part of the pupil of the right eye. There is also chocolate around his mouth!

- The child may prevent diplopia by closing one eye.
- Even though in the initial phase diplopia may be present, when asked the child may simply say that "my eyes have gone funny".

Examination

Work from front to back. Do not disturb the evidence as certain signs can be "destroyed" by the examination, e.g. pupil dilation.

General Examination

Observe the child generally. Important facial signs are easily missed, such as a compensatory head posture. Causes of this (abnormal head posture or torticollis) include:

- Ocular – squints (often paralytic) to maintain single

vision; nystagmus to improve acuity; ptosis and visual field defects to optimize the use of the visual field.
- Non-ocular – tight sternomastoid muscle in the neck; deafness; spinal disorders.

Compare both sides of the face looking for both symmetrical anomalies and asymmetries. Decide first which is the abnormal side and which structure is abnormal – this is not always as simple as it sounds!

Ophthalmic Examination

Organization is essential. Remember that, ophthalmoscopic signs often do not correlate well with vision.

Vision. Use the most appropriate, and *sensitive* test for the age and stage of development. Depending on circumstances meaure:

- Distance vision. From each eye, and if reduced:
  (a) Use a pin-hole (1 mm). If due to a refractive error, acuity should improve.
  (b) Measure the vision of both eyes together, as in certain types of nystagmus this may be considerably better than each eye individually.
- Near vision. This is important in older children and vital for education.

Orbits/eyelids/globes. Compare the two sides of the face looking for subtle symmetrical anomalies. Microphthalmos, or more correctly microcornea, can give a clue to timing. Eye shrinkage after severe intraocular inflammation is obvious, otherwise reduced corneal size indicates incomplete eye growth and is seen in many developmental anomalies, but not in retinoblastoma.

Eye movements. This has been discussed above (see p. 240).

Anterior segment. Look specifically for three features:

- Size – enlargement may indicate congenital glaucoma (Figure 17.4), and reduction can be due to a growth failure or shrinkage (see above).
- Clarity of the media – early cataracts and corneal oedema (e.g. glaucoma) can be difficult to identify. The simplest way to see these is through an ophthalmoscope held about 10 in. away from the eye.
- Interocular symmetry of all the above signs.

In addition, look for redness. Conjunctival infection is an important sign of inflammation.

Finally, look for the light and near responses of the pupils, but also note the following points. Asymmetry between the two pupils (>0.4 mm, anisocoria) is pathological, and indicates an efferent defect. Differentiating

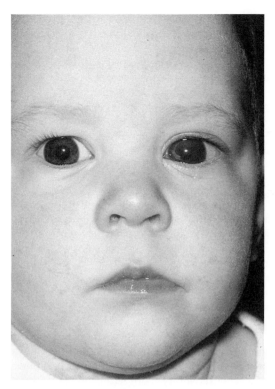

Figure 17.4   Congenital/infantile glaucoma of the left eye. The left cornea is slightly enlarged, and the light reflex fuzzy compared to the right. Some tearing is evident, and conjunctival injection. Glaucoma in infancy may present with minimal symptoms and signs.

between light and near responses can be difficult in practice as the child will naturally look toward the light thereby inducing a near response. As pupil fibres for the light reflex leave the visual pathway before the lateral geniculate nucleus, the light reflex is abnormal only in disorders of the anterior visual pathway, and not in cortical blindness. It is also normal if the media are opaque (e.g. a white cataract), unless there is underlying retinal or optic nerve pathology.

Posterior segment. This includes the vitreous, retina and optic disc and a detailed examination requires pupillary dilatation with:

- Cyclopentolate or tropicamide eyedrops 0.5% in neonates and 1.0% infants only after 3 months.
- Phenylephrine eyedrops 2.5%. 10% should not be used in neonates as it can cause hypertension. In practice 2.5% phenylephrine is adequate for all purposes.
- Atropine is a long-acting (7–10 days) mydriatic agent and should only be used when prolonged dilatation is

required, such as in the treatment of certain inflammatory diseases, and very occasionally in cycloplegia for refraction. Use 0.5% in infants and 1.0% after 3 months. Ointment is preferred because of reduced systemic absorption. Atropine should not be used in neonates.

Other Investigations

Measurement of Intraocular Pressure

It is possible to measure intraocular pressure in a neonate using a hand-held tonometer, but in children less than 4 or 5 years old tonometry has usually to be done under general anaesthesia. Recently, hand-held "puff" tonometers have been developed which are convenient and time saving and make it possible to avoid some examinations under general anaesthesia.

Electrophysiology

Three electrophysiological investigations are frequently used in paediatric ophthalmology: the electroretinogram (ERG), electro-oculogram (EOG) and the visually evoked potential (VEP). While technical details are not relevant here, every paediatrician should know their strengths and limitations. At the outset it is important to emphasize that they are complementary to, but not a substitute for, a meticulous clinical evaluation.

Electro-oculogram (EOG)

The EOG is the standing potential between the cornea and retina. It is generated by the retinal pigment epithelium which lies just beneath the retinal photoreceptors, and is therefore affected early on in conditions affecting the rods and cones such as retinitis pigmentosa. The EOG is recorded by moving the eye from side to side over a standard excursion (30°) in the dark, and then in the light, and comparing the two. In normals the light peak to dark trough difference is around 200%. Because young children are unable to make a series of standard eye movements, the EOG can only be measured after about 6–7 years of age. The EOG provides information on the outer layers of the retina (retinal pigment epithelium) and like the ERG is a mass response.

Indications for this test include, the investigation of retinal problems, particularly the early stages of retinal dystrophies such as retinitis pigmentosa and Best's disease. It has been used in the past to investigate possible drug toxicity such as desferrioxamine or chloroquine toxicity. It is almost always performed with an ERG, and the two together have complementary localizing value.

Electroretinogram (ERG)

The ERG is generated by the retinal bipolar and Muller cells, but is dependent on functioning retinal photoreceptors. It requires an electrode to be placed on, or close to the surface of the eye, such as a corneal contact lens, gold-foil eyelid electrode, carbon fibre on the cornea/conjunctiva, or electrode on the eyelid or forehead skin. The size of the ERG depends on electrode placement, and in the case of the skin is so small that averaging over a number of stimuli is required to elicit a useful ERG. A single stimulus is sufficient when a corneal electrode is used. The ERG is recorded in response to a bright flash of light at either 2 or 30 Hz (flicker ERG). The former reflects rod and cone activity, whereas the latter is a measure of cone function alone. Using these two frequencies, rod and cone function can be differentiated, and this is useful in practice, although isolated rod activity can only be recorded under scotopic conditions. In most circumstances, an ERG can be obtained without sedation, but it may be part of an examination under anaesthesia (see below) (Figure 17.5).

In clinical practice the ERG is the major test of retinal function, and being a mass photoreceptor response is not sensitive to focal retinal lesions. The ERG is dominated by the activity of the retinal rods and it is not a measure of acuity, indeed a normal ERG can be obtained in a legally blind patient. It can be abnormal (with the EOG) long before any ophthalmoscopic signs are visible (e.g. Leber's amaurosis) and is a vital and sometimes quite specific diagnostic aid. An example of the last is a flicker ERG in the photosensitive child due to achromatopsia (Figure 17.6). Thus there are a number of conditions in which the ophthalmic signs are minimal and the diagnosis can only be made by an ERG (Figure 17.7).

Visually Evoked Potential (VEP)

The VEP measures the visual response from the retina (ganglion cells) along the visual pathway to the cortex, and is thus dependent on a functioning retina and an intact visual pathway. Scalp electrodes, overlying the visual cortex, pick up the response to either a flash (luminance) or patterned stimulus. The VEP undergoes considerable maturational changes. In early infancy the VEP has a large voltage and is relatively simple, but by about 3 months of age, the waveform becomes more complex, and the latency of the major positive peak also shortens. The VEP, especially the flash VEP, is prone to considerable variability, both within and between individuals. It is also influenced by state, and can be grossly abnormal in children suffering fits. Unlike the robust ERG, the VEP is affected by arousal state and anaesthesia (i.e. the background EEG), and for this reason is not included in the battery of tests for an examination under anaesthesia. Of all the electrophysiological investigations the VEP is the most controversial, with clinical views oscillating from tremendous enthusiasm for its use in a

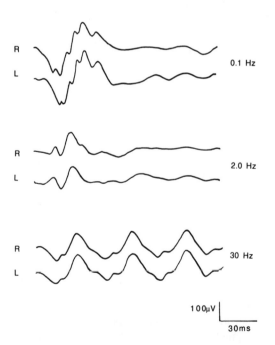

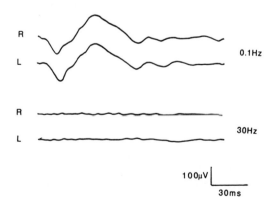

Figure 17.5 Normal ERG at 1, 2 and 30 Hz. The ERG at 1 and 2 Hz consists of an initial downward deflection (a wave) followed by a much larger b wave reflecting both rod and cone activity. At 30 Hz the response consists of a more sinusoidal waveform and depends entirely on cone activity.

Figure 17.6 ERG in achromatopsia. A reasonable ERG was obtained at 0.1 Hz but this disappeared at 30 Hz. The major feature to note is the presence of a response at low frequencies which is always absent at 30 Hz.

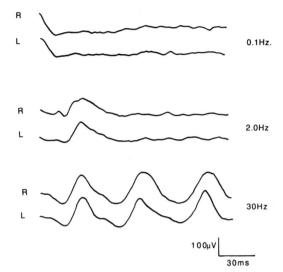

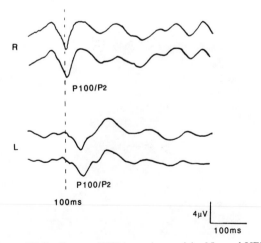

Figure 17.7 ERG in congenital stationary night-blindness. A rare cause of nightblindness, in which the retina appears normal. At 0.1 Hz there is a downward deflection of the a wave, but no b wave. At 2.0 Hz the b wave is present but smaller than normal (it is measured peak-to-peak, not from a baseline).

large range of clinical problems, through to a virtual complete negation of any clinical value, the latter partly because of the wide range of findings in cortical blindness.

The flash VEP is simply an indication of visual pathway maturation and conductivity, but cannot, because it has no definable features, be used to measure visual acuity (Figure 17.8). On the other hand, by varying pattern size

(checks or gratings) the VEP can be used to measure acuity. Techniques are used including pattern-reversal or pattern onset (Figure 17.9). Recently a variation of pattern-reversal the sweep VEP has been introduced to measure acuity. The sweep VEP uses a high stimulation rate (steady state) with the rapid sweeping through a large range of stimuli, and an estimate of acuity. As yet quantifying visual acuity by VEP methods is a research technique, and is currently possible in very few centres. On the other hand, qualitative use of the VEP is widespread.

Despite the problems mentioned above the VEP is an important non-invasive clinical tool. Because of the high concentration of ganglion cells at the macula the VEP is affected by macular disorders, but is not sensitive to peripheral retinal disorders. In cortical visual impairment, its value is more controversial as both normal and abnormal responses have been obtained, and the same holds true for delayed visual maturation (see later). It is above all an excellent test of optic nerve function and this is one of its major indications. In optic nerve disease the VEP is characteristically delayed and the amplitude reduced but, although certain features may suggest a particular aetiology, they are not pathognomic, should be proposed only tentatively, and not be considered in isolation from the clinical findings. The VEP is the only way to diagnose (providing the appropriate paradigm is used) misrouting of the visual pathway at the chiasm which occurs in albinism. It also has value as a baseline measure in progressive neurological conditions. Finally, the pattern VEP, using a range of check sizes, can be most useful in diagnosing functional (hysterical) visual loss.

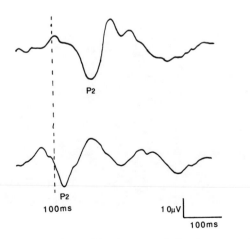

Figure 17.8 Flash VEP in normal development. In infancy the major positive peak (P2) does not appear at its mature latency of 100 ms but much later, and this shortens during the first few months of life.

Figure 17.9 Pattern VEP in optic neuritis. Normal VEP to a patterned stimulus obtained from the right eye. The major positive peak is now called P2 or P100, as that is its normal mature latency. The VEP from the left eye is delayed due to unilateral optic neuritis.

Summary of Electrophysiology

The EOG, ERG and VEP are complementary investigations, each assessing a different part of the visual pathway. All three have considerable value, are complementary to the clinical examination, and in many cases in children a diagnosis cannot be made without them. Electrophysiological tests help the clinician determine whether the basis of a problem lies in the retina or more posteriorly, and if the retina is involved, which part. While it is important to attempt to quantify these tests, they must be interpreted with caution, and, if in doubt, repeated. There are few falsely normal results, but falsely abnormal results are common.

Indications for electrophysiology include:

- *Infant who may be blind*:
  (a) ERG*
  (b) Although variable in delayed visual maturation and cortical visual impairment, VEP can provide a clue to a widespread neurological disturbance.
- *Nystagmus*:
  (a) ERG for a retinal dystrophy;*
  (b) VEP to diagnose visual pathway misrouting in albinism.
- *Retinal dystrophy*: ERG and EOG.
- *Evaluating visual pathway maturation and function*, e.g. opaque media, due to cataract, trauma, etc.: ERG and VEP.

*EOG can be used as an adjunct to the ERG in older children and adults, but is not included in the list as it cannot be performed in infants and young children.

- *Optic nerve disorders*:
  (a) ERG, to exclude subtle retinal dystrophy which may not have been visualized ophthalmoscopically;
  (b) VEP.
- *Functional visual loss*: VEP.
- *Baseline measurements in possibly progressive neurological disorders* – here it is important to differentiate retinal and neurological functions: ERG and VEP.

Ultrasound Scan

This technique enables the anatomical structures of the eye to be studied and measured. Ophthalmic ultrasound uses frequencies of around 10 000 Hz. The ultrasound probe is placed close to the cornea through a water bath, or usually in children, against the eyelid. It enables the study of the interior of the eye for masses or retinal detachment in the presence of opaque media (Figures 17.10 and 17.11). Ultrasound is also useful to study the consistency of an intraocular mass, for instance looking for tissue calcification in a possible retinoblastoma. The role of ultrasound to visualize the optic nerve as it passes through the orbit has largely been supplanted by other techniques such as CT and MRI scanning. Ultrasound can also accurately measure the dimensions of the eyeball.

Photography

The value of photography to document clinical signs has been mentioned. Fundus photography is notoriously difficult except in older children, but if possible it is an invaluable method of documenting clinical findings. If

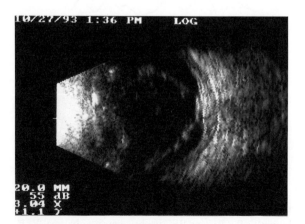 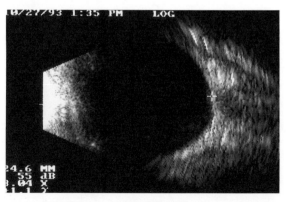

Figure 17.10 Ultrasound scans in normal and retinal detachment. The right eye is normal with an axial length of 24.6 mm. The left eye contains a retinal detachment and is smaller (only 20.0 mm). Despite a difference in eye length the corneae are of equal diameter, so this difference is not visible from the examiner's perspective. The retinal detachment is a sequela of severe retinopathy of prematurity, but did not occur until 4 years of age.

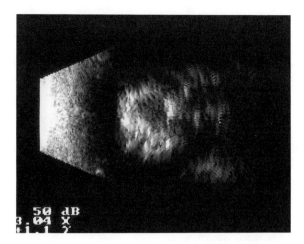 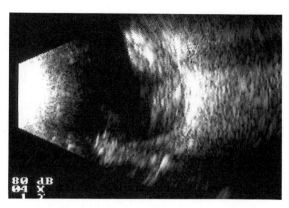

Figure 17.11   Ultrasound scans in leucocoria. Solid tumours in each eye, that on the right occupying the posterior part of the globe, and the left extending forward to fill most of the vitreous cavity.

photography is necessary in younger children it is often undertaken as part of an examination under anaesthesia (EUA). The use of fluorescein angiography is infrequent even in an EUA. If necessary the dye can be introduced orally instead of the more usual intravenous route, and this is used occasionally to aid in the diagnosis of papilloedema.

Examination Under Anaesthesia

This was frequently resorted to in the past, but is now an infrequent event because of the development of simple electrophysiology, methods of measuring acuity (ACP), and improved ophthalmoscopy. However an EUA is still sometimes necessary. A grossly abnormal ERG can be an indication. In this instance, it is essential to be absolutely certain that the ERG finding is correct, and confirmation obtained under "ideal" conditions of an EUA is advisable. Repeated EUAs are still sometimes required for the measurement of intraocular pressure in the review of infantile glaucoma (see above).

A PROBLEM-BASED APPROACH

The purpose of this section is to discuss patterns of investigation starting with the presenting symptom or sign. The problem facing clinicians is mainly one of identification, and management will not be covered. Conditions are grouped into broad categories. Inevitably some sit uncomfortably in a particular group, but hopefully this approach will be helpful to the clinician. Only selected clinical details will be given. For a comprehensive review the reader is referred to Taylor (1990). It will

be obvious that some ophthalmic signs, such as nystagmus and optic atrophy are literally just signs, and are not diagnoses in themselves.

Leucocoria

The white pupil, or leucocoria, is one of the most important clinical signs (Figure 17.3) as some of its causes are potentially lethal, or have severe consequences for sight. These devastating consequences can often be prevented by prompt treatment. Causes of leucocoria include:

- *Tumours*:
  (a) *Retinoblastoma* is the commonest ocular malignancy in childhood. *Bilateral cases* are inherited as an autosomal dominant trait, and in the absence of a positive family history are considered to be due to a new mutation. Children with learning difficulties with a deletion of 13q have a high incidence of retinoblastoma. *Unilateral* cases are more likely to be sporadic (85%). Retinoblastoma may present at any time in childhood with leucocoria, squint, glaucoma, etc. It may be obscured by haemorrhage, inflammatory signs, etc.
  (b) *Other tumours*. Astrocytic hamartoma is a retinal phakoma seen in tuberous sclerosis and less frequently in neurofibromatosis. Often multiple and distributed along retinal vessels, they can grow very slowly, but do not require treatment. These lesions can be confused with retinoblastoma.
- *Cataract* (see later).
- *Retinopathy of prematurity* (see later).

- *Developmental anomalies*:
  - (a) Persistent primary hyperplastic vitreous.
  - (b) Retrolental masses and retinal dysplasias: Norrie's disease, incontinentia pigmenti, and vitreoretinopathies.
    (a) and (b) cover a wide range of conditions presenting as either leucocoria or retinal folds. The classification is unsatisfactory and many are inherited.
  - (c) Coloboma.
- *Inflammations*: due to infections – endophthalmitis, toxocariasis and toxoplasmosis.
- *Coat's disease*: mostly unilateral and affects boys far more than girls; only very rarely is it inherited. The average age of presentation is 8 years but it may occur at other times, even rarely in infancy. The Coat's lesion consists of telengiectatic retinal vessels, extensive lipid exudation and retinal detachment. The major differential diagnosis is between Coat's and retinoblastoma.

Clinical Evaluation

Evaluation of leucocoria is urgent. Take a family history as many of these conditions can be familial. Unilaterality or bilaterality is suggestive of, but does not absolutely exclude, any of the conditions. Inspection should differentiate cataract from other causes. Time of presentation can be helpful as cataract and developmental anomalies are present at birth, retinopathy of prematurity by 3 months after term, and inflammation and Coat's disease at any time in childhood. Retinoblastoma can present from birth onwards. Microphthalmos is a frequent feature of retinopathy and developmental abnormalities, and if the eye becomes atrophic in inflammatory conditions.

Special Tests

Ocular ultrasound is essential for many cases, especially if retinoblastoma is a possibility, because it enables the posterior segment of the eye to be scrutinized even in the presence of haemorrhage or other opacity. The finding of calcium in the tumour by ultrasound is very suggestive of retinoblastoma. Other tests include fluorescein angiography in early cases and CT scan when the media are opaque. Leucocoria is one of the major indications for examination under anaesthesia. If an examination under anaesthesia is to be undertaken this is the logical time to perform ultrasound.

Referral

Specialist ophthalmic and sometimes multidisciplinary investigations are necessary. All cases of leucocoria should be referred as a matter of urgency to a paediatric ophthalmologist. Retinoblastoma should be managed by a team including a paediatric oncologist and an ophthalmologist. The genetic implications of many of these conditions should not be ignored.

The Watery (including the Red) Eye

This is a frequent reason for referral, mostly during infancy. By knowing the possible aetiologies, most cases can be diagnosed relatively simply. Causes of watery eye include:

- With a "white" eye: congenital blockage of the nasolacrimal system.
- With a "red" eye:
  - (a) Congenital glaucoma.
  - (b) Inflammations – conjunctivitis, keratitis, uveitis, endophthalmitis.

Clinical Evaluation

First differentiate the "white" and "red" eyes as the latter require urgent investigation and treatment. The presenting features of congenital glaucoma may range from the very subtle (mild corneal clouding and enlargement) (Figure 17.4) to severe photophobia (see below) and a red enlarged, watery eye(s).

Referral

Congenital nasolacrimal obstruction almost always resolves spontaneously by 9 months of age and referral to an ophthalmologist is only necessary if that fails to occur. All cases of red watery eye need urgent ophthalmic referral and some will require an examination under anaesthesia.

Children who are Unduly Sensitive to Light and Dark

Infants and children who are unduly sensitive to either bright or dim illumination may have serious eye problems. Causes of light sensitivity include:

- "Red" eye:
  - (a) Cornea and anterior segment – congenital glaucoma (the corneal oedema causes this symptom), keratitis, and uveitis.
- "White" eye:
  - (a) Cornea – cystinosis – corneal crystalline deposits.
  - (b) Lens – cataract.

(c) Lack of ocular pigmentation – albinism.
(d) Retina – retinal dystrophies affecting cones, such as achromatopsia.

Clinical Evaluation

Urgent specialist investigation is required if there is a red eye. All cases of photosensitivity require a slit-lamp examination, as this is normal only in those with a retinal dystrophy.

Photosensitivity without a red eye is a diagnostic dilemma. Cystinosis and cataract can be diagnosed in most cases by ophthalmoscopy at about 10 in. away from the eye, otherwise slit-lamp biomicroscopy is necessary. The possibility of albinism must be considered in any child with nystagmus, particularly if photosensitive, and this is not always a simple diagnosis to make. Cone retinal dystrophies are uncommon, but must be suspected in a child with photosensitivity, nystagmus, reduced acuity, or colour blindness. The diagnosis can only be confirmed by an ERG at 2 and 30 Hz (to test cone function differentially).

Special Tests

Slit-lamp examination should be done in all cases. An ERG is essential in those in whom an obvious cause has not been identified and must be undertaken if a cone disorder is a possibility.

Nightblindness (Nyctalopia)

This indicates retinal rod dysfunction and occurs in many potentially severe retinal problems. The causes are:

- Retinitis pigmentosa and related conditions.
- Congenital stationary nightblindness (rare).
- Vitamin A deficiency: malnutrition, malabsorpton, or chronic liver disease.

Clinical Evaluation

Nightblindness may be a difficult symptom to elicit, and the child who is asked whether he or she can see at night may seriously doubt the sanity of the clinician. It can be suggested by a parent commenting that the child is more frightened of the dark than a sibling, is the only child to insist on a night light, etc. The visual fields should be assessed for constriction, a characteristic of established rod disorders.

Special Tests

For visual-field assessment, an ERG should be performed in all cases, and an EOG if the patient is old enough.

Children with Special Needs

There are special groups of children who have a high incidence of ophthalmic problems which can pass unnoticed. Some affect the child and require treatment and support, while others may have genetic implications.

Learning Difficulties

Unfortunately for the child with both severe learning difficulties and visual impairment, the latter can pass unnoticed. Consequently, the child may not receive the appropriate support, thus limiting the effectiveness of other management measures.

Around 30–50% of children with neurodevelopmental abnormalities also have ophthalmic problems which include: cortical visual impairment/complicated delayed visual maturation (see later); optic atrophy; refractive errors (usually hypermetropia but also sometimes myopia); and squint and other eye movement problems.

Treatment

While the basic condition is untreatable, important help may be given by treatment of the refractive error, squint, and occasionally other ophthalmic problem. Most importantly, understanding the visual capability of a child is an enormous help to parents and carers.

Clinical Evaluation

Ideally, all children with neurodevelopmental problems should have a full ophthalmic examination, including vision and refractive assessment. The need for review is determined by the findings.

Special Tests

The acuity card procedure is often more helpful in measuring vision than traditional means. The need for other tests is indicated by the clinical situation.

Hearing Impairment

Sensory neural hearing loss can be due to a variety of aetiological factors, including genetic causes and about 40% of these children also have a visually significant eye problem. Some problems are progressive, resulting in blindness. The causes are:

- *Retinitis pigmentosa-like retinopathy*:
  (a) Usher's syndrome.
  (b) Refsum's disease.
  (c) Cockayne's syndrome.

(d) Alstrom's syndrome, etc.
Retinitis pigmentosa-type picture of nightblindness, visual field constriction and blindness.

- *Congenital rubella*: in this instance the pigmentary retinopathy does not behave like retinitis pigmentosa and does not cause severe bilateral visual loss.
- *Prematurity*.
- *DIDMOAD*: diabetes insipidus, diabetes mellitus, optic atrophy and deafness. Onset in youth or later.
- *Others*: this abbreviated list should also include metabolic, chromosomal, infective and neurodegenerative causes.

Clinical Evaluation

Every deaf child should have an ophthalmic assessement which includes taking a history of nightblindness, measuring visual acuity and the visual fields (simple confrontation for constriction) at the very least. Probably there should be at least two to three assessments before the age of 16 years.

Special Tests

Visual field analysis should always be performed. The clinician must have a low threshold to perform an ERG to determine if there is a retinal problem as this is the only definitive method of diagnosing Usher's syndrome or other retinal dystrophy, or excluding rubella.

Premature Birth and the Visual System

The immediate concern with preterm birth is retinopathy of prematurity (ROP), however other long-term ophthalmic sequelae will also be mentioned.

Retinopathy of Prematurity

Despite meticulous neonatal care ROP is currently not entirely preventable. Indeed with the increased survival of the very immature neonate the incidence of severe ROP is increasing. The survival rates for infants < 1000 g birthweight is about 50–60% and these infants have an incidence of severe ROP of approximately 20%. The classification of acute ROP is shown in Table 17.4. The classification of the sequelae (cicatricial ROP) is not covered here. All maximum stage 1 and 2 ROP resolves without adverse consequences. The term severe ROP refers to stage 3 or more and is *almost* confined to babies < 1250 g birthweight. "Threshold" ROP (Table 17.4) because it carries a risk of blindness, of about 50% if untreated, is chosen as the indication for surgical inter-

Table 17.4 International classification of retinopathy of prematurity

Stage 1 Demarcation line
Thin white line, lying within the plane of the retina and separating avascular from vascular retinal regions

Stage 2 Ridge
The demarcation line has increased in volume to extend out of the plane of the retina. Isolated vascular tufts may be seen posterior to the ridge

Stage 3 Ridge with extraretinal fibrovascular proliferation
This may be:
(a) Continuous with the posterior edge of the ridge
(b) Posterior, but disconnected, from the ridge
(c) Into the vitreous

Stage 4 Retinal detachment – subtotal
(a) Extrafoveal
(b) Involving the fovea

Stage 5 Retinal detachment – total
Funnel:

Anterior	Posterior
open	open
narrow	narrow
open	narrow
narrow	open

"Plus" disease: signs of activity which can accompany any stage and include retinal vessels (tortuosity and engorgement of the vessels at the posterior pole), iris (vascular engorgement and rigidity), and vitreous (haze)

Threshold ROP: stage 3 with five continuous or eight cumulative clock hours. Associated with "plus" disease

vention. Treatment by cryotherapy or laser therapy reduces the unfavourable outcome of "threshold" by about 50% and consequently screening for ROP is now essential.

ROP Screening

The purpose is to identify severe ROP requiring treatment, i.e. "threshold" disease. Screening should be done in all neonates of < 1500 g birthweight and ≤ 31 weeks gestation. With no accurate predictors of severe disease, all the above are included regardless of sickness criteria and the amount of supplemental oxygen given. Larger babies requiring oxygen may also be examined, but this is not strictly necessary.

The onset and progression of ROP are both largely determined by postmenstrual age (PMA) rather than by neonatal events. The mean age for the onset of threshold ROP is 37.7 weeks PMA (5th and 95th percentiles 33.6

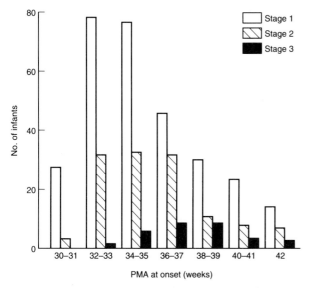

Figure 17.12 Age at onset and progression of ROP. Postmenstrual age at development of ROP stages 1, 2 and 3 in 572 neonates. No ROP developed until the 30th week, although 201 babies were ≤27 weeks and 345 were ≤29 weeks gestational age. Onset and progression are largely determined by postmenstrual age. The single infant who developed stage-3 ROP at >46 weeks had not been examined for 4 weeks previously. The screening protocol must identify infants with stage-3 ROP. Reproduced with permission of Churchill Livingstone.

and 42.0 weeks PMA, respectively). Unfortunately, the time window available for effective treatment is only about 2–3 weeks, and this determines the screening protocol.

The screening protocol comprises:

- Infants ≤25 weeks gestational age (GA):
  (a) 6–7* weeks postnatally; and then
  (b) fortnightly until 36 weeks PMA, or until vascularization is in zone 3.
- Infants 26 to ≤31 weeks GA:
  (a) 6–7* weeks postnatally; and then
  (b) 36 weeks PMA, or within a week or two of this age, if the baby is to be transferred to another hospital, or to be discharged to home around this time.

Many babies only require one examination. Logistically it is simpler to include at least one examination before discharge from hospital as this enables the clinician to determine the need for review. Timing is

*In the original publication of the Working Party, 7 weeks was the recommended age at for the first examination. This has been broadened to 6–7 weeks.

vital, one too early has no value, and after discharge may be too late for treatment. The need for review is dictated by individual clinical criteria.

Screening for ROP is still not undertaken in all centres, and neonatologists can facilitate this development. Co-ordination is required to ensure that neonates transferred between units are screened at the correct time.

Ophthalmic Sequelae of Preterm Birth

ROP Related

Not all ROP responds satisfactorily to treatment and the sequelae range from the visually insignificant to total blindness, this last being associated with leucocoria. Stage-3 ROP, even if treated, may result in myopia which develops in early childhood. Deterioration of vision due to retinal detachment can occur at any time after severe ROP. The long-term outcome of treatment for severe ROP is not yet known.

Non-ROP Related

Preterm babies are more likely to suffer from myopia as teenagers, squint (10–15% at <1500 g birthweight), optic atrophy, or cortical visual impairment.

Cataract

Cataract is a major cause of visual impairment in childhood, which meticulous surgical treatment can reduce but not eliminate. The presence of a cataract may also have important systemic implications and the appropriate work-up is essential. There are far too many causes to list individually, therefore only certain major categories are given here (see Table 17.5).

Clinical Evaluation

As with so many eye disorders, the clinical appearance can be quite misleading with respect to function. Measure visual functions carefully and perform a full ophthalmic examination. If the pupil response is abnormal there may well be an underlying retinal or optic nerve lesion. As some cases require urgent treatment, and the eye may also harbour a serious ocular disorder, all cataracts should be referred to a paediatric ophthalmologist as a matter of urgency.

Special Tests

There may be an important ocular condition (e.g. tumour) behind the cataract. As this often cannot be visualized, ocular ultrasound and/or ERG are frequently necessary.

Table 17.5   Aetiology of cataract

Isolated anomaly – this includes at least 50% of cataracts in childhood:
(a) Sporadic
(b) Inherited, usually as a dominant trait, other patterns are known. Many of these cataracts are associated with microphthalmos

Intrauterine infection:
(a) Rubella
(b) Toxoplasmosis

Chromosomal abnormalities:
(a) Trisomy 21
(b) Trisomy 18

Ocular disorders:
(a) Trauma
(b) Ocular inflammation/uveitis, juvenile rheumatoid arthritis, endophthalmitis
(c) Severe widespread ocular disorders. Severe ROP, aniridia, retinitis pigmentosa, etc.

Metabolic disorders:
(a) Galactosaemia
(b) Galactokinase deficiency
(c) Diabetes mellitus
(d) Lowe's syndrome

Skeletal disorders:
(a) Stickler syndrome
(b) Conradi syndrome
(c) Hallerman-Streiff syndrome

Dermatological disorders:
(a) Atopy
(b) Cockayne syndrome

Central nervous system disorders:
(a) Marinesco-Sjögren syndrome
(b) Norrie's disease
(c) Zellweger's syndrome

Optic Atrophy

Optic atrophy is a sign and not a diagnosis. It may be due to a condition directly affecting the optic nerve (primary optic atrophy), or consecutive to long-standing retinal disease (see Table 17.6).

Clinical Evaluation

The appearance of the optic disc alone does not indicate visual function. Narrowing of the retinal arterioles may offer a clue to the presence of retinal pathology. All children with optic atrophy should have a full ophthalmic and neurological assessment. Examination of available family members is important, as dominant optic atrophy may be subclinical and its finding in a relative obviates the need for extensive neurological investigations.

Table 17.6   Aetiology of optic atrophy

Compressive

Optic neuritis
Unlike in adults, in children it is usually bilateral. Despite the severe loss, recovery is the rule, and the outlook is excellent for most. It may be infectious in origin

Retinal disease
Optic atrophy often occurs in chronic widespread retinal conditions such as retinitis pigmentosa. A subtle distinguishing feature from primary atrophy is narrowing of the retinal arterioles at the optic disc

Hereditary
(a) Autosomal dominant optic atrophy. Quite common, but is not usually apparent until around school age
(b) Recessive optic atrophy (Behr's) may present in the first year of life with mild mental retardation, hypertonia and ataxia
(c) DIDMOAD syndrome includes diabetes mellitus, diabetes insipidus, optic atrophy and deafness. The optic atrophy is a constant feature of this condition which develops in teenage years and in some cases is probably inherited by a mitochondrial mechanism
(d) Leber's optic neuropathy. A mitochondrial abnormality which usually commences in young adults

Intra-uterine neurological disease
Optic atrophy may follow intrauterine infections, asphyxia and cerebral malformations

Perinatal damage
Can result from events such as birth asphyxia

Inflammatory
Meningoencephalitis, etc.

Metabolic
Including the neurodegenerative lipid storage diseases (e.g. Batten's disease), Leigh's subacute necrotizing encephalopathy and osteopetrosis

Trauma

Special Tests

Both the ERG and VEP are useful, the former to exclude retinal disease and the latter to aid the identification of subtle optic nerve involvement, and also to provide a crude estimation of function.

The Infant or Child who Appears not to See Well

Every paediatrician will be consulted at some time about an infant or child who appears not to see well. Quantitative assessment of vision is difficult and many signs are subtle or absent, even in a blind infant. Therefore a strategy for evaluation is required. Classification of the infant who appears not to see well is as follows.

- **Abnormal ocular examination**
  (a) *Cornea* – corneal opacities and other anterior segment malformations obvious on examination.
  (b) *Lens* – cataract, dislocated lenses, etc.
  (c) *Vitreous and retina* – leucocoria, ROP and other retinal problems.
  (d) *Optic nerve* – optic atrophy, optic nerve hypoplasia and colobomas affecting the optic disc.
- **"Normal" ocular examination**
  (a) *Unidentified abnormal.* Many retinal and optic nerve conditions have very subtle signs, thus optic atrophy and optic nerve hypoplasia sufficient to cause blindness may not be identified.
  (b) *Leber's amaurosis.* This retinal dystrophy is inherited as an autosomal recessive trait and produces a severe visual impairment. Apart from the indirect sign of nystagmus, Leber's amaurosis may produce almost no visible signs.
  (c) *Achromatopsia.* Congenital absence of retinal cones which produces reduced vision, photophobia, colour blindness, nystagmus and an absence of specific ocular signs.
  (d) *Delayed visual maturation (DVM).* This term denotes an infant, blind from birth who subsequently improves, the amount of improvement depending upon other factors such as coexistent neurological or ocular problems. In clinical practice many clinicians restrict the term DVM to type-1 DVM because in this situation the picture is not complicated by any other ocular or neurological problem. Unfortunately life is not quite so simple, and DVM is now recognized as a broad clinical spectrum.

  Type 1: DVM as an isolated anomaly. Apart from the severe visual defect the infant is normal. Improvement is complete and rapid within the first six months of life. Some of these infants have suffered perinatal problems.

  Type 2: DVM with obvious and persistent neuro-developmental problems. In these infants improvement is limited, and governed by the severity of the neurological problem. It is characteristically slow, often taking many months.

  Type 3: DVM associated with infantile nystagmus and albinism. Infants in this group are blind in early infancy, and at that time do not have nystagmus. Around the time of visual improvement the nystagmus commences. Rapid improvement of vision occurs within 6 months, but this is not complete and completely normal vision is not achieved.

  Type 4: DVM with severe congenital, bilateral structural ocular abnormalities such as optic nerve hypoplasia, Leber's amaurosis, colobomas, etc. (but excluding albinism). *Some* infants with severe ocular disorders exhibit very limited improvement which is very useful to the children, although they remain legally blind. *In practice differentiating type 4 from other types does not pose a problem.*

  (e) *Cortical visual impairment (CVI).* "CVI" is preferred to the term "cortical blindness", as many infants exhibit some improvement of vision. The child with CVI has reduced vision, and a normal eye examination including pupil responses. The causes of CVI are: prenatal (malformations, intrauterine infections, ischaemia, etc.); perinatal (ischaemia and other neurological catastrophies, including infections); or acquired (infections, trauma, cardiac arrest, neurodegenerative disorders, etc.).

Clinical Evaluation

Careful assessment of vision, the ideal situation for the acuity cards. The pupil light reflex must be assessed and is abnormal in retinal and optic nerve, but not in cortical, problems. All children should be seen by both an ophthalmologist and a paediatrician.

Special Tests

Most cases require electrodiagnostic tests, except perhaps for the child whose visual deficit can be *fully* explained by a corneal opacity, cataract, etc. However, even in these last two instances there may be an associated retinal problem. The most important electrodiagnostic test is the ERG, which is:

- Normal in: Disorders of the anterior segment; DVM types 1, 2 and 3; CVI; optic nerve abnormalities.
- Abnormal in: Leber's amaurosis and other retinal dystrophies.
- Normal or abnormal in: DVM type 4, as this may be due to a retinal or optic nerve abnormality.

The flash VEP is also frequently used in DVM, but here its value is less well defined. In type-1 DVM during the phase of blindness, both normal and abnormal responses have been recorded. The VEP is abnormal in optic nerve disorders, but not always in CVI.

Nystagmus

Nystagmus is a sign and not a diagnosis, and is encountered by all clinicians. The causes of nystagmus are listed in Table 17.7.

Table 17.7   Causes of nystagmus

Physiological nystagmus
Caloric, rotational and optokinetic nystagmus

Central nervous system conditions
The association of nystagmus and CNS disorders is well known, and is a feature of brain-stem, cerebellar and vestibular lesions. Some specific types have localizing value

Sensory-deprivation nystagmus
Bilateral reduced vision in infancy and early childhood (before 6 years) causes nystagmus. Any condition of the anterior visual pathway sufficient to preclude normal visual development can do this, such as opacities of the media, aniridia, and optic nerve pathology, but disorders of the posterior visual pathway such as cortical visual impairment do not.
    Sensory nystagmus ranges from the slow wandering movements seen in total blindness to the rapid oscillation indistinguishable from idiopathic infantile nystagmus, albinism, etc.

Congenital (infantile) nystagmus
Often also called motor nystagmus. The term is reserved for nystagmus presenting in infancy in which other ocular (i.e. sensory) abnormalities have been excluded. It may be sporadic, or inherited as a dominant, recessive or X-linked disorder. The nystagmus is binocular, symmetrical and horizontal in all positions of gaze, except for a rare vertical variant

Special nystagmus types
Certain types of nystagmus have important neurological implications and localizing value, such as see-saw, downbeat, upbeat, dissociated (as in internuclear ophthalmoplegia), ocular bobbing, and retraction nystagmus

Spasmus nutans
This syndrome consists of nystagmus, head nodding and torticollis, and commences at 4–18 months of age and usually resolves within 1–2 years. Not all features are present at one time. It can be grossly asymmetrical and either horizontal or vertical. Spasmus nutans can be associated with intracranial tumours

Asymmetric nystagmus
Asymmetry between the two eyes may be due to blindness of the oscillating eye, to spasmus nutans, and/or a chiasmal tumour.

Clinical Evaluation

Nystagmus may be the first sign of a serious neurological or ocular disorder which cannot always be clinically differentiated. All cases should have a full ophthalmic and paediatric-neurological assessement.

Special Tests

Unless there are compelling reasons for not doing so (albinism, or strong family history of nystagmus), all children with nystagmus should have an ERG at 2 and 30 Hz to test rod and cone function individually. The need for neurological investigations must be judged according to each case.

Amblyopia

Amblyopia is the commonest visual disorder of childhood affecting 2–5% of the population. It is defined as a reduction of visual acuity not explained by physical examination which persists after correction of its cause. Its causes are: refractive error, squint and form deprivation (any lesion obstructing the visual pathway such as, ptosis or haemangioma of the eyelid, cataract, opacity in the vitreous, etc.). Usually it is unilateral, but it can affect both eyes.

Amblyopia is thus caused by any "obstruction" to visual development. The sensitive period for its development is in infancy and early childhood, and similarly the possibility of successful treatment is also confined to this period – success is rare after about 6 years of age. Thus preschool screening programmes are in place in many countries.

Clinical Evaluation

Early identification is the key issue, and much of the visual screening in childhood is directed to this end (see Table 17.9). Amblyopia is a diagnosis of exclusion. All squints should be referred for full orthoptic and/or ophthalmic examination. The magnitude of the squint is immaterial to its potential for causing amblyopia.

Any child harbouring a lesion which might result in form deprivation should be referred for full ophthalmic assessment as a matter of urgency as this type of amblyopia is particularly severe.

Amblyopia which is not associated with either a squint or form deprivation presents the greatest identification problem. This is usually due to a unilateral refractive error (anisometropia). Bearing in mind the relative insensitivity of vision screening tests in the preschool child (see earlier) the clinician must be very sensitive to *any slight* difference of acuity between the two eyes: if in doubt repeat again very soon.

Squint

The incidence of squint is 1–2%. The paediatrician must be aware of any ophthalmic and systemic associations. While most have no "sinister" connotations, a squint may be the first sign of a serious ocular or systemic condition. The classification of squint is given in Table 17.8.

Clinical Evaluation

Take action immediately. Test acuity for amblyopia. Every child should have a full orthoptic and ophthalmic

---

Table 17.8   Classification of squint

Isolated anomaly – by far the most common type of squint
(a) Neonatal: the eyes of neonates frequently appear to diverge. This resolves over the first month or so of life
(b) Infantile esotropia, formerly known as a congenital convergent squint. The word "congenital" is incorrect as the onset is between 3 and 9 months
(c) Paralytic squint: not rare, particularly a 4th nerve palsy, usually without systemic association

Ocular disorders – visually impaired eyes may diverge or converge

Systemic conditions
(a) Prematurity – children born prematurely have an increased risk of developing a squint (10–20%) and the risk is especially high in those with severe ROP or who have suffered neurological damage
(b) Acute CNS disorders – both concomitant and paralytic squints can occur in acute neurological disorders due to: raised intracranial pressure, tumours, trauma, degenerative and inflammatory diseases
(c) Learning difficulties – children with these disorders have a high incidence of squint
(d) Brain-stem disorders – a number of brain-stem anomalies such a Duane's and Mobius' syndrome are associated with squint and other eye movement abnormalities
(e) Muscle disease – this is infrequent, but it is important not to forget myasthenia. Other muscle conditions are rare

Orbital disorders
These are infrequent, but squint may be the presenting sign of a rhabdomyosarcoma and is frequent in craniostenosis.

---

examination, the latter including ophthalmoscopy. The possibility of an underlying ocular or systemic disorder should always be considered. However, because of the infrequency of these associations, not every child should be so scrutinized.

Special Tests

These are only indicated if there is the possibility of associated ocular or neurological pathology.

OPHTHALMIC SCREENING

A plan for the screening of children is outlined in Tables 17.9 and 17.10.

Table 17.9   Overview of screening for ophthalmic problems in childhood:* All children

---

Birth
Screening for: leucocoria (e.g. retinoblastoma and cataract); congenital abnormalities
Procedure: use ophthalmoscope looking for red reflex

6 weeks
Screening for: visual awareness and squint
Procedure: take a history and examine

7–8 months
Screening for: visual defects and strabismus
Procedure: ask about vision and look for squint†

3–4 years
Screening for: amblyopia and squint
Procedure: test vision and look for squint

School entry
Screening for: amblyopia and refractive errors
Procedure: test visual acuity using Snellen chart

8 years
Screening for: visual defects and refractive errors
Procedure: test visual acuity using Snellen chart

11 years
Screening for: visual defects and colour vision
Procedure: test visual acuity and colour vision

---

*This information has been culled from several sources and simply provides an overview of screening for ophthalmic problems in childhood. Not all are currently undertaken everywhere. Deliberately, professional issues, such as who performs the various tests have been omitted, as there are considerable local variations.
†Many squints present between screening examinations (at any age); refer appropriately.

Table 17.10   Ophthalmic screening for special groups of children*

Preterm neonates
Screening for retinopathy of prematurity and be aware of sequelae of prematurity†

Juvenile chronic arthritis (JCA)
High risk – pauciarticular disease with onset before 6 years, ANA positive
Medium risk – polyarticular and ANA positive, or pauciarticular and ANA negative
Low risk – systemic JCA, B27 associated with JCA, or any JCA starting after 11 years

(a) All groups – initially by an ophthalmologist
(b) High risk – every 4 months for year 1 and then 6 monthly for 5 years
(c) Low risk – screen annually
(d) Screening to continue for 10 years after onset of JCA, or until 12 years of age, whichever is the shorter

Diabetes mellitus
Screening for diabetic retinopathy to start at puberty, and then annually

Learning difficulties†
Should screen for a range of ophthalmic problems

Hearing impairment†
Screening should be undertaken about 2–3 times before 16 years and should include visual acuity, visual fields, and in certain instances an ERG

*See footnote to Table 17.9.
†See text for details.

SUGGESTED READING

General Texts

Fielder AR (in press) Disorders of vision. In: Levene MI, Lilford R, Bennett MJ, Punt J (eds) *Fetal Neurology and Neurosurgery*, 2nd edn. Churchill Livingston, Edinburgh.

Isenberg SJ (ed) (1989) *The Eye in Infancy*. Year Book Publications, Chicago.
Taylor D (ed) (1990) *Pediatric Ophthalmology*. Blackwell Scientific, Boston.

Vision Abnormalities and Measurement of Vision

Fielder AR, Mayer DL (1991) Delayed visual maturation. *Sem Ophthalmol* 6: 182–193.
Fielder AR, Best AB, Bax MCO (1993) *Clinics in Developmental Medicine vol. 128: The Management of Visual Impairment in Childhood*. MacKeith Press, Cambridge.
Sonksen PM (1993) The assessment of vision in the preschool child. *Arch Dis Child* 68: 513–516.
Van Hof-van Duin J (1989) The development and study of visual acuity. *Dev Med Child Neurol* 31: 543–552.
Heckinlively JR, Arden GB (1991) *The Principles and Practice of Clinical Electrophysiology of Vision*. Mosby, St Louis.

Squint

Fielder AR (1989) The management of squint. *Arch Dis Child* 64: 413–418.
Mein J, Trimble R (1991) *Diagnosis and Management of Ocular Motor Disorders*, 2nd edn. Blackwell Scientific, Oxford.

Retinopathy of Prematurity

Fielder AR, Levene MI (1992) Screening for retinopathy of prematurity. *Arch Dis Child* 67: 860–867.

Screening Protocols

Hall DMB (ed) (1992) *Health For All Children*, 2nd edn. Oxford Medical Publications, Oxford.

18
Rheumatology

T R Southwood

INTRODUCTION

The diagnosis, differential diagnosis and monitoring of rheumatic diseases in children can be challenging. Appropriate laboratory investigations are important in this process, but should never be used as a substitute for meticulous clinical assessment. In fact, the utility of the investigations is dependent on the quality of the clinical information accompanying the investigation request.

At present, there are three main areas in which laboratory investigations are important. Firstly, investigations are useful to exclude "non-rheumatic" disease from the differential diagnosis of rheumatic symptoms and signs. For example, a sterile joint aspirate helps to rule out septic arthritis, and a normal bone marrow biopsy usually excludes leukaemia. Secondly, investigations may support the diagnosis of a specific rheumatic disease, although this usually requires a combination of several investigations. For instance, the diagnosis of systemic lupus erythematosus (SLE) is strongly supported by the combination of high titre antinuclear antibodies (ANA), antibodies to double stranded (native) DNA, and evidence of complement consumption. Finally, when used for monitoring a rheumatic disease, investigations may provide a guide to disease activity and its consequences through imaging modalities including magnetic resonance imaging (MRI), ultrasound, and radionucleide scanning, and indirect assessments such as the acute phase protein response.

There are, however, some caveats to the use of investigations in paediatric rheumatology. As a group, the chronic rheumatic diseases are characterized by the relatively non-specific pathological processes of chronic inflammation and autoimmunity. There are few, if any, laboratory tests which yield results pathognomonic of a rheumatic disease. In general, abnormal results from a combination of several investigations have more diagnostic power than those from any one investigation in isolation. Conversely, normal results rarely exclude the diagnosis of a rheumatic disease. For example, normal radiographs, erythrocyte sedimentation rate (ESR) and full blood count, and absent autoantibodies and rheumatoid factor do not exclude juvenile chronic arthritis. Juvenile dermatomyositis (JDM) may occur in the presence of normal muscle enzyme levels and a normal muscle biopsy, and SLE is occasionally ANA negative. For monitoring rheumatic disease also, the results of investigations must be interpreted cautiously. Many tests are too insensitive to reflect changes in disease activity. They may yield results which are too non-specific to be interpretable, or the investigations themselves may be too invasive (or expensive) to be used repetitively.

The chapter is divided into three sections; the first discusses the major investigations used in rheumatic disease, and where possible their sensitivity and specificity. The second deals with the appropriate use of these investigations in the context of common clinical situations, including joint swelling and musculoskeletal pain. The final section outlines suitable investigations for the diagnosis and monitoring of specific rheumatic diseases including juvenile chronic arthritis, systemic lupus erythematosus, and dermatomyositis. The characteristic results of these investigations are also discussed in relation to each disease.

INVESTIGATIONS USED IN PAEDIATRIC RHEUMATOLOGY

The investigations used in paediatric rheumatology can be split into those which directly assess the disease process in affected tissues, and those which indirectly measure the disease through indices of inflammation or consequences of the disease. The first includes tissue biopsy, synovial fluid aspiration, arthroscopy, electrophysiological studies, and various imaging techniques. These investigations are particularly important for defining the nature and extent of disease at diagnosis, and perhaps are less useful for monitoring the disease process. In contrast, indirect measurements of disease, including inflammatory indices, biochemical markers, and immune responses to foreign or self antigens, are generally more useful for monitoring the progress of the illness.

Direct Assessment of the Rheumatic Disease Process

Tissue Biopsy

The histology of most rheumatic disease is characterized by non-specific inflammation. For this reason, and because it is relatively invasive, biopsy is uncommonly used to assess rheumatic disease in children. For example, in most chronic arthritides the findings on synovial biopsy are non-specific and unhelpful in either making a diagnosis or monitoring the course of disease. There are several conditions in which biopsy findings are relatively specific, but even in these situations the combination of clinical features and less invasive laboratory features often renders the biopsy unnecessary. In dermatomyositis for example, muscle biopsy is reserved for patients with atypical disease. However, tissue biopsy has its undoubted uses in rheumatic diseases including SLE (renal biopsy), vasculitis (biopsy of skin, nasal mucosa or other affected organs), amyloidosis (rectal biopsy), Sjögrens syndrome (salivary gland biopsy), tuberculous or foreign body arthritis (synovial biopsy), and the differential diagnosis of acute synovitis (bone marrow biopsy). Advances in immunohistological techniques, such as *in-situ* hybridization and monoclonal antibody staining, may improve the specificity of biopsy analysis in the future.

Synovial Fluid Analysis

Synovial fluid aspiration and microbiological analysis are used to differentiate septic from other forms of arthritis. Most younger children need general anaesthesia for the procedure, and hip aspiration requires fluoroscopic or ultrasonographic guidance. Older children may only need sedation with or without local anaesthesia for large joint aspiration. The diagnosis of septic arthritis requires the demonstration of viable intra-articular infectious agents, by Gram staining, microscopy and culture of synovial fluid or tissue. Septic synovial fluid will often appear purulent to the naked eye, but neither this appearance, its low viscosity, nor its high cellular content are reliable guides to the presence of infection. For example, sterile synovial fluid aspirated from children with chronic arthritis may have a turbid appearance, low viscosity, and leucocyte counts in excess of 20 000 cells/ml, due to

chronic inflammatory changes. In both conditions, the synovial fluid glucose levels will usually be lower than the normal range (the normal range is equivalent to the serum level ± 10%).

There are several other diagnostic advantages to aspiration of the swollen joint. Aspiration of blood raises the possibility of a traumatic effusion, or more rarely coagulation disorders, pigmented villonodular synovitis, or a synovial haemangiomatous malformation. Crystal induced arthropathy is very rarely seen in children, but occasionally gout (diagnosed by polarizing light microscopic demonstration of birefringent uric acid crystals) may occur as a complication of chemotherapy for neoplasia, or as part of an inherited disorder of metabolism such as the Lesch–Nyhan syndrome. In the research laboratory, synovial fluid lymphocyte proliferation assays have implicated bacterial and viral antigens in the pathogenesis of chronic arthritis, and such investigations may have a clinical role in the future.

Arthroscopy

Advances in fibreoptic technology have enabled a reduction in arthroscope dimensions to a size suitable for paediatric use. Visualizing the synovial cavity directly can be a highly specific and sensitive technique for the diagnosis of acute joint dysfunction suspected to be of mechanical origin. In the knee, meniscal tears, the plica syndrome (redundant synovial folds), and intra-articular loose bodies, can be detected and occasionally treated arthroscopically. Arthroscopy also enables the operator to choose a suitable site for synovial tissue biopsy if required. Unfortunately, the technique leaves appreciable scars (e.g. around the patella after knee arthroscopy). Indications include recurrent joint locking or giving way, suspected foreign body synovitis or other rare causes of synovitis such as sarcoidosis. In general it is not indicated for investigation of juvenile chronic arthritis (JCA) unless interference with joint function by intra-articular loose bodies is suspected.

Electrophysiological Studies

The use of electrophysiological studies in paediatric rheumatology is usually confined to the investigation of muscle weakness with electromyography. The electromyogram (EMG) is usually abnormal in juvenile dermatomyositis, but it is not always needed to make the diagnosis. However, if one of the major clinical features, proximal muscle weakness and typical skin rash, are missing, or if the muscle enzymes are not elevated, then an EMG is indicated. The EMG is an uncomfortable procedure, and should be avoided in children unless absolutely necessary. Other electrophysiological studies which are occasionally used include nerve condition studies for investigation of peripheral neuropathy and electroencephalograms (EEG) for assessment of cerebral vasculitis and SLE.

Imaging in the Rheumatic Diseases

Magnetic Resonance Imaging

Magnetic resonance imaging (MRI) is proving to be a very exciting development for the investigation of rheumatic disease. Variations in pulse sequences, field strengths, surface coils and contrast materials allow bone, cartilage, synovium, tendon, muscle, and neural tissue to be visualized using MRI in much greater detail than with other imaging techniques. In general, structural abnormalities are better visualized using T1 weighted images (e.g. bone erosions), whereas changes in tissue composition are better seen using T2 weighted images (e.g. muscle oedema in dermatomyositis). The use of medium bore MRI (rather than whole body machines) and surface coils for limbs and peripheral joints have improved image resolution, and contrast material (e.g. gadolinium) helps to distinguish between inflamed synovium and synovial effusion. At present, there is insufficient knowledge of the sensitivity and specificity of this technique to warrant its use for the diagnosis and monitoring of most paediatric rheumatic conditions. Further disadvantages for investigation of children are its rather frightening noise, the occasional need for intravenous administration of contrast material, and the need to remain stationary for long periods of time. Small children will usually require sedation for the procedure, although the time taken to obtain images is decreasing with increasing sophistication of the machinery. In the future, MRI is likely to be of great use for assessing the progress of arthritis, dermatomyositis, CNS lupus, and large vessel vasculitis.

Plain Radiographs

Radiographs have a role to exclude fractures, local tumours, osteonecrosis, congenital structural abnormalities of bone, and acquired epiphyseal disorders such as slipped upper femoral epiphysis. When used for the investigation of limb dysfunction, radiographs of the affected site are often most useful when compared with a similar field of the unaffected side. Plain radiography has also been used for the assessment of the pericarditis seen in systemic onset JCA, the polyserositis of SLE, and the muscle oedema and subcutaneous calcification of dermatomyositis. It is less useful for monitoring the progress of most rheumatic diseases. Even in JCA most radiographic features occur late in the disease process, and may not be reversible with treatment. These include joint space narrowing due to cartilage erosions and radiographically detectable bone erosions. The advantages of plain radiography are ready availability and brief imaging time.

Diagnostic Ultrasound

Real-time ultrasound is a particularly useful modality for the investigation of hip disease; even small effusions can be visualized and needle placement for joint aspiration facilitated. Other sites of fluid accumulation may also be visualized, such as popliteal cysts (Baker's cysts) and muscle abscesses. Echocardiography is particularly valuable for demonstrating effusions and cardiac function in systemic onset JCA and SLE, and coronary aneurysms in Kawasaki's disease. Recently, the combination of real time and Doppler ultrasound has proved useful in the investigation of large vessel vasculitis, for the estimation of blood vessel wall thickness and compliance. The advantages of ultrasound scanning in children are its non-invasiveness, rapidity and availability. However, obtaining good quality images requires considerable technical skill, as does interpretation of the results.

Radionucleide Scanning

The diagnosis of several clinical situations may be aided by radionucleide scanning (scintigraphy). The technetium99 bone scan is useful in the differential diagnosis of localized and generalized musculoskeletal pain syndromes, as it may highlight areas of inflammation on the blood pool phase, or increased bone metabolism on the delayed bone images. Gallium67 scanning is used less frequently, but may be useful for revealing clinically covert inflammatory foci or neoplastic lesions. Highly specialized single photon emission computed tomography (SPECT) scanning may help to detect inflammatory foci in the central nervous system (e.g. cerebral SLE). Although still a research tool, radiolabelled serum amyloid A protein can now be used for the detection of amyloidosis. Scintigraphy has one obvious disadvantage in children; it requires intravenous access for administration of the radiopharmaceutical.

Computerized Tomography (CT)

CT scanning in musculoskeletal disease is currently the investigation of choice for defining bony lesions such as osteoid osteoma and other bone tumours. In other areas it has been superseded by MRI, even though it is more readily available and cheaper. Disadvantages of its use in young children are similar to MRI; it may need sedation and venous access is required for contrast material. There is now little indication for standard tomography in paediatric rheumatology.

Angiography

Although highly invasive, contrast angiography remains useful for the investigation of vasculitis. Particular uses include defining the extent of Takayasu's arteritis and the coronary artery involvement of Kawasaki's disease. Advances in the techniques of diagnostic ultrasound and MRI may eventually supplant this investigative modality.

Thermography

Thermography is largely a research tool, but it is highly effective for demonstrating differences in the skin temperature overlying normal and abnormal joints/limbs in JCA and the localized idiopathic pain syndromes such as reflex sympathetic dystrophy. The evolution of disease activity in localized scleroderma can be serially documented using this investigation; the degree of inflammation at the leading edges of skin lesions is reflected by changes in the skin temperature. Refinements of the equipment are improving the sensitivity of the technique; at present detectable differences in skin temperature of 0.2°C or less are possible. Unfortunately, thermography is not widely available, and requires expensive equipment, a temperature controlled environment, and considerable technical skill.

Clinical Photography

Serial photographs documenting rheumatic clinical features are often valuable for recording disease progress; for example, the evolution of skin abnormalities in vasculitis and localized scleroderma are perhaps best monitored using photography.

Indirect Investigations for Rheumatic Disease

The Acute Phase Response

Hepatic production of proteins in response to an inflammatory stimulus is known as the acute phase response, and measurement of this response is one of the most frequently used investigations in paediatric rheumatology. C-reactive protein (CRP) levels, the erythrocyte sedimentation rate (ESR), plasma viscosity, and the platelet count are all widely used. If one or more of the acute phase reactants are found to be elevated at the onset of disease, serial measurements may provide a useful guide to the progress of disease. However, the acute phase response is non-specific and is not helpful in pinpointing the cause of acute or chronic inflammation. The sensitivity of these investigations for detecting inflammation is also variable; patients with clinically active inflammatory disease such as JCA, SLE or dermatomyositis, may have normal results.

The response time of the individual acute phase reactants following inflammatory stress is relatively predictable, and may be useful clinically. The CRP changes most rapidly; it is detectably elevated within 6 h of an inflammatory stimulus, peaks by 24–48 h and settles rapidly within 2 days of the resolution of inflammation. Elevation of the ESR is detectable next, peaking after 3–4 days and settling over 7–10 days. The platelet count is the most sluggish of the acute phase reactants. It begins to rise approximately one week after an inflammatory stimulus, and will often remain persistently elevated for several weeks in the absence of inflammation. A factor in deciding which test should be routinely employed for measurement of the acute phase response is the rapidity with which results are available. Simple office-based kits for the determination of CRP are now available which provides a reasonably reliable result within a few minutes of taking the blood, whereas an ESR result takes at least 1 h (the time to perform the investigation). The ESR may be falsely elevated in the presence of anaemia, and falsely low in polycythaemia.

The Blood Film and Full Blood Count (FBC)

Abnormalities on visual inspection of the blood film are critically important in the differential diagnosis of musculoskeletal pain. Leukaemia, other haematological malignancies, and the haemoglobinopathies may all present in this way. Virtually every permutation of blood cell number can be induced by rheumatic disease, including anaemia, leukocytosis, leukopenia, thrombocytosis and thrombocytopenia. Anaemia may be secondary to chronic inflammation, iron deficiency or haemolysis. Leukocytosis may be prominent in systemic-onset JCA, vasculitis, Kawasaki's disease and as a result of corticosteroid therapy. Eosinophilia may be seen in Sjögren's syndrome, fasciitis, vasculitis and sarcoidosis. Thrombocytosis is usually an indicator of an active acute phase response. Cytopenia in the rheumatic diseases is usually an indicator of an autoimmune process such as SLE (mainly lymphopenia), or drug toxicity, especially secondary to slow-acting antirheumatic drugs and cytotoxic therapy.

Autoantibodies and Rheumatoid Factors

Antinuclear antibodies (ANA) are a broad group of auto-antibodies directed against different components within the nucleus of the cell. At least 5% of normal children have detectable circulating ANA, and they may be induced by a wide variety of acute and chronic inflammatory conditions including viral infections, neoplasia, and rheumatic disease. The lack of specificity of ANA limits their diagnostic use, although high titre ANA are found in 95% of SLE patients, and the presence of ANA in subgroups of JCA is a risk factor for the complication of chronic anterior uveitis. In some cases, the particular components of the nucleus to which the ANA are directed can be further defined. SLE is associated with antibodies against specific nuclear antigens including double stranded DNA, Sm, Ro/SSA, and La/SSB.

Other autoantibodies of some clinical use include rheumatoid factors for the subclassification of JCA, ANCA (antineutrophil/cytoplasmic antibodies) in vasculitis, anticardiolipin antibodies in thrombotic episodes mainly associated with SLE, anti-Scl-70 antibodies in progressive systemic sclerosis, anti-centromere antibodies in CREST syndrome (Calcinosis–Raynaud's phenomenon–oesophageal dysfunction–sclerodactyly–telangiectasia), and anti-RNP (ribonucleoprotein) antibodies in mixed connective tissue disease. Juvenile dermatomyositis is associated with ANA rather than the autoantibodies found in adult forms of polymyositis such as anti-Jo-1 and anti-Mi antibodies.

Biochemistry

Serum biochemistry profiles are generally not useful for the diagnosis of rheumatic diseases. One exception is juvenile dermatomyositis, in which muscle enzymes, including creatine phosphokinase, aspartate transaminase and lactate dehydrogenase, are usually elevated. In monitoring rheumatic disease, however, biochemistry does have an important role. Serum electrolytes, urinalysis, liver enzymes, and renal function tests are useful for detecting disease-related complications and drug toxicity. Determination of urinary VMA levels may be useful for the diagnosis of neuroblastoma, which may present with joint swelling.

Serology and other Screens for Infection

Many infectious agents have been implicated clinically in the initiation and exacerbation of various rheumatic diseases, but it is very rare to culture viable micro-organisms from the rheumatic lesions themselves. Evidence supporting the role of infection in these diseases is usually provided by extralesional culture of infectious agents, or the demonstration of specific immune responses to those agents. Investigations include throat swab microscopy and culture, faecal cultures, blood cultures, and antibody titres to infectious agents. In general, useful results from serology are more likely if the suspected infectious agent is specified in the investigation request; asking for "viral and bacterial titres" in a child with arthritis is unlikely to yield useful information. In a few research departments, cell-mediated immune responses to infectious agents can be assessed using lymphocyte proliferation assays.

HLA Typing

Many of the rheumatic diseases appear to have a genetic basis; they are associated with a set of genes on the short arm of the sixth chromosome known as the major histocompatibility complex (MHC). Tissue typing can determine the patients HLA type, which reflects in part the genetic composition of the MHC. This is largely a research tool, but one clinical application is the determination of the HLA-B27 status in children with chronic arthritis, especially those with an older age of disease onset or a family history of ankylosing spondylitis. Such information may increase the accuracy of prognostication and potentially influence the choice of therapy.

Immune Complexes and Complement Consumption

The assessment of parameters of complement consumption (C3, C4 and CH50) and circulating immune complexes have a role in monitoring SLE. They are rarely abnormal on routine testing in other connective tissue diseases, even though some degree of complement activation probably occurs in most. Several products of complement activation and degradation can be measured, but the techniques used are not widely available at present.

Urinalysis

Urinalysis is such a simple screening investigation that it should be performed regularly for every child with rheumatic disease. Most rheumatic diseases have been associated with renal abnormalities, including JCA, SLE, vasculitis, systemic sclerosis and mixed connective tissue disease. Many of the drugs used in rheumatic disease also have the potential for renal side-effects.

INVESTIGATING THE CHILD WITH RHEUMATIC SYMPTOMS AND SIGNS

The aim of this section is to provide a practical sequence of investigations to help the clinician make a diagnosis in a child who presents with rheumatic or musculoskeletal symptoms and signs. Three relatively common clinical situations are dealt with in more detail in this section; acute joint swelling, the limping child/hip pain, and back pain. There is obviously diagnostic overlap between these clinical situations, which is reflected in the investigational plans.

Acute Joint Swelling

Acute joint swelling in a child requires urgent clinical assessment and investigation (Table 18.1). The diagnostic possibilities vary depending on the age of the patient, but three to exclude swiftly irrespective of age are septic arthritis, leukaemia and other haematologic malignancy, and non-accidental injury.

Septic Arthritis and Osteomyelitis

The child with septic arthritis usually appears very unwell, with high fever, a warm, swollen, tender joint and pseudoparalysis (markedly restricted range of joint movement). If these features are absent, then septic arthritis is less likely, but in general any child with an acute monoarthritis should have the joint aspirated urgently and synovial fluid sent for microscopy, Gram stain, and culture. In septic arthritis, approximately 50% of aspirates are positive on Gram stain unless the child has received antibiotics. The synovial fluid white cell count is an unreliable guide to septic arthritis, but antigens from the infecting organism may be detected by specific latex agglutination tests. Eighty percent of children with untreated septic arthritis have culture positive synovial

Table 18.1   Acute joint swelling

Key investigations
Joint aspiration, synovial fluid microscopy and culture
Blood cultures
Plain radiographs of the affected area
Full blood count, visual examination of the blood film
Acute phase response: ESR, CRP, or plasma viscosity

Other investigations which may be useful
Bone scan
Antistreptococcal antibody titres
Culture of faeces, microscopy and culture of CSF
Antinuclear antibody titres
Creatine phosphokinase, aspartate transaminase, lactate dehydrogenase
Immunoglobulin levels
Joint arthroscopy, synovial biopsy
Bone marrow aspiration
Abdominal ultrasound, urinary VMA level

VMA, vanillyl mandelic acid.

aspirates. Cultures from blood or extra-articular sites are positive in the vast majority of the remainder, including CSF (positive in a third of patients < 3 years of age). The organism causing the septic arthritis tends to vary depending on the age of the child; the more common neonatal pathogens include *Staphylococcus aureus*, *Escherichia coli*, *Candida* and *Streptococcus*, from infancy to 2 years of age *Haemophilus influenzae* predominates, and after 2 years *S. aureus* and streptococci are more frequent.

Twenty per cent of children with septic arthritis also have osteomyelitis, but in addition osteomyelitis adjacent to a joint may result in a sympathetic effusion in the absence of intra-articular sepsis. The metaphysis of a long bone is the usual site of sepsis, and can often be best determined by clinical examination revealing a well localized area of pin-point tenderness. The most sensitive screening investigation for an osteomyelitic focus is the bone scan, as plain radiographic changes occur relatively late. As access to MRI scanning becomes easier, it may become the investigation of choice. MRI has been demonstrated to be superior to indium-labelled leukocyte scans for the localization of osteomyelitic foci. Definitive diagnosis requires aspiration of subperiosteal pus, although a bone biopsy is occasionally needed. Rarely, the lesion fails to resolve and chronic osteomyelitis results. Plain radiographs may reveal a radiodense sclerotic sequestrum in the middle of a poorly defined radiolucent lesion.

Repeated major infections suggest that the child may be immunodeficient, and require further investigations as outlined in Chapter 12. However, the child with IgA deficiency may develop joint swelling in the absence of demonstrable sepsis; approximately 5% of children with acute or chronic joint swelling are IgA deficient, compared with 1 in 500 of the normal population.

Leukaemia and other Haematologic Malignancies

Leukaemia may present with musculoskeletal symptoms in up to 40% of cases, and the diagnosis is usually suspected on full blood count (see Chapter 1). Plain radiographs may reveal metaphyseal lucent lines, periosteal elevation and occasionally erosions around the metaphyses; a bone scan may also show increased linear uptake consistent with periostitis. Very rarely, children with musculoskeletal symptoms may have a "preleukaemic" condition. The initial full blood counts and even bone marrow aspirates are normal and the diagnosis of leukaemia may be delayed by months. Neuroblastoma should also be considered in the younger child with one or more swollen joints, and the diagnosis of lymphoma in the older child or adolescent with similar problems.

Non-accidental Injury (see Chapter 11)

The joint swelling of non-accidental injury will usually be due to traumatic haemorrhage, epiphyseal fracture or periostitis. Non-accidental injury may be suggested by a radiographic skeletal survey showing multiple sites of skeletal damage in various stages of resolution, including fracture lines, callus formation, periosteal reaction, and bony deformity. The diagnosis may also be supported by bone scan findings of several sites of increased uptake of radionucleide.

Reactive Arthritis

Reactive arthritis (arthritis occurring within 2 weeks after a defined episode of extra-articular infection) is one of the commonest causes of acute arthritis in children. Investigations to delineate the source of the infection will obviously be guided by the clinical findings. The commonest sites of infection include the gastrointestinal tract and the pharynx; supporting investigations include faecal culture (for *Salmonella*, *Yersinia*, *Campylobacter* or *Shigella*), throat swab microscopy and culture, and anti-streptococcal antibody titres. Post-streptococcal arthritis, in the absence of other features of rheumatic fever, is well recognized, but a small proportion of children with this problem may eventually develop rheumatic carditis.

Lyme arthritis is probably a form of reactive arthritis, as the pathogenic organism *Borrelia burgdorferi* has only rarely been isolated from joint tissues or synovial fluid. The disease may be difficult to diagnose clinically, as one or more of the characteristic clinical features (erythema chronicum migrans, neuropathy, cardiac conduction defects, and episodic arthritis) may be absent. The diagnosis usually relies on the detection of borrelia specific antibodies, but these tests are not widely available. Results also require considerable expertise in interpretation; currently it is unclear which of the borrelia antigens are clinically significant.

Viral agents which have been associated with childhood arthritis and are detectable serologically include influenza, rubella, coxsackie B, herpes (chicken pox, CMV and EBV), mumps, parvovirus B19, hepatitis B, the endemic mosquito transmitted alphaviruses (such as Ross River virus), and adenovirus. Mycoplasma has also been associated with several arthritic patterns, including oligoarthritis and polyarthritis. Elevated serological responses to mycoplasma, and increased cold agglutinins, are important laboratory features.

Osteochondritis

Tender swelling over the tibial tuberosity, particularly in an adolescent boy, usually indicates Osgood Schlatter's disease. Occasionally the clinical features may be mistaken for arthritis of the knee itself. While the clinical observation is usually sufficient to make the diagnosis, a lateral plain radiograph of the knee indicating increased thickness of the soft tissues anterior to the tuberosity may help to confirm it. Apparent radiographic fragmentation of the tuberosity is difficult to differentiate from the normal process of ossification. Anteroposterior radiographs will also help to exclude benign and malignant tumours occurring around the joint.

Bleeding Disorders

Rarely, boys (and even more uncommonly girls) with bleeding diatheses may present initially with a swollen, painful joint. Joint aspiration will reveal the haemarthrosis, and bleeding and clotting studies will confirm the diagnosis (see Chapter 1).

Tumours

Intra-articular and periarticular tumours are rare causes of joint swelling; more common features of these conditions are musculoskeletal pain and limb dysfunction. Plain radiography is the initial investigation of choice, but bone scans, CT scans and MRI all have important roles in delineating the lesion. Osteoid osteoma is a relatively common benign bone tumour, which is usually confined to the diaphyses of the long bones, and occasionally the spine (see Hip Pain, p. 264 and Back Pain, p. 266). Other benign lesions which may present with joint swelling include osteochondroma, chondroma, fibrous cortical defects, bone cysts, and eosinophilic granuloma. Malignant tumours are rare in childhood, but include Ewing's sarcoma and osteosarcoma. Differentiation between the various tumours of the joint usually requires histological examination of a suitable biopsy.

Foreign Body Synovitis, Sarcoidosis, Tuberculous Arthritis

These disparate conditions can be diagnosed by arthroscopy and synovial biopsy. Intense inflammation often surrounds a foreign object such as a rose thorn, and bony destruction may be visible on plain radiographs. Sarcoidosis is characterized by histologic findings of non-caseating granuloma in lymph nodes as well as synovium. Supporting investigations include a chest radiograph showing hilar lymphadenopathy, elevated angiotensin converting enzyme levels, hypercalciuria and a positive Kveim test. Tuberculous arthritis also results in a granulomatous synovitis with prominent giant cells; in almost all cases the tubercle can either be cultured, or visualized as an acid-fast bacillus on Zeihl–Neelsen staining.

Connective Tissue Diseases

The diagnosis and monitoring of the connective tissue diseases will be considered in detail in the following section. Several may present with acute joint swelling, including juvenile chronic arthritis, systemic lupus erythematosus, dermatomyositis, vasculitis and mixed connective tissue disease.

Localized Idiopathic Musculoskeletal Pain Syndrome

Dramatic localized musculoskeletal pain without an apparent cause is not uncommon in children. Occasionally the affected area will be held fixed in a bizarre posture and become swollen and purplish in appearance; a condition known as reflex sympathetic dystrophy. The syndrome is usually associated with stress stemming from learning difficulties, the pressure of overachievement, or occasionally physical or mental abuse. Investigations are usually directed at excluding underlying organic pathology, but there is a risk that continued testing to exclude very rare diagnoses may actually perpetuate the stress and resultant pathology. Important investigations include plain radiographs of the affected area, a bone scan, a full blood count and a measure of the acute phase response. Plain X-rays may demonstrate patchy osteopenia, and the bone scan may show either increased or decreased uptake of radionucleide. The full blood count and acute phase proteins should be normal.

The Child with Hip Pain or Limping in the Absence of Joint Swelling

Hip pain and limping secondary to hip disease are common childhood complaints. Investigations have a very important role to play in the differential diagnosis of these symptoms, as the hip joint is difficult to assess clinically (Table 18.2). Most of the investigations used to

Table 18.2   Hip pain or limping without joint swelling

Key investigations
Ultrasound examination of the hips
Joint aspiration, synovial fluid microscopy and culture
Plain radiographs (including lateral views) or MRI
Bone scan, with pin-hole views of the hips
Full blood count, visual examination of the blood film
Acute phase response: ESR, CRP, or plasma viscosity

Other investigations which may be useful
Plain radiographs or MRI of the spine and lower limbs
Abdominal ultrasound examination
CT scanogram for leg length discrepancy

assess the swollen joint are also applicable to the hip, but the interpretation of the results requires some knowledge of the range of hip pathology.

Septic Arthritis and Osteomyelitis

The hip is second only to the knee as the most frequent site of joint sepsis; it is of particular importance in neonates. The diagnosis of the condition has been discussed in detail in the previous section, but for the hip in particular, greater emphasis is placed on ultrasound examination for observing increased synovial fluid volume and facilitating needle placement for joint aspiration. Raised intra-articular pressure is likely to compromise the vascular supply to the femoral head, and avascular necrosis is a well-recognized consequence of sepsis. Plain radiographs of the hip are useful for detecting this complication (see below).

Transient Synovitis of the Hip (Irritable Hip)

This self-limited condition of childhood may represent a form of reactive arthritis, although it has not been strongly linked to any specific infectious agent. The child usually appears well apart from mild fever and limitation of hip movement at the extremes of joint range. The hip ultrasound often demonstrates increased synovial fluid volume, a feature which may also be suspected from widening of the affected joint space on plain radiography. The full blood count is usually normal but measures of acute phase proteins may be elevated. The frequency of avascular necrosis of the femoral head following irritable hip is increased, occurring in approximately 2% of cases.

Avascular Necrosis of the Femoral Head (Perthes Disease)

Children on corticosteroids and pre-adolescent boys are most at risk for avascular necrosis of the femoral head, a disease which is usually confined to the 5–10 year age group. MRI is probably the most sensitive investigation, demonstrating subchondral changes well before the characteristic radiographic findings of increased head density, fragmentation and reduced height secondary to subchondral fracture. Late features include remodelling and flattening of the ossifying femoral head. The bone scan is likely to show reduced radionucleide uptake by the affected head, which may be best visualized using pinhole views.

Slipped Upper (Capital) Femoral Epiphysis

Slipped upper femoral epiphysis is more frequent in obese children and pre-adolescent boys. Almost all cases are seen in young people between the ages of 10 and 20 years. Plain radiographs are the investigation of choice; the frog-leg lateral view is more sensitive than routine anteroposterior views for detecting early slipping. The upper femoral epiphysis is displaced posteriorly and inferiorly, and avascular necrosis may be an added complication. The condition is bilateral in 25% of cases.

Mechanical Disorders: Hypermobility and Leg Length Discrepancy

There are no specific investigations for hypermobility (Table 18.3), which is one of the more common causes of paediatric hip pain. Occasionally, hypermobile joints are associated with generalized musculoskeletal pain, and rarely may be part of an inherited abnormality of connective tissue such as Marfan's syndrome or Ehlers–Danlos syndrome. In Marfan's syndrome, echocardiography may reveal increased diameter of the aortic root, a change which may precede dissecting aneurysm of the aorta.

A leg length discrepancy from whatever cause may result in hip pain. One of the best methods for quantifying the discrepancy is the "CT scanogram" where a single longitudinal radiographic "slice" of the femora and tibiae is performed and measured accurately. Plain radiographs may substitute for this technique, but usually result in a greater exposure to radiation.

Osteoid Osteoma and Other Tumours

The greater trochanter and neck of femur are among the commonest sites for the benign condition of osteoid

Table 18.3 The diagnosis of hypermobility in children

Generalized hypermobility
Three or more of:
(a) Passive hyperextension of the fingers so that they lie parallel to the forearms (with the wrists extended maximally)
(b) Passive apposition of the thumbs to touch the surface of the forearms (with the wrists flexed maximally)
(c) Hyperextension of the elbows > 10°
(d) Hyperextension of the knees > 10°
(e) Flexion of the trunk with the knees straight until the palms of the hands touch the floor

Localized hypermobility
Any of the above, or either of:
(a) Pes planus
(b) Ankle valgus

Note: the range of movement of joints varies with age; young school age children tend to be more mobile than adolescents. The diagnosis of hypermobility in prepubertal patients should be made with caution.

osteoma. Lesions in these areas will usually result in nocturnal leg or hip pain, which may be relieved dramatically by aspirin. The bone scan is the most sensitive investigation for the early detection of osteoid osteoma, demonstrating a well-localized area of increased technitium uptake. Plain radiographs may be normal initially, but will eventually show a radiolucent nidus surrounded by a sclerotic margin. There may be some adjacent periosteal reaction. It is possible that MRI will eventually prove to be a more sensitive technique for detecting this and other tumours.

Ewing's sarcoma is a highly malignant bone tumour occasionally found in the diaphysis of the femur. Plain radiographs demonstrate a lytic lesion lying in the medullary cavity, lacking the sclerotic margin of the osteoid osteoma, and associated with marked periosteal reaction (onion skinning). Metastatic bone disease may also present with hip pain, and neuroblastoma is the most common primary lesion. The bone scan is the most sensitive technique for detecting the multiple areas of increased uptake associated with this condition.

Referred Pain (Intra-abdominal or Back Pathology)

The differential diagnosis of hip disease is made more difficult by the deep anatomical placement of the hip, and its relative proximity to the spine, knee, pelvis and abdomen. In unusual or recalcitrant cases which remain undiagnosed, other sites of pathology should be sought. Sacroiliac joint disease, including osteomyelitis and chronic inflammation may result in pain referred to the hip. This is best investigated with CT scans or MRI, although even these techniques are not infallible. Unsuspected intra-abdominal abscess or tumour, renal pathology or pelvic pathology giving rise to hip pain may be revealed by an abdominal ultrasound or gallium-labelled white cell scan. Localized bony lesions of the spine are discussed in the following section.

Chronic Inflammatory Disease

Isolated hip pain or disease is a surprisingly rare presenting complaint in children who develop chronic arthritis. In almost all cases of JCA affecting the hip initially, there will be other clinical evidence of synovitis. During the course of JCA, the hips can undoubtedly be a major cause of disability. The diagnosis of ankylosing spondylitis, or the precursor disease "seronegative enthesopathy and arthropathy" (SEA syndrome) should be considered in patients who present during late childhood or adolescence. An important clinical feature of the SEA syndrome is enthesitis, defined as tenderness over the bony insertions of tendon, muscle or joint capsule. A bone scan may indicate increased uptake in affected areas, which may include the greater trochanter and give rise to complaints of hip pain. Other investigations for JCA are considered in a following section.

The Differential Diagnosis of Back Pain

In contrast to adults, chronic back pain is uncommon in children, and often associated with definable pathology (Table 18.4). The back itself is composed of a complex series of potentially painful synovial joints (the posterior apophyseal joints) which are obviously not as accessible to clinical examination as peripheral joints. Other structures which may give rise to pain include the periosteum of the vertebrae, the intervertebral disks, the paravertebral musculature and soft tissues, the sacroiliac joints and the spinal cord and nerve roots. The back is a common site of referred pain, particularly from retroperitoneal organs and posterior thoracic structures. In addition, pain resulting from back pathology may be referred to the abdomen, chest, limbs or head, depending on the level of the lesion.

Discitis

The most frequent cause of back pain in young children is discitis. The child will often have been unwell with a preceding upper respiratory tract infection, and usually presents with fever and difficulty walking as well as back pain. The child may sit in the typical tripod position with the back held in extension and the arms thrust backwards onto the bed. Interesting physical signs include the relief of the back pain if the child is picked up and supported

Table 18.4   Back pain

Key investigations
MRI
Plain radiographs: anteroposterior and lateral views
Bone scan
Full blood count, visual examination of the blood film
Acute phase response: ESR, CRP, or plasma viscosity
Lumbar puncture and CSF for Gram stain, culture,
    protein and sugar levels

Other investigations which may be useful
CT scan with contrast myelography
Abdominal ultrasound
Ultrasound examination of the hips
Sacroiliac joint CT scanning
HLA B27 determination

---

under the axillae, and the finding of localized tenderness in the lumbar region. The most useful investigation is the bone scan, indicating increased uptake into the vertebral bodies on either side of the inflamed lumbar (in over 90% of cases) intervertebral disk. The ESR or other estimation of the acute phase response is usually elevated. The aetiology of discitis is thought to be infectious, but blood cultures are usually negative and a disk biopsy unnecessary. Not uncommonly the affected disk becomes visibly narrower on plain radiography during the recovery phase, and this may be the explanation for ongoing back pain.

Osteomyelitis of the Vertebral Body and Sacroiliac Joint Sepsis

Infection of a vertebral body or a sacroiliac joint is rare. The clinical features of the former are similar to discitis, except the child is usually markedly febrile and appears toxic. The latter may present with indolent back pain. The investigation likely to show the earliest abnormalities is the bone scan, with increased uptake in the inflamed site. Visible destruction of either is usually a late radiographic feature, and the definitive diagnosis requires culture of the organism from a subperiosteal aspirate, sacroiliac joint aspirate, or blood cultures. Occasionally open bone biopsy will be required. The organisms most commonly cultured include *Streptococcus*, *Staphylococcus*, and *Haemophilus*.

Osteochondritis (Scheuermann's Disease)

Back pain associated with a dorsal kyphosis is the most common clinical manifestation of Scheuermann's disease. Most patients are in their mid-adolescent years; there is a slight female preponderance. The diagnosis is made on inspection of a lateral radiograph of the kyphosis, which usually reveals anterior wedging of 2–3 adjacent vertebral bodies accompanied by irregularity of the anterior vertebral margin. The pathology is unknown, but it appears to involve a disturbance of ossification of the cartilagenous vertebral end-plates.

Histiocytosis and Osteoid Osteoma

Tumours of the spinal column, spinal cord or nerve roots are painful but rare conditions in children. Osteoid osteoma may affect the vertebral facets, pedicles or spinous processes, osteoblastoma may involve the vertebral arch, and eosinophilic granuloma more often affects the vertebral bodies. Although these lesions may be visualized on bone scans or plain radiographs, CT or MRI scanning is usually required, together with bone biopsy, for accurate diagnosis of the nature and extent of the disease.

Spondylolysis, Spondylolisthesis, Intervertebral Disc Herniation and Diastematomyelia

Both congenital spondylolysis (a defect in the pars inter-articularis) and spondylolisthesis (spondylolysis with the upper vertebral body displaced forward) may lead to low back pain particularly in adolescents. The characteristic feature of spondylolysis on lateral plain radiographs is a "Scottie dog with a broken neck" appearance; the ears are formed by the posterior facets, and the neck by the pars interarticularis. Intervertebral disc herniation is very rare in children. Valsalva manoeuvres such as coughing, sneezing, or straining at stool may aggravate the symptoms, and the diagnosis may be made by MRI of the affected area. The child with progressive back pain and any superficial markings suggestive of intraspinal pathology (skin dimpling, hairy naevus, spinal sinus) should have an MRI examination to rule out diastematomyelia.

Fibromyalgia and Hypermobility

There are no investigations which confirm fibromyalgia, the diagnosis resting instead on the clinical features of generalized idiopathic musculoskeletal pain, a history of stress, and multiple soft tissue trigger points. The bone scan is probably the best screening investigation to rule out organic pathology. Increased joint laxity (hypermobility) of the lower limbs is occasionally associated with back pain in the presence or absence of fibromyalgia.

Juvenile Ankylosing Spondylitis, Enthesitis and Sacroiliitis

Like the hip, it is rare for chronic arthritis to present initially with back pain. The sacroiliitis of ankylosing spondylitis is very unusual in children, but a peripheral arthritis in association with enthesitis, especially in older boys, may precede this disease. The symptoms may be reproduced by hyperextension of the spine, which places the posterior facet joints (the only spinal joints which are synovial in nature) under stress. Plain radiographs of the sacroiliac joints may reveal lateral border sclerosis, which is likely to be the first investigational abnormality found. Unfortunately, interpretation of sacroiliac radiographs is fraught with difficulty before the SI joints fuse, and even CT scans and MRI may be too insensitive. Hopefully, advances in MRI technology will redress this unsatisfactory state of affairs.

INVESTIGATIONS IN THE DIAGNOSIS AND MONITORING OF PAEDIATRIC RHEUMATIC DISEASE

Juvenile Chronic Arthritis

The diagnosis of juvenile chronic arthritis (JCA) rests on two factors: the presence of persistent peripheral joint swelling for at least 3 months, and the exclusion of other diseases. In joints such as the hip, spine, or shoulder in which swelling is difficult to ascertain clinically, the presence of joint pain, restricted joint range of movement, and muscle spasm around the joint is sufficient to make the diagnosis of arthritis. The investigations which are used to rule out other diseases have been discussed under the differential diagnosis of joint swelling. Once the diagnosis of JCA is made, the disease is subclassified on the basis of disease features during the first 6 months of disease; oligoarticular onset (≤ 4 joints involved), polyarticular onset (> 4 joints involved), and systemic onset (with prominent extra-articular manifestations such as daily spiking fever, an evanescent, salmon-pink rash, lymphadenopathy, organomegaly, and serositis). Within the oligoarticular onset group there are at least two further subgroups including patients with juvenile psoriatic arthritis, and the spondyloarthropathies; usually boys with an older age at onset of arthritis. Unfortunately, there are no laboratory results which are pathognomonic of JCA, but several which may help to confirm the presence of inflammation, document the extent and severity of the disease, and monitor the disease process (Table 18.5).

Table 18.5   Juvenile chronic arthritis

Initial investigations
Exclude other diseases (see previous sections)
Plain radiographs of the affected joints
Acute phase response: ESR, CRP, or plasma viscosity
Haematology
Antinuclear antibodies: test and retest 6 months apart
Rheumatoid factor (polyarticular JCA only): test and
   confirm as for ANA
HLA B27 in late onset JCA (> 6 years of age)

Monitoring disease progress
Slit lamp biomicroscopy: 3–6 monthly in high risk cases
Full blood count: 3–6 monthly*
Acute phase response: 3–6 monthly
Urinalysis: 6 monthly*
Serum electrolytes, liver function tests: 6 monthly*
Radiographs (possibly MRI) of affected joints 1–2 yearly
Therapeutic drug level monitoring

*Monthly if slow-acting antirheumatic drugs are used.

Acute Phase Response

Measures of the acute phase response are abnormally elevated in 60–70% of JCA patients at diagnosis. C-reactive protein levels and the ESR (Westergren method) are usually moderately increased (CRP 15–60 mg/l, NR < 6, ESR 25–80 mm, 1st hour NR < 20); very high levels are seen in polyarthritis, systemic onset JCA, and the arthritis of inflammatory bowel disease. The ESR is also varied with the degree of anaemia; the more severe the anaemia, the greater the ESR.

If elevated initially, either the ESR or the CRP may be useful for monitoring the progress of the disease and response to treatment. The decision about which investigation to use should be based on local availability and rapidity of reporting, but the CRP has some advantages; it has greater sensitivity to change than the ESR, and requires a smaller volume blood sample (finger prick). Persistent elevation of the acute phase proteins and inadequate clinical response to non-steroidal anti-inflammatory medication are indications for considering the addition of slow-acting antirheumatic drugs to the therapeutic regimen. The platelet count is occasionally the only haematologic indication of inflammation (thrombocytosis of $> 1000 \times 10^9/l$ is not uncommon), but is quite insensitive to change. These parameters are usually monitored 3–6 monthly. In the child whose arthritis has settled clinically, normalcy of the acute phase response is an indication for reducing or withdrawing treatment.

Radiography and MRI

MRI is more sensitive than plain radiography, and is likely to become one of the investigations of choice for the differential diagnosis and monitoring of JCA. Joint effusions and proliferative synovitis are easily visualized; inflamed synovium is best imaged with intravenous contrast material (gadolinium). Cartilage erosions can be documented and total cartilage volume quantified. Accurate assessment of these parameters is likely to provide a guide to therapeutic decision-making in the future.

However, until MRI becomes more accessible and less costly, plain radiographs will continue to have an important role. The key radiographic "end-point" is the presence of bony erosions of the joints, but this is rarely seen until after 2 years of persistent arthritis and is preceded by several other features. Soft tissue swelling around the joint, joint space widening and the displacement of fat lines secondary to joint effusion are the first changes to be observed. These are followed within the first few months by periarticular osteoporosis, visible when at least 30% of

bone mineral density has been lost. Occasionally, periosteal new bone formation is seen, especially if digital tenosynovitis is present, and may result in abnormally wide phalanges. A reduction in cartilage volume due to erosion is manifest as joint space narrowing, but is a relatively late change (after 6 months to a year of persistent inflammation). Joint space is relatively easily documented in unilateral joint disease by comparison with the unaffected opposite joint. For example, the wrist joint space is best observed by comparing the distance from the bases of the metacarpals to the distal end of the radius; this represents a summation of carpal cartilage loss. Disturbances of limb growth can be documented radiographically; lower limb large joint involvement (especially the knee) before the age of nine years is likely to lead to overgrowth of the limb, whereas after this age, and for the digits, premature epiphyseal fusion and shortening is more often seen. Horizontal growth arrest lines are often visible even in the absence of frank growth disturbance, especially around the knees and wrists.

In many cases of JCA, bony erosive joint disease is not apparent. Subchondral cyst formation may precede frank erosions, but the interpretation of joint radiographs in children is complicated by the fluffy appearance of the maturing normal epiphyses. In addition to the search for marginal joint erosions, specific sites which should be carefully inspected include the tibial spines, ulnar styloid processes, bases of the metacarpal and metatarsal bones, and carpal bones. Ankylosis of the posterior elements of the cervical spine may occur, and is obviously a contra-indication to overvigorous neck physiotherapy! Plain radiographs of the affected joints are usually repeated on a 1–2 yearly basis to assess disease progression. Rarely, resolution of erosions can be documented radiographically.

Haematology

The most common abnormalities observed in JCA are anaemia and thrombocytosis. The anaemia is usually secondary to chronic inflammation, and begins with a normocytic, normochromic pattern. With persistent disease a microcytic hypochromic pattern is occasionally seen, and in these cases a low or low–normal serum ferritin level may suggest iron deficiency (ferritin is an acute phase protein and usually mirrors the extent of inflammation). Marked anaemia (7–10 mg/dl) and leukocytosis (polymorphonuclear) are often prominent features of systemic onset JCA.

Autoimmunity, Slit-lamp Biomicroscopy

Antinuclear antibodies (ANA) are found in 30–80% of early onset (< 6 years) oligoarticular JCA, although they may be found in other subgroups as well. The actual autoantigen against which ANA are directed is unknown; a homogeneous nuclear staining pattern is usually observed on indirect immunofluorescence which is partially accounted for by anti-histone antibodies. The presence of ANA should be confirmed by testing on at least two occasions about 6 months apart, as ANA are expressed transiently in 5% of normal children and many other acute or chronic inflammatory paediatric diseases. Its importance in JCA lies in its association with chronic iridocyclitis, a clinically silent and potentially blinding complication. All children with JCA should have at least one technically satisfactory slit lamp ocular examination, and those at sufficient risk of chronic iridocyclitis (all except ANA negative systemic onset JCA, rheumatoid factor positive JCA, or spondyloarthritic forms) should be enrolled in an ongoing screening programme (3–6 monthly). (See Table 17.10, p. 256.)

Rheumatoid factors (IgM-anti IgG antibodies) are commonly associated with rheumatoid arthritis in adults, but testing for these in children is often inappropriately performed. Rheumatoid factor tests should not be used to screen for JCA, being neither sensitive (it is absent in over 90% of chronic childhood arthritis) nor specific (it may be present in many acute viral and bacterial illnesses, as well as chronic lung, liver and other inflammatory diseases). It is useful to determine rheumatoid factor *after* a diagnosis of polyarticular JCA has been made; the persistent presence of this autoantibody is associated with a poor prognosis compared with rheumatoid factor negative JCA. Investigations for other rheumatoid factors (IgG, IgA, "hidden" IgM) are performed in research institutions, but have not yet proved to be clinically useful.

HLA Typing

The genetic basis of juvenile chronic arthritis is not fully understood, and in most cases HLA typing has little clinical relevance. One possible exception is children with a spondyloarthropathy or clinical features which suggest this disease pattern (older age of onset, male, presence of enthesitis). In these children, determining the HLA-B27 status may have therapeutic implications; B27 positive individuals have a greater risk of developing ankylosing spondylitis during adult life and should be instructed about back exercises and care.

Systemic Lupus Erythematosus

Paediatric systemic lupus erythematosus (SLE) usually presents during the adolescent years (Table 18.6). It is a

Table 18.6 Systemic lupus erythematosus

Diagnosis
Autoantibodies: ANA, anti-DNA, -Sm, -Ro/SSA, -La/SSB, -cardiolipin
Complement consumption: C3, C4, CH50, circulating immune complexes
Haematology: full blood count
Acute-phase response: ESR and CRP
Renal studies
Investigation of affected organ systems as indicated

Monitoring disease progress
Autoantibody titres
Full blood count
Acute phase response: ESR and CRP
Complement consumption
Serum electrolytes, liver function tests
Urinalysis

disease of protean manifestations, but most common are non-specific constitutional symptoms (lethargy, fever, weight loss), nephritis, arthritis, photosensitive skin rash, hepatomegaly, splenomegaly, lymphadenopathy, and anaemia.

Autoantibodies

Autoantibody formation is the hallmark of SLE. Antinuclear antibodies (ANA) are sensitive markers for the disease (elevated in 95% of SLE patients), although they lack specificity, as they are found in normal children and those with other acute and chronic inflammatory conditions. Determining the antigenic specificities of the ANA often yields information which is more useful for the diagnosis and monitoring of SLE. The nucleus contains many potential antigens, including native (double-stranded) DNA, histones (the structural proteins which package DNA), and various "extractable" nuclear antigens (ENA) (these can be eluted from nuclear material). Extractable nuclear antigens include Sm, Ro (identical to SSA), La (identical to SSB), and RNP; the odd system of nomenclature relates either to the first two letters of the names of the patients in whom the antigens were originally described (Sm: Smith), the disease with which the antigens were first associated (SSA: Sjogren's syndrome associated A antigens), or the actual name of the antigen (RNP: ribonucleoprotein).

Anti double-stranded DNA antibodies (antinative DNA) are found in the majority of paediatric lupus patients, especially those with active nephritis, and only rarely in other diseases. Anti-Sm is also virtually specific for SLE but is not sensitive, being found in only 40% of cases; in these patients it correlates with CNS disease. The autoantibody titres in any individual patient may be very useful for disease monitoring. Initial aggressive drug therapy can be aimed not only at improving the patient's clinical state, but also at normalizing the autoantibody titres. Occasionally, rising autoantibody titres may precede a flare in clinical disease activity, and may warrant reinstitution of more aggressive treatment. For these reasons, the patient's autoantibody status is usually monitored at each clinic visit.

The neonatal lupus syndrome is a rare but interesting disease associated with transplacental passage of antibodies to Ro/SSA and La/SSB. The infant usually presents with at least one of: cardiac conduction defect (usually complete heart block), photosensitive rash, or haematological abnormalities (thrombocytopenia, haemolytic anaemia, lymphopenia). Apart from the cardiac conduction defects which are permanent, the clinical manifestations of the syndrome are transient (<6 months) in keeping with the natural half-life of maternal antibodies in the neonatal circulation. In about half of cases, the mother does not complain of connective tissue disease symptoms.

There are many other autoantibodies associated with SLE, including anticardiolipin antibodies, which may predict thrombotic events and recurrent abortion, anti-neutrophil cytoplasmic antibodies associated with vasculitis, antihistone antibodies found in drug-induced lupus, and rheumatoid factors. Tissue autoantibodies, such as antithyroid antibodies, are also common.

Complement

Complement levels are often useful for monitoring SLE, especially when considered in association with auto-antibody titres. C4 levels are most frequently depressed, either through immune complex mediated activation of the classical complement pathway, or rarely because of an inherited complement component deficiency (C2 or C4). C3 levels may also be low, although less commonly than C4. The total haemolytic complement level is reflected by the CH_{50}; this is usually below the normal range. Investigations to quantify complement component degradation products, such as C3d and C3e, are research tools at present but appear to be more sensitive than standard tests and may become more widely available in the future.

Circulating immune complexes are thought to play an important role in the disease pathogenesis. They may be measured by various laboratory techniques; such assays are clinically useful for monitoring disease activity especially if other investigations are equivocal. The deposition of immune complexes, or the formation of in situ immune complexes, can be demonstrated by renal biopsy. Rarely, the lupus band test (from a biopsy of non-exposed, non-lesional skin) is useful for the diagnosis of atypical lupus.

Haematology

Abnormalities of the full blood count are very commonly found in SLE. Anaemia is a feature in approximately 50% of patients, and is caused by either chronic inflammation, iron deficiency or haemolysis. Testing for IgG anti-red-cell complement fixing antibodies (Coombs' antibodies) and serum ferritin levels (which are likely to be low or low–normal in iron deficiency) may help to ascertain the cause. Leukopenia (white blood cell counts of $<4.5 \times 10^9/l$) and more specifically lymphopenia (lymphocyte count $<1.5 \times 10^9/l$) is noted in two-thirds of patients. Occasionally, children with idiopathic thrombocytopenic purpura may develop SLE; thrombocytopenia (platelet count $<150 \times 10^9/l$) is an important manifestation of lupus, although it is rarely severe enough to warrant platelet transfusion. Assays for factor VIII related antigen, a marker of endothelial cell damage which is raised in vasculitis, may be useful for monitoring this complication.

Acute Phase Response

Measurement of both ESR and CRP should be recorded at the time of diagnosis of lupus. The ESR is usually raised, but paradoxically the CRP may be normal unless there is an intercurrent infection; this discrepancy may be useful for monitoring lupus.

Renal Investigations: Urinalysis, Renal Function Tests, Renal Biopsy

Nephritis is a major cause of morbidity and mortality in children with SLE, and it is present at diagnosis in 70% of patients. The urinary sediment, urinary protein/creatinine ratio (normal <20), and serum urea and creatinine levels should be tested at every clinic visit. A renal biopsy is usually only indicated if there are persistent abnormalities in at least one of these screening investigations. The classification of renal histopathology is difficult and largely beyond the scope of this chapter. Clinically significant glomerulonephritis is either proliferative (focal, segmental or diffuse) or membranous (characterized by thickened capillary walls).

CNS Investigations: CSF, MRI, SPECT Scan and EEG

The management of cerebral lupus is one of the most challenging areas of paediatric rheumatology. The child with this complication is usually very unwell, and warrants virtually every available CNS investigation, even though there are no pathognomonic test results, and considerable controversy currently surrounds which tests are the most sensitive and specific. Cerebrospinal fluid microscropy and culture to exclude infection should be undertaken on all patients in whom the diagnosis is suspected; CSF electrophoresis may reveal oligoclonal bands consistent with lupus-associated local immunoglobulin production. The electroencephalogram is usually abnormal, showing either a diffuse increase in slow waves, or focal abnormalities. If readily available, MRI is probably more sensitive for documenting lesions than the CT scan. Cerebral vasculitis is suggested by the findings of multiple areas of cerebral oedema and infarction. Radionucleide scanning (SPECT scan) is also reported to be very sensitive, but is not widely available.

Juvenile Dermatomyositis

Juvenile dermatomyositis can often be diagnosed on clinical grounds alone, but investigations are important to help make the diagnosis if the presenting features are atypical, and for monitoring disease progress (Table 18.7). The underlying pathology is a small vessel vasculitis which has a predilection for muscle and skin. Classical clinical features include a progressive proximal myopathy which often affects the neck and abdominal flexor muscle groups first and most severely, and a characteristic dermatitis. The dermatological manifestations may begin with periorbital, facial and less commonly peripheral oedema. Typical dermatitis includes a violaceous heliotrope of the upper eyelids and symmetrical erythematous scaling plaques over the dorsal surfaces of the elbows, small joints of the hands and anterior surfaces of the knees. Important acute compli-

Table 18.7   Juvenile dermatomyositis

Diagnosis
Muscle enzymes: CPK, AST, LDH
Electromyography
Muscle biopsy
Magnetic resonance imaging
Haematology and the acute phase response
Pulmonary function tests as indicated
Oesophageal and swallowing studies as indicated

Monitoring disease progress
Muscle enzymes: CK, AST, LDH
Spirometry/pulmonary function tests
Haematology and acute phase response
MRI
Radiography for calcinosis

cations include respiratory muscle weakness, respiratory failure, and disorders of swallowing leading to aspiration. Joint contractures and calcinosis are later complications.

Muscle Enzymes

Characteristically the creatine phosphokinase (CPK) (in particular the MB isoenzyme) is increased above the normal range by a factor of 10–20 in acute dermatomyositis. Elevations of aspartate transaminase (AST) and lactate dehydrogenase (LDH), two less specific muscle-associated enzymes, are often less marked. Rarely, none of the muscle enzymes are increased at any stage during the disease. However, in most clinical situations, serial monitoring of the enzymes is the most valuable laboratory guide to disease activity, and should be checked at each clinic visit. Increases in muscle enzymes may precede worsening disease. However, the interpretation of such a finding in a patient who is clinically improving is confused by the fact that increasing vigorous exercise is associated with transient rises in enzyme levels.

Electromyography

The electromyograph (EMG) is only necessary if the diagnosis of the disease is in doubt. The changes are those of myopathy and denervation; typically polyphasic, low amplitude, short duration action potentials (myopathy) are found, together with irregular sharp waves and fibrillations (denervation). The EMG is of doubtful use in monitoring the progress of the disease. It is an uncomfortable procedure for which smaller children may require sedation. Care should be taken to avoid potential muscle biopsy sites when obtaining the EMG, as it may induce artefactual changes.

MRI

MRI may have an important role in the diagnosis and monitoring of JDM. Muscle oedema can be visualized as increased signal using T2 weighted images, and quantified using muscle/fat signal ratios. Changes seen on serial imaging appear to directly reflect alterations in disease activity. Perhaps the most important role for MRI at present is in the selection of potential sites for muscle biopsy; images often show patchy disease.

Muscle Biopsy

The muscle biopsy is usually only indicated if the presenting features of the patient are atypical. It has the advantages of excluding other causes of myopathy, and perhaps providing prognostic information, but the disadvantage of needing to be performed under a general anaesthetic, and postoperative scarring. The use of needle muscle biopsy may circumvent these problems. MRI probably has a role in selecting a site for biopsy; usually the quadriceps muscle is selected. Typical changes include perifascicular group atrophy and evidence of small vessel and capillary vasculitis. There is often variation in muscle fibre size due to fibre degeneration and regeneration. Some degree of inflammatory cell infiltrate is usually seen. Electron microscopy shows sarcomeric disruption and myofibril degeneration.

Pulmonary Function Tests

Spirometry or more formal pulmonary function tests may be abnormal in children with JDM due to respiratory muscle weakness. For the acutely unwell child, serial spirometry may provide a more objective assessment of muscle weakness than clinical muscle strength testing of the limbs.

The Diagnosis of other Paediatric Rheumatic Diseases

Vasculitis

Vasculitis is not an uncommon paediatric pathology; Henoch Schöenlein Purpura, Kawasaki's disease, SLE, dermatomyositis, postviral vasculitis, as well as the rarer classical vasculitides (Wegener's, Churg–Strauss, Takayasu's arteritis) are all linked by underlying inflammation of the blood vessels. The diagnosis of the commoner diseases is usually based on clinical features, but the rarer conditions almost invariably require tissue biopsy. The association of antineutrophil cytoplasmic antibodies (ANCA) with vasculitis is now well recognized, although their role in diagnosis and monitoring requires elucidation. For vasculitis involving larger vessels, the combination of real time and Doppler ultrasound is a valuable technique which may eliminate the need for angiography. Laboratory monitoring of this group of diseases is dependent on the site and extent of organ system involvement, but in most cases measures of the acute phase response will provide an indication of disease activity, as will factor-VIII-related antigen levels.

Scleroderma

Most scleroderma in children is localized in nature; in these cases the main object of laboratory investigation is to rule out systemic involvement. Skin biopsy is rarely required for the diagnosis or monitoring of these conditions. The presence of antinuclear antibodies, particularly of the anti-Scl 70 specificity, is found in progressive systemic sclerosis. Anticentromere antibodies are associated with the CREST syndrome. Serial pulmonary function tests, which typically reveal reduced vital capacity and slowed gas diffusion, may be useful for monitoring progressive systemic disease.

The monitoring of the localized forms of scleroderma (linear scleroderma and morphea) is perhaps best accomplished with serial clinical photographs of the affected sites. Thermography is a research investigation which helps to quantify the degree of inflammation at the leading edge of the lesions. The findings may influence therapeutic decision making; for example, intravenous corticosteroids may be helpful to damp down prominent leading edge inflammation.

Mixed Connective Tissue Disease

The clinical features of this group of conditions are highly variable, but usually elements of at least two of chronic arthritis, SLE, dermatomyositis and scleroderma are present. One of the most characteristic clinical features, although not specific for the disease, is the presence of extensor digital tendon nodules; the dorsal surfaces of the hands are particularly affected. Investigations are tailored to the most prominent disease features, and broadly follow the guidelines given in the preceding sections. The autoantibody most closely linked with mixed connective tissue disease is ANA, particularly of the anti-RNP specificity.

REFERENCES

Cassidy JT, Petty RE (1990) *Textbook of Pediatric Rheumatology*, 2nd edn. Churchill Livingstone, New York.

Jacobs JC (1992) *Pediatric Rheumatology for the Practitioner*, 2nd edn. Springer-Verlag, New York.

Rosenberg AM (1993) Investigations in children with chronic arthritis. In: Southwood TR, Malleson PN (eds) *Chronic Arthritis in Children and Adolescents*. Baillière Tindall, London.

19
Genetic Disorders

P A Farndon

THE IMPORTANCE OF GENETIC DISEASES

The majority of genetic diseases are individually rare but they contribute substantially to childhood mortality and morbidity. About 40% of UK childhood mortality is attributable to genetic diseases, and at least 1 in 20 individuals under the age of 25 years develops a serious disease with an important genetic component.

There may be wider implications for a family when a genetic disease has been diagnosed in a child. Many members may be at risk of being affected themselves or of being carriers. In order to give families accurate genetic information, a combination of traditional clinical skills and specialist tests is required.

TYPES OF GENETIC DISEASE

Genetic diseases can be classified into the five main categories (see Table 19.1). Clinical information may suggest which of these five mechanisms is operating in an individual family, allowing confirmation by specialist laboratory tests.

Genetic diseases, by definition, are caused wholly or in large part by altered gene structure, regulation, or function. These alterations can be caused by several mechanisms ranging from a single base change in one gene to the deletion or rearrangement of a large amount of DNA involving many genes. Some of these alterations can have a demonstrable effect on the phenotype, and are detectable by observing dysmorphism or other physical signs, or by measuring levels of enzymes or metabolites.

This mainly indirect approach can now be supplemented by laboratory techniques which can be used to examine directly the structure of chromosomes or sequences of DNA. Genetic laboratory investigations are

Table 19.1 Types of genetic disease (note that a genetic disorder may present differently in different members of the same family, and disorders which are clinically similar may follow different patterns of inheritance in different families)

	Diagnostic tests
Single gene (Mendelian) Incidence 1% Numerous though individually rare Clear pattern of inheritance High risk to relatives Examples: neurofibromatosis, congenital adrenal hyperplasia, haemophilia	Pedigree analysis Clinical examination Clinical investigation Biochemical analysis DNA analysis
Chromosomal Incidence 0.6% Mostly rare Usually no clear pattern of inheritance and low risk to relatives (except for inherited rearrangements) Examples: Down, Edwards, and Turner syndromes	Chromosomal analysis
Multifactorial Single congenital malformations (incidence 3–4%) Common adult disorders (10% of adults) No clear pattern of inheritance Complex interaction of genes and environment Low or moderate risk to relatives Examples: pyloric stenosis, neural tube defects, schizophrenia	Clinical examination Clinical investigations Biochemical analysis

continued

	Diagnostic tests
Mitochondrial	Pedigree analysis
Can be caused by	Clinical examination
abnormalities of DNA in	Clinical investigations
mitochondrion itself, or in a	Histopathology
nuclear gene	DNA analysis
Variable pattern of inheritance:	
matrilineal transmission highly	
suggestive	
Affected men do not have	
affected children	
Many patients have new	
mutations	
Examples: Leber's optic	
atrophy, myoclonic epilepsy	
with ragged red fibres (MERRF)	
syndrome	
Mutations occurring in somatic	Clinical examination
cells	Chromosomal analysis
Mechanism for some cancers,	DNA analysis
and mosaicism	Histopathology

requested in paediatrics for two main indications: during the investigation of "syndromes", and when a diagnosis of a single gene disorder has been made or is suspected.

CLINICAL INVESTIGATIONS

Clinical investigations are used to evaluate the phenotype. A genetic mechanism may be suggested by the family pattern of affected people, the precise diagnosis, or specific tests. Recording the family tree is a vital first step in determining the genetics of a disorder and, with practice, takes only a few minutes.

Family Trees (the Pedigree)

The best (and easiest) way to record genetic information about a family is to draw a pedigree. A family tree is constructed as follows:

1. Build up the tree from the "bottom", starting with the affected child and siblings. "Please give me the names of your children, and their dates of birth in order of their ages, starting with the eldest first".
2. Choose one of the parents (usually the mother) and ask about her siblings and their children, and then her parents, moving from generation to generation.
3. Add information on the paternal side of the family.
4. Use clear symbols, e.g. circles for females, squares for males. Colour in the symbol if the person is affected.

5. Put a sloping line through the symbol (from the bottom left-hand to the top right-hand corners) if the person has died.
6. Record names, dates of birth and maiden names.
7. Ask for miscarriages, stillbirths or deaths in each partnership. For each partnership ask: "How many children have you had? Have you lost any children?"
8. Ask about consanguinity: "Are you and your partner related; are there any surnames in common in the family?"
9. Date and sign the pedigree.

When the diagnosis is already known (for example, an autosomal recessive condition), it may not be necessary to record personal details about all the family members in as much detail as would be required for an unknown disease.

Record at least basic details about both sides of the family, even if a disorder appears to be segregating on one side. In particular, ask about female relatives and their sons on the maternal side of the family if an X-linked disorder is suspected, but remember that many cases of the more serious X-linked diseases are new mutations. This can make it difficult to counsel parents unless reliable carrier detection is available.

The presence of consanguinity does not prove autosomal recessive inheritance, but makes it more likely. The absence of other affected members does not mean that the disorder is not genetic!

Examine the parents of a child with an apparently sporadic autosomal dominant disorder (for example neurofibromatosis or tuberous sclerosis) carefully to detect clinically extremely mild expression in a parent, before concluding that the child has a new mutation.

Carrier detection for X-linked disorders can be very difficult. Whether a female shows signs of the condition, either physically or on laboratory testing, depends on the particular disease and also on the chance pattern of X chromosome inactivation in that individual.

Investigation of a Syndrome

The procedure is as follows:

1. Take a detailed history, including pregnancy, birth and development details.
2. Draw out a family tree.
3. Note any particular patterns of behaviour (personality, feeding, sleeping).
4. Perform a detailed systematic physical examination recording measurements, including height, weight, head circumference, and eye measurements (inner canthal, interpupillary and outer canthal distances).

If you are not familiar with the precise technically descriptive words describe the appearance of the child in simple unambiguous terms, or draw a picture of the anomaly.

5. Plot the measurements on centile charts for age and sex. Note discrepancies (for instance, an outer canthal measurement above 97th centile whilst head circumference is on the 10th centile confirms hypertelorism). Repeated measurements will be helpful in demonstrating dysharmonic growth.

6. Ask for permission to take photographs. Note that in many syndromes (e.g. Williams and Noonan syndromes) the phenotype changes with age.

7. Examine the parents to determine whether a dysmorphic sign in the child is a familial characteristic unrelated to the syndrome.

8. Organize investigations (usually metabolic or cytogenetic). Remember that dysmorphic features are part of some metabolic disorders, for instance Zellweger's syndrome, mucolipidosis or mucopolysaccharidoses.

9. Consult the literature. Using a combination of the most unusual physical signs or behavioural characteristics, search in a book of syndromes or one of the computerized databases. Begin with very unusual characteristics and widen the search if no syndromes are suggested. For example, using the non-specific example of low-set ears as the only criterion will result in a list of over 250 syndromes. Consult the original literature when a possible match is found. Although the written description may appear to match, comparing the patient's appearance with photographs in the reference may prove otherwise.

10. Assess the risk. In the absence of a specific syndromic diagnosis, an empirical recurrence risk of 3–10%, depending upon the particular features, may be given.

Other Clinical Investigations

Other investigations, e.g. imaging or eletrophysiological tests) may be required to confirm a diagnosis or may be useful in determining if apparently unaffected family members show minor signs.

LABORATORY INVESTIGATIONS

Laboratory investigations involve direct examination of the genetic material. Examination of chromosome structure by light microscopy has become increasingly detailed, but direct gene analysis is now possible for many diseases using DNA technology.

The Provision of Specialist Genetic Investigations

Cytogenetic and molecular investigations and their interpretation can be complex, and are performed in specialist laboratories, which in the UK are organized regionally. The laboratories are always pleased to discuss diagnostic problems.

The laboratories work in close collaboration with consultant clinical geneticists who are clinicians with specialist training in genetics. They offer diagnosis, genetic counselling, and risk estimation, and will see patients to organize appropriate tests and explain the results. Many health districts have a genetic clinic staffed by specialists from the regional centre.

Cytogenetic Investigations

These are used to study the structure and function of chromosomes.

Preparation of the Karyotype

The 46 chromosomes in human somatic cells consist of 22 pairs of autosomes and two sex chromosomes (X and Y), and contain sufficient DNA to code for up to 100 000 genes. Chromosomes are normally visible only during cell division. Although some tissues have sufficient numbers of dividing cells for direct study (bone marrow, chorionic villus material, and meiotic divisions in the testis), routine chromosome analysis is carried out on cultured lymphocytes, fibroblasts and amniotic fluid cells.

A minimum of 0.5 ml whole blood in heparin is required from a baby, but 2 ml is preferred and 5 ml should be taken from older children and adults. The sample should be sent to the laboratory as soon as possible, but may be posted. Cytogenetic analysis is not possible on stored blood spots (Guthrie cards) or formalin fixed tissues.

Lymphocytes are stimulated with phytohaemagglutinin to give large numbers of dividing cells. The cell cycle is synchronized and division blocked in metaphase by adding colchicine which prevents the movement of chromosomes on the spindle. The cells are harvested when they are between late interphase and early metaphase, and swollen by treatment with a hypotonic solution to separate the chromosomes on the metaphase plate for staining and examination by microscopy.

Giesma staining (G-banding) is the technique used routinely to produce a pattern of light and dark bands which is specific for each chromosome. Other staining procedures emphasize different segments or features and can be helpful in determining the clinical significance of morphological changes. For instance, C-banding emphasizes the heterochromatic regions found at the centromere.

Karyotyping is a labour-intensive investigation for the microscopist as high resolution (or extended) chromosome preparations reveal over 850 bands. In preparations of excellent quality, more than 1100 bands may be seen. Occasionally only a limited analysis may be possible because of poor elongation of the chromosomes. The sample should be repeated if clinical features strongly suggest a chromosomal syndrome.

The Cytogenetic Report

The karyotype of a cell is reported in an internationally agreed format giving a precise description of an abnormality. Its three parts are each separated by a comma: the total number of chromosomes seen, the sex chromosome constitution, and the abnormalities or variants.

Breakpoints involved in structural rearrangements are described according to the chromosomal short (p) or long (q) arm involved, the region of that arm, and then by band or subband(s) within that region or band. The region is denoted by a digit 1–4, the band by a digit 1–8, and the subband by a digit following a decimal point. For example, band Xq27.3 is found on the long arm of the X chromosome, in region 2, band 7, and subband 3. Some examples are listed below:

46,XY	normal male.
46,XX	normal female.
47,XX+21	female with trisomy 21.
45,X	Turner syndrome.
47,XXY	Klinefelter syndrome.
46,XY,fraX(q27.3)	male with fragile X syndrome.
46,XX,del (5) (p25)	female with a deletion of short arm of chromosome number 5, cri du chat syndrome.
46,XY,t(3p21.2;10q1.1)	Balanced translocation in a male: one breakpoint on the short arm of one chromosome number 3, region 2, band 1, subband 2, and the other breakpoint on the long arm of one chromosome number 10 at region 1, subband 1.

Classification of Chromosomal Anomalies

Chromosomal anomalies include numerical abnormalities of whole chromosomes (e.g. trisomies) or structural

abnormalities such as duplications, deletions or translocations. Indications for chromosomal analysis are in Table 19.2.

As a chromosome contains thousands of genes, aberrations will affect multiple organ systems, causing congenital malformations and mental retardation.

Chromosomal analysis is unlikely to be helpful in patients with a single congenital malformation, a known single gene disorder, or a recognized non-chromosomal syndrome.

Chromosomal Anomalies – Practical Points

Normal Lymphocyte Chromosomes in a Child with Features of a Chromosomal Anomaly

- Consider karyotyping the parents to exclude a parental balanced translocation. Some translocations are easier to detect in the balanced form in a parent than in the unbalanced form in a child.
- Consider a skin biopsy for culture and karyotyping in children with normal lymphocyte chromosomes who have dysmorphic features, asymmetry, growth failure, developmental delay, or pigmentary disturbances to detect chromosomal mosaicism.

Two cell lines are present in somatic mosaicism – usually one with a normal and one with an abnormal chromosomal complement. The proportion of each cell line can vary from tissue to tissue, and the number and distribution of cells with the abnormal karyotype will reflect the severity of the phenotype, physically and mentally. It can be very difficult to predict the outcome when mosaicism is found at prenatal diagnosis. Examples include Pallister–Killian syndrome (12p tetrasomy) which is viable only in mosaic form, and hypomelanosis of Ito.

Table 19.2   Indications for chromosome analysis

Dysmorphic features suggestive of a chromosomal syndrome
Multiple congenital abnormalities and/or dysmorphic features
Suspected contiguous gene disorder (deletion syndrome)
Unexplained mental retardation
Family study of structural chromosomal anomaly
Assisting diagnosis and prognosis in leukaemia
Recurrent miscarriages
Unexplained stillbirth
Female with unexplained short stature
Ambiguous sexual development

Clinical Effects of Structural Chromosomal Anomalies

The karyotype will allow an assessment of the amount of chromosomal material in monosomic or trisomic form, but this does not necessarily predict the degree of disability as some small deletions can have major deleterious effects. Broadly, more serious effects can be expected from deletion than duplication of chromosomal material.

Translocations

A translocation results from the transfer of material between chromosomes, requiring breakage of both chromosomes with repair in an abnormal arrangement. If the exchange results in no loss or gain of DNA or disruption of genes, the translocation is balanced. The individual is clinically normal but is at risk of having a chromosomally abnormal baby with an unbalanced form of the translocation. The abnormalities, and the risk, depend on the chromosome fragments present in monosomic or trisomic form. Sometimes spontaneous abortion is inevitable; in other cases a child with multiple abnormalities is born alive. Relatives should be offered investigations to identify carriers of the balanced translocation so that genetic information and prenatal diagnosis can be offered.

Down Syndrome

Arrange chromosomal analysis in clinically diagnosed cases of Down syndrome to exclude a translocation which could give high risks of recurrence.

Parents of Children with Trisomies

As virtually all parents of children with regular trisomies have normal chromosomes, it is not usually necessary to perform parental karyotypes unless the pedigree suggests that a translocation may be segregating.

Parents of Children with Structural Chromosome Anomalies

The parents of children with structural chromosome anomalies should have chromosomal analysis to determine if the anomaly is inherited or *de novo*.

Leukaemia

Cytogenetic investigations are helpful in assessing prognosis and the likely response to treatment. The primary chromosomal event (e.g. a specific translocation) appears to be associated with the basic biology of particular types of leukaemia. When additional chromosomal aberrations

occur, they herald a worsening prognosis, and such abnormalities may precede clinical evidence of relapse or disease acceleration.

Congenital Malformations and Dysmorphic Features

Minor anomalies are of no functional significance, but when several are present an accompanying more serious congenital malformation should be sought. Minor external anomalies are usually found in the face, ears, hands and feet, but before ascribing significance to a minor anomaly determine whether it is also found in other family members. Almost any minor defect can be found in a family; several in combination should raise the possibility of a dysmorphic syndrome or chromosomal anomaly.

Deletions (and Inversions or Duplications) of Chromosomal Material

Duplications and deletions of even apparently small segments of chromosomes can result in severe phenotypic effects. Small deletions have been identified by microscopy in syndromes of previously unknown origin (for example some patients with Prader–Willi syndrome).

Contiguous Gene Syndromes

DNA techniques can identify deletions too small to be identified by conventional light microscopy (see below). Where such a deletion involves several genes, the resulting syndrome is called a "contiguous gene syndrome" and can be expected to give mental handicap, multiple congenital abnormalities and/or dysmorphic features. A patient with several single gene disorders is likely to have a deletion affecting genes lying close together on the chromosome. Miller–Dieker syndrome (chromosome 17p deletion) is an example.

Recurrence Risks

The recurrence risk for another chromosomally abnormal child is generally low if the previous child has a regular trisomy (usually 1:100) or other *de novo* structural abnormality. The parents may still wish to undertake prenatal diagnosis. Carriers of translocations should be referred to the genetic clinic, as the risk of a child with serious malformations may be high.

DNA Investigations

Over 2000 genes have been cloned, and the approximate chromosomal positions of many more are known. DNA techniques can now offer precise diagnostic information and risk estimation for many families by tracking the inheritance of disease genes within a family, or detecting the presence of a specific mutation. Identification of genes associated with increased susceptibility to diseases such as asthma is underway. Our understanding of the mechanism of cancer (stepwise mutation in several genes) relies heavily on techniques of DNA analysis. DNA techniques in cytogenetics (molecular cytogenetics) can give clinically valuable information by identifying the precise nature of chromosomal anomalies in complex cases.

The Value to Families of DNA Techniques

DNA techniques can allow:

- Confirmation of diagnosis (especially helpful in diseases where clinical features can be equivocal).
- Carrier testing (especially where biochemial testing is not available or the results may be equivocal).
- Presymptomatic diagnosis so that surveillance can be instituted (for instance in familial adenomatous polyposis coli).
- Precise estimation of risk.
- Prenatal diagnosis.

Each family has to be individually assessed because some techniques rely on the family structure and the necessary DNA samples being available.

How the Techniques are Used

DNA techniques are used in two main ways: to follow the inheritance through a family of a stretch of DNA which is very close to, or contains, the disease gene (gene tracking); or to identify directly a mutation in the gene, which in some cases may be a complete or partial deletion of the gene. In clinical practice, therefore, the techniques can be used to:

- Detect a mutation to confirm a diagnosis (e.g. a deletion in Duchenne muscular dystrophy).
- Offer families carrier testing, presymptomatic diagnosis, and prenatal diagnosis.

Diseases for which DNA diagnosis may be available are listed in Table 19.3.

Samples

DNA can be extracted from cells with nuclei, most usually lymphocytes, and can be stored frozen from many years. For investigations involving Southern blot

Table 19.3 Diseases for which DNA diagnosis may be available by gene tracking or direct mutation detection

Adrenoleukodystrophy
Adult polycystic kidney disease
α_1-Antitrypsin deficiency
Alport syndrome
Becker muscular dystrophy
Congenital adrenal hyperplasia
Cystic fibrosis
Duchenne muscular dystrophy
Familial adenomatous polyposis coli
Familial hypercholesterolaemia
Fragile X syndrome
Freidrich's ataxia
Haemophilia A and B
Hereditary motor and sensory neuropathy
von Hippel–Lindau disease
Huntington's disease
Marfan syndrome
Multiple endocrine neoplasia
Myotonic dystrophy
Neurofibromatosis
Ornithine transcarbamylase deficiency
Phenylketonuria
Retinoblastoma
Sickle cell disease
Spinal muscular atrophy
Tay Sachs disease
Thalassaemia

Note: family studies with DNA from at least one affected person are required for some of these diseases.

analysis, 10 ml whole blood is required. Investigations using probes for which polymerase chain reaction (PCR) primers are available need only small amounts of DNA – from a blood spot on a Guthrie card for instance. It may be possible to extract DNA which can be used for PCR amplification from fixed pathological specimens if no other specimens are available.

The Basis for DNA Tests

DNA molecules consist of two strands, held together by weak hydrogen bonds in a double-stranded helix. The order in which amino acids are assembled into proteins is encoded in the sequence of the bases in the centre of the helix. As the bases can pair only in certain combinations (e.g. adenine with thymine, and guanine with cytosine) the sequence of bases along one of the DNA chains determines the sequence of bases along the other. A denatured double strand (i.e. made into two single strands) must reassemble in its former configuration because of the pairing constraints of the bases. Diagnostic

DNA tests utilize this property of DNA. A single-stranded DNA molecule will rejoin only with its naturally occurring complementary DNA strand or with synthetic copy of the complementary DNA strand's base sequence – a DNA "probe".

Gene Tracking

When the chromosomal location of a gene is known, DNA sequences situated next to or within the disease gene can provide markers (for instance, restriction fragment length polymorphisms or microsatellite markers) for the normal and disease genes.

Restriction Fragment Length Polymorphisms (Figure 19.1)

The very long molecules of DNA are reduced to thousands of smaller fragments using restriction enzymes which cleave the DNA at specific sites. These sites vary in

position from person to person because of DNA sequence variation occurring naturally in the population. Markers generated in this way are called restriction fragment length polymorphisms (RFLPs) because they are generated by differences in lengths of DNA between restriction enzyme sites.

The DNA fragments are separated according to their sizes by electrophoresis and transferred to a nylon membrane (Southern blotting). The DNA is denatured and a DNA probe used to find the DNA sequence of interest.

A probe used in diagnosis is a length of single-stranded DNA, the sequence of which lies in close proximity to the disease gene. It is radiolabelled and hybridized to the DNA fragments on the nylon filter. When it finds the copy of its sequence, the two strands join to reform a double helix, a radioactive signal on the nylon filter marking its position.

The normal and disease genes may be on different lengths of DNA, which can be detected because of the

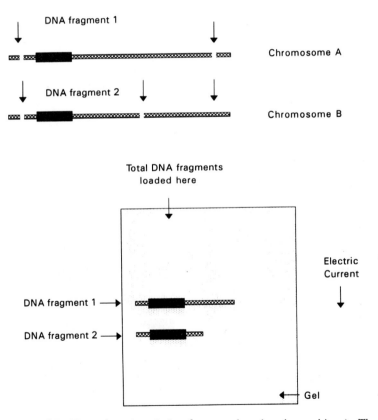

Figure 19.1   The generation of DNA markers (restriction fragment length polymorphisms). The two homologous chromosomes are labelled A and B. The arrows represent the sites at which the enzyme cuts. The black box represents a DNA sequence detected by a DNA probe. Chromosome A has cutting sites which result in the probe detecting a fragment (1). Chromosome B has a sequence variation which has resulted in a shorter fragment (2). These fragments are separated by electrophoresis and, after hybridization with the radiolabelled DNA probe, give two bands on the autoradiograph.

different positions on the gel after electrophoresis (see Figures 19.2–19.4). By scoring the fragment patterns of the affected family members, it is possible to deduce which fragment is being inherited with the disease gene. Unfortunately some RFLPs are not very informative, depending on the frequency of the alleles in the general population, and so diagnosis is not always possible.

The error in the test (as in all "gene tracking") is related to the distance between the DNA probe and the disease gene, as the "marker" could move away from the disease gene at meiosis as a result of crossing-over (recombination). This error is the recombination rate observed in a large number of families between the probe and the disease gene.

Microsatellite Markers

Microsatellite markers are very useful diagnostically because they have many alleles, which makes them potentially informative in nearly all families. They consist of multiple repeats of a dinucleotide sequence, often of 10 to more than 30 copies. Microsatellites have many possible alleles of different lengths, depending upon the number of dinucleotide repeats present on the homologous chromosomes.

Microsatellite polymorphisms are best detected by the polymerase chain reaction (PCR) which can amplify a specified area of DNA by up to a factor of 10^6. It is designed to make multiple copies of a piece of DNA. Part of the precise DNA sequences at each end of the area to be studied have to be known, and copies of these sequences synthesized (primers). The DNA sequence which is to be copied is denatured and the primers annealed to the separated strands. A polymerase enzyme adds bases sequentially to the end of the primer to synthesize a new strand using one of the original strands as a template, starting at the primer. At the end of the first cycle, there are two copies of the original target DNA. Each of the

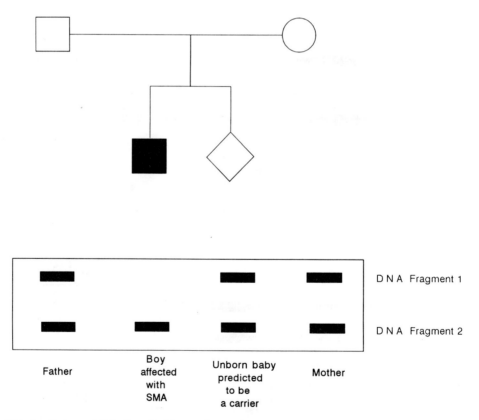

Figure 19.2   This family has a child affected with spinal muscular atrophy (SMA). A probe closely linked to the disease locus in available. Both parents have two detectable bands (1 and 2) but their son, who is affected with SMA, shows only one (2). As the marker is known to be very close to the disease gene, the SMA gene must be on the parental chromosomes which give fragment 2. In the next pregnancy the fetus was shown to have two bands (1 and 2) and, therefore, is predicted to be a carrier, but not affected by SMA. Note that for gene tracking, DNA from the affected person and family studies are required.

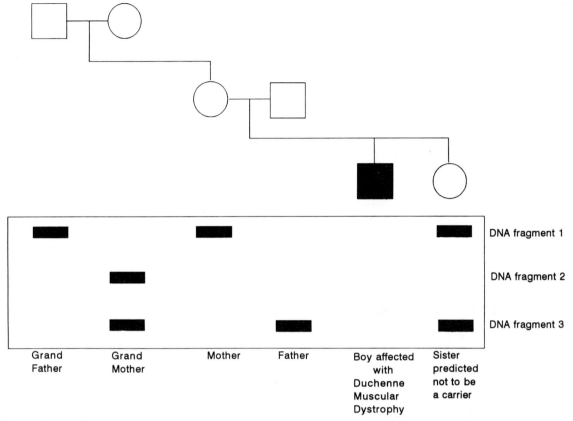

Figure 19.3   A family with Duchenne muscular dystrophy caused by a deletion of the dystrophin gene. The DNA probe being used is part of the coding sequence of the dystrophin gene. Note that the affected boy does not appear to have inherited a band from his mother, and that she herself does not appear to have inherited either band 2 or 3 from her own mother, as the autoradiograph shows only band 1 (which she has inherited from her father). One explanation is that the deletion of the dystrophin gene occurred during the formation of the egg from which the affected boy's mother developed. She is a carrier of the disease, but her mother is not. The DNA probe is unable to hybridize with the DNA from the affected boy's X chromosome to produce a band on the autoradiograph because that area of the gene has been deleted. The affected boy's sister has inherited band 1 from her mother and band 3 from her father. Therefore she is not a carrier from the deletion which her brother has.

four strands, after denaturation, can then act as a template for synthesis of more copies. The process is repeated for about 20–30 cycles of denaturation.

Diagnosis by Demonstration of Gene Deletion

In some families a deletion of part of a gene can be demonstrated by Southern blotting (the signal is absent, or the length of a fragment is shorter than normal) confirming diagnosis and allowing prenatal diagnosis.

Diagnosis by Direct Detection of Mutation

When the coding sequence of a gene is known, the precise mutation in a particular family may be characterized, and used directly for diagnosis in that family (e.g. familial adenomatous polyposis, mutations in cystic fibrosis caused other than by δ-F508). Some diseases (e.g. fragile X syndrome, myotonic dystrophy) have been shown to be due to a small sequence of DNA within or close to a gene being repeated many times resulting in disruption of the gene itself or of its control mechanism.

Storage of DNA

DNA should be stored from children with lethal conditions (usually autosomal recessive) where the gene has been localized and DNA diagnosis for other family members relies on linked markers. An important example is spinal muscular atrophy. Regional labora-

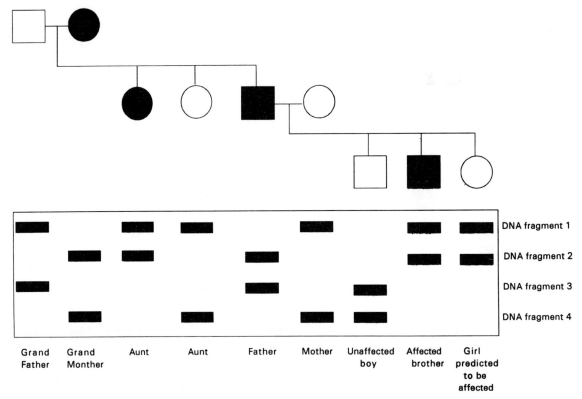

Figure 19.4   A family with autosomal dominant Marfan syndrome and the results of DNA marker tests using a probe on chromosome 15 which is situated in close proximity to the gene for the syndrome. By comparing the band patterns of affected and unaffected members, it can be seen that every affected member has inherited band 2, which is therefore a predictive marker for the disease gene. The girl (right), who has equivocal physical signs, is predicted to be affected and warrants regular surveillance for ophthalmic and cardiac complications.

tories have special facilities for long-term storage of DNA.

Molecular Cytogenetics

DNA techniques have been especially useful in diagnosis of syndromes involving small deletions of chromosomal material. The clinical effects are likely to be caused by the affected person being monozygous for several genes.

Light microscopy can at best visualize chromosome bands representing about 2 million bases of genomic DNA. This is much larger than the size of even moderately sized genes (the DNA code for the cystic fibrosis transmembrane regulator gene is 250 000 bases long).

Fluorescent *in situ* Hybridization (FISH)

After routine analysis of metaphase spreads, the DNA of the intact chromosomes on the microscope slide is dena-

tured. A cloned DNA sequence of known chromosomal location is tagged with a fluorescent dye and allowed to anneal to its complementary sequence. There will be two signals, in the correct positions on each homologous chromosome, if the normal two copies of the sequence are present and the chromosomes are structurally normal.

A deletion is confirmed if only one homologous chromosome has a fluorescent signal. FISH can identify the precise breakpoints of translocations. By using probes from several chromosomes sequentially, the origin of very small additional chromosomes (marker chromosomes) detected at prenatal diagnosis can be identified, giving useful information about prognosis.

TECHNIQUES AVAILABLE FOR PRENATAL DIAGNOSIS

Options available to families at risk of genetic disorders include:

- presymptomatic tests to institute surveillance or early treatment.
- having no (more) children.
- accepting the risk.
- prenatal diagnosis.
- adoption.
- artificial insemination by donor or *in vitro* fertilization and embryo transfer.

Prenatal diagnosis can give couples information on which they are able to make decisions. Many couples at high risk will embark on a pregnancy only if prenatal diagnosis is available. About 93% of prenatal tests give reassurance. The limitations of the tests should be fully discussed, as should the fact that a normal result from a test for a specific disease gives no information about other possible abnormalities, from which the fetus might be at the same risk as the general population. If the pregnancy is ended, the complete products of conception should be sent to the laboratory for diagnostic confirmation.

As tests and techniques for prenatal diagnosis are constantly changing, families should be encouraged to seek advice before each pregnancy to determine if new advances have occurred. Technical advances regarding prenatal diagnosis include:

- The development of chorionic villus sampling (CVS) in the first trimester.
- The use of DNA techniques in detecting specific disorders.
- Early amniocentesis (at 13 weeks).
- High-resolution ultrasound scanning.

Tests used in prenatal diagnosis are:

- Chromosomal analysis for:
  (a) Family history of chromosomal abnormality, either a parent with a balanced structural anomaly, or a previous child with a chromosomal abnormality.
  (b) Pregnancies shown to be at higher risk for a chromosome abnormality as a result of prenatal serum screening tests or maternal age (over 35 years).
  (c) Confirmation of fetal sex in X-linked conditions.
- DNA analysis for single gene disorders (where the family is informative).
- Biochemical analysis for certain metabolic disorders. Enzyme assay may be performed on cultured cells or direct metabolite assay may be done on the supernatant.

These tests can be performed on samples obtained by CVS or amniocentesis, depending on the particular disorder. For some metabolic disorders and subtle chromosome abnormalities, tests can be carried out only on samples obtained at amniocentesis.

Prenatal Diagnostic Procedures

Chorionic Villus Sampling

Chorionic villus sampling (CVS) is usually performed at about 10 weeks gestation. The usual procedure is transabdominal, as the transcervical route carries a higher rate of miscarriage. Under ultrasound guidance a fine needle is passed through the abdominal wall into the placenta and tissue gently aspirated. Each aspiration can yield about 5–30 mg tissue which can be used for fetal sexing, fetal karyotyping, biochemical studies and DNA analysis.

Direct chromosomal analysis is possible within 24 h, but results are not usually reported until analysis has been completed on cultured cells (within 7–10 days).

The miscarriage rate following CVS is estimated to be between 1 : 50 and 1 : 100. This figure includes all pregnancies lost up to 28 weeks of pregnancy in women who have had CVS.

Amniocentesis

Amniocentesis is a routine out-patient procedure and 10–20 ml liquor is aspirated. The procedure is performed usually around 16 weeks as the ratio of viable to nonviable cells is maximal. In some centres it is being offered at about 13 weeks.

For most tests amniotic fluid cells have to be cultured. Results of chromosome analysis may take up to 3–4 weeks. Results of biochemical analysis on the fluid itself may be available earlier, but if culture is required it may take much longer.

There is a small risk (about 1%) of miscarriage associated with amniocentesis, in addition to the risk (2.5%) at 16 weeks gestation of spontaneous miscarriage.

Fetal Blood Sampling

Fetal blood sampling is performed for clarification of an abnormal result found on CVS or amniocentesis (e.g. chromosomal mosaicism) or when abnormalities are detected by ultrasound scan which may suggest a chromosome disorder. The procedure is not usually performed before around 19 weeks, and can be performed at a much later gestation. The risk of miscarriage as a result of the test is about 1%.

Fetoscopy

Fetoscopy is the endoscopic visualization of part of the fetus, usually performed at about 18–20 weeks, for fetal skin biopsies, fetal blood sampling or fetal liver biopsy.

Ultrasound Scanning for Congenital Abnormalities

Abnormalities may be recognized during routine scanning of apparently normal pregnancies. Detailed ultrasound examination by a specialist service may be indicated for some dysmorphic syndromes where specific signs may be expected, usually beginning at about 18–19 weeks gestation.

PRESYMPTOMATIC AND CARRIER TESTING OF CHILDREN

The consequences of performing carrier tests on children should be considered carefully. Stigmatization must be avoided. It is a widely held view that children should not be tested for carrier status before the age at which they can make the decision for themselves and can understand the implications of the test and the subsequent genetic consequences. It is likely that the request will come from a family with an affected member and so the consequences of the disease may be well known. Misconceptions about the genetics of the condition must be explored; some carriers of autosomal recessive traits do not appreciate that they are at risk only if their partner is also a carrier.

The person tested may not need to act on the information about carrier status for many years, and so the result should also be sent to the general practitioner for the primary care health records. Regional genetics units may operate a review and recall system (often called a "genetic register") specifically to offer carrier testing. Most units provide this service for sisters of boys affected with Duchenne muscular dystrophy, for example, as well as other diseases.

Genetic testing for presymptomatic disease may be indicated if surveillance for serious complications or preventative therapy can be instituted, but should be discussed fully with the parents and a senior colleague before proceeding. There is a widespread view that predictive testing for adult onset diseases such as Huntington's disease should not be contemplated until the child is able to take an informed decision.

GENETIC TESTS IN SPECIFIC DISEASES

α-Thalassaemia Mental Retardation Syndrome (X-linked)

This syndrome has characteristic dysmorphic features including telecanthus, epicanthic folds, flat nasal bridge, midface hypoplasia, "carp shaped" mouth with full lips, enlarged protruding tongue, and head circumference less than third centile. Genital anomalies include cryptorchidism and severe dysgenesis, and hypospadias. Mental handicap is very severe with absent or very limited speech. The diagnosis can be confirmed in boys with severe undiagnosed mental retardation, characteristic face, genital and skeletal abnormalities, by demonstrating red cells containing HbH inclusions after incubation with 1% new methylene blue in saline. It is an X-linked condition which causes down-regulation of the synthesis of α-globin synthesis. Carriers have rare HbH inclusions.

Cystic Fibrosis

This autosomal recessive disease is caused by mutations in the cystic fibrosis transmembrane conductance regulator gene located at 7q31. The highest incidence is in Northern Europeans, with a carrier frequency of about 1:20. It is far less common in other racial groups, for instance in black and oriental populations. Over 190 mutations have been identified.

In Northern Europeans the three commonest are a 3 base pair deletion at position 508 (δ-F508) (76%) and two point mutations (G551D, 3–5%; and G542X, 3–5%) which together account for about 85% of mutations. There is a north–west to south–east gradient in Europe, δ-F508 being most common in Scandinavia. The background of a person should be taken into account in population testing.

Homozygosity of δ-F508 is associated with severe disease including pancreatic insufficiency. There is no clear correlation of genotype with lung function.

Direct mutation detection or gene tracking with intragenic or extragenic probes allow prenatal diagnosis and carrier detection.

Carrier Risks

It may be possible to give absolute carrier risks to members of a particular family when the cystic fibrosis mutations are known. When testing a member of the general population, however, a negative test does not exclude carrier status absolutely, but it can reduce the risk considerably. This is because not all CF mutations can be identified: in Great Britain the proportion of CF mutations which can be detected routinely is about 85%. Consequently, only 72% of couples in the general population at a 25% risk of having a child with CF can be identified. The residual risk of having an affected child is about 1 : 500 if a mutation can be identified in one partner but not in the other. Note that these figures will change depending upon the numbers of mutations screened, and assuming that there is no family history of CF.

Prader–Willi Syndrome

Most patients with Prader–Willi syndrome have a deletion of the paternal homologue of chromosome 15. They have only a maternal contribution for the critical area of the chromosome 15q11–13. Occasionally patients with the same phenotype have no deletion, but have inherited both copies of chromosome 15 from their mother (uniparental disomy). The child and both parents should have blood sent to the cytogenetics laboratory for comparison of the banding patterns of this area if the diagnosis is strongly suspected, as 50–60% of patients have a cytogenetically detectable microdeletion. It may be necessary to undertake molecular studies using DNA probes to determine submicroscopic deletions and chromosome rearrangements of this area.

Similarly, about 50% of patients with Angelman syndrome show a microdeletion cytogenetically at 15q12, the deletion being of maternal material. DNA techniques may reveal a deletion in others. The recurrence risk for Angelman syndrome with a *de novo* deletion is low, but familial recurrences have occurred in families where no deletion has been found on cytogenetic or DNA testing.

Fragile-X Syndrome

This X-linked syndrome is the commonest inherited cause of mental handicap. It is named after the cytogenetic appearance of the X chromosome on lymphocyte culture under special conditions; a gap appears in the chromosome near the tip of the long arm in 5–50% of cells.

DNA analysis has shown a sequence of three bases (CGG) which is repeated many times in the first exon of the FMR-1 gene at Xq27.3. The sequence is repeated 6–54 times in a "normal" FMR-1 gene, but the number of repeats is unstable, and can increase from generation to

generation during female meiosis or in somatic cell division.

Men and women with a gene with 60–230 repeats are said to have a "premutation": they are mentally and cytogenetically normal. The variable number of repeats can be detected by DNA techniques, as shown in Figure 19.5.

A premutation in a man or woman gives a fragment of increased size on Southern blotting. The full mutation is detected as a smear in the high molecular weight region. PCR amplification techniques are being developed to size the number of repeats accurately which will be important in screening carriers.

Clinically normal men with the premutation pass on the premutation to all their daughters, who may pass it on intact (with no clinical effect) or with expansion to the full mutation (causing mental handicap in a male). Women who inherit the full mutation on one X chromosome may be normal, or show mild (about 30%) or moderate (about 1%) mental handicap.

For initial diagnosis, blood from a clinically affected man should be analysed for the cytogenetic marker. DNA will be required subsequently for confirmation of the mutation and for family studies. Families should be referred to the genetic clinic for the DNA tests. Note that other forms of X-linked mental retardation exist.

Huntington's Disease

There is general consensus that children should not be tested for late-onset genetic disorders such as Huntington's disease. However, direct DNA diagnosis is available by demonstrating an increased number of triplet repeats in the gene on chromosome 4p which may be useful in the rare cases of juvenile onset disease. The diagnosis in other affected family members should be confirmed by demonstrating the mutation.

A patient requesting a presymptomatic test agrees to follow an internationally agreed protocol before DNA testing is performed, which can be arranged through the regional clinical genetics service.

Duchenne Muscular Dystrophy (DMD)

Duchenne and Becker muscular dystrophy are due to mutations in the same gene (dystrophin) at Xp21. About 65% of boys with DMD have deletions (the size and position of which vary from patient to patient) and, therefore, every boy with X-linked muscular dystrophy should have DNA analysis. The diagnosis is confirmed if a deletion in a coding sequence is found. There appear

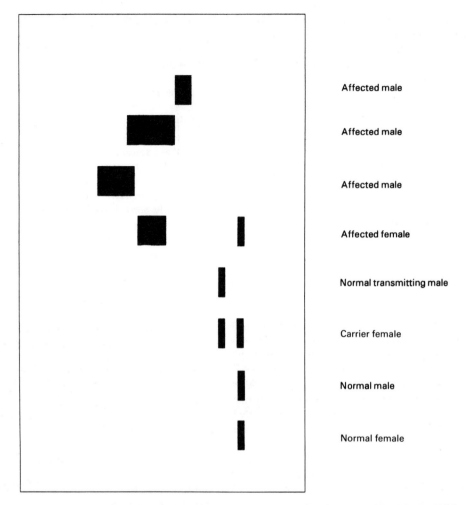

Figure 19.5 DNA analysis in the fragile-X syndrome. (1) Normal man (one band in normal position). (2) Man with the premutation. (3) Affected man – a smear of fragments (caused by somatic instability of the mutation). (4) Normal woman (one band in normal position). (5) Carrier woman – a fragment and the premutation. (6) Affected woman showing the full mutation – a fragment and a smear.

to be two deletion hotspots, one at the 5' end of the gene, between exons 6 and 7, and another more centrally, between exons 44 and 45. There is little correlation between the extent of the deletion and clinical severity. Some men with mild Becker muscular dystrophy have large portions of the gene deleted, whilst some boys with severe DMD have relatively minor deletions. Other molecular pathology includes partial duplications and point mutations. The clinical severity appears to be correlated with whether the molecular defect interrupts the reading frame; if a deletion interrupts a codon the rest of the gene will be read out of frame causing an incorrect sequence of amino acids in the protein. Molecular path-

ology which alters only one amino acid, or removes a sequence of several amino acids will allow the rest of the molecule to contain the correct sequence of amino acid residues.

Two-thirds of mothers of isolated boys are carriers. Detection of carriers using serum creatine kinase (CK) levels is not wholly reliable, as the normal and carrier distributions overlap. A normal result does not mean that a woman is not a carrier. Three estimations of CK are required, and the absolute value converted to a relative risk. CK testing is not reliable in pregnancy. Carrier risks are calculated from pedigree, CK and gene tracking information and so families should be referred to the genetic clinic. Most regional genetics centres have a genetic register to offer carrier testing to girls at risk in their late teenage years.

Prenatal diagnosis may be possible by gene tracking or by direct detection of the mutation, depending upon the family.

Spinal Muscular Atrophy

It is vital to save DNA from affected children, as prenatal diagnosis may be possible in future pregnancies by linked markers. It appears that the childhood spinal muscular atrophies types I–III are linked to markers on chromosome 5 in most families, but not necessarily all.

DiGeorge, Velocardiofacial (Shprintzen), and Conotruncal Syndromes

What were thought to be three separate syndromes now appear to be a contiguous gene syndrome, the common cause being deletion of material from chromosome 22q11. There is overlap of features between them, which include cardiac anomalies, dysmorphic facies, thymic hypoplasia, cleft palate and hypocalcaemia. (It has been suggested that this group be given the acronym "CATCH 22", which may be appropriate as an *aide-mémoire* to professionals, but may cause distress to some parents. Perhaps "22q11 deletion syndrome" may be preferable.)

Eighty-three per cent of DiGeorge syndrome patients, 68% of patients with Shprintzen syndrome, and 29% of patients with sporadic non-syndromic conotruncal anomalies have deletions of 22q11. Information on the natural history and variability of this contiguous gene syndrome is being collected.

SUGGESTED READING
General Overviews of Medical Genetics

Connor JM, Ferguson-Smith MA (1993) *Essential Medical Genetics*, 4th edn. Blackwell, Oxford.
Hodgson SV, Maher ER (1993) *A Practical Guide to Human Cancer Genetics*. Cambridge University Press, Cambridge.
Kingston HM (1989) *ABC of Clinical Genetics*. British Medical Association, London.

Information about Recurrence Risks

Harper PS (1993) *Practical Genetic Counselling*, 4th edn. Wright, London.

Syndrome Diagnosis

Buyse ML (ed) (1990) *Birth Defects Encyclopaedia*. Center for Birth Defects Information Services/Marston Book Services, Dover, MA/Oxford.
Gorlin RJ, Cohen MM, Levin LS (1990) *Syndromes of the Head and Neck*, 3rd edn. Oxford University Press, Oxford.
Hall JG, Froster-Iskenius UG, Allanson JG (1989) *Handbook of Normal Physical Measurements*. Oxford University Press, Oxford.
Winter RM, Baraitser M (1991) *Multiple Congenital Anomalies*. Chapman & Hall, London.

Overview of the Use of Molecular Techniques

Brock DJH (1993) *Molecular Genetics for the Clinician*. Cambridge University Press, Cambridge.

20

Neonates

G Stewart and T L Turner

INTRODUCTION

In this chapter we use a problem-orientated approach as this is the presentation faced by the clinician. It is not possible to consider all the many problems presented by the newborn infant and some are covered in other chapters but we shall consider the following:

- *Respiratory disorders*
  Tachypnoea.
  Apnoea.
  Cyanosis.
  Stridor.
- *Blood disorders*
  Excessive bleeding.
  Pallor.
  Plethora.
- *Jaundice* (see also Chapter 8).
- *Neurological problems*
  Abnormal movements (jitteriness and seizures).
  Floppy infants.
  Abnormalities of head size.
- *Potential infection*.
- *Miscellaneous disorders*
  Abdominal masses.
  Anuria and oliguria.
  Vomiting and diarrhoea.
  Delayed passage of meconium.
  Persisting metabolic acidosis.
  Ambiguous genitalia (see also chapter 3).
  Thyroid disease.

We recognize that the above approach is not exhaustive, but it represents the more common difficulties met in neonatal practice.

Since the total blood volume of the infant, particularly preterm, lies in the range 85–100 ml/kg body weight, it is relatively easy to exceed a 10% blood loss by sampling and hence to produce hypovolaemia. It is therefore important to restrict the volumes of blood needed for analysis to the absolute minimum necessary. To achieve this, co-operation with laboratory colleagues is essential and co-ordinated investigations can do much to reduce excessive blood losses.

It is also imperative to prevent other investigational risks such as hypothermia, induction of apnoea, hypoventilation and hypoglycaemia during handling for procedures such as imaging, cardiological investigation and lumbar puncture. Constant awareness of the potential physical and psychological effects of painful investigations and the steps which may reduce or abolish these risks is necessary. The value of careful preparation for investigation cannot be overemphasized since good planning can alleviate many potential problems. On the other hand, investigating the newborn is in some respects easier than in the older child or adult. For example, the open anterior fontanelle and lack of subcutaneous fat make ultrasound imaging easy. Ready access to the vascular bed through the umbilicus can also prove a very positive advantage.

As in other clinical situations, the planning of appropriate investigations has its roots in a directed and adequate history coupled with an accurate clinical examination. Evaluation of an infant's illness will require information on maternal health both before and during pregnancy and on family and social history.

Accurate information on perinatal events is paramount and usually requires access to the maternal case record and discussion with the obstetrician and midwife. Neonatal medicine cannot be practiced in a vacuum. All of these factors taken together with the clinical findings will allow the clinician to formulate a differential diagnosis and choose investigations accordingly.

RESPIRATORY DISORDERS

The Tachypnoeic Infant

Investigation involves:

- History and clinical examination, including body temperature.
- Surface swabs.
- Blood culture.
- Chest X-ray.
- Arterial blood gases.

Babies often breath rapidly during the first few hours of life (40–60 breaths/min). This is the period during which fetal lung fluid is being absorbed. Tachypnoea may also occur in infants who have been allowed to become hypothermic. If there is no history to suggest congenital infection or aspiration and the infant is otherwise well with no evidence of cyanosis then observation alone is acceptable. If the respiratory rate has not fallen below 40 breaths/min by 4 h of age, a chest X-ray may provide the diagnosis: for example diaphragmatic hernia, air leak or aspiration. However, the appearance of the chest X-ray may not be diagnostic and infection must be considered. A blood culture should be taken and appropriate antibiotic treatment prescribed.

If there is no obvious pulmonary cause of respiratory distress then congenital heart disease must be excluded. Investigations which may be helpful include an electrocardiogram (ECG) and, if possible, echocardiography. If echocardiography is not available then a hyperoxia test (see below) may be helpful. If there is a fixed shunt, the arterial oxygen tension will not increase significantly. The causes of tachypnoea are summarized in Table 20.1.

Table 20.1 Causes of tachypnoea

Respiratory distress syndrome
Congenital pneumonia
Overwhelming sepsis (group B *Streptococcus*, other congenital pneumonias)
Transient tachypnoea of the newborn
Pneumothorax
Pneumomediastinum
Pneumopericardium
Persistent pulmonary hypertension of the newborn
Meconium aspiration
Congenital lobar emphysema
Pulmonary hypoplasia
Diaphragmatic hernia

The Apnoeic Infant

The investigation and diagnosis of causes of apnoea is summarized in Table 20.2.

Apnoea must be distinguished from periodic breathing. Periodic breathing is sometimes normal, whereas apnoea is associated with serious illness. Clinical observation may allow differentiation between obstructive apnoea when respiratory effort continues, and central apnoea when respiratory effort is absent.

Short-lived apnoea occurs in normal infants with greatest frequency in the first week of life during active sleep. Posture such as neck flexion may provoke apnoea. Significant apnoeas are almost always accompanied by bradycardia or cyanosis. Apnoea in the second week of life or later should always be investigated. Infection may be the cause of apnoea and it should be remembered that apnoea of prematurity is a diagnosis of exclusion.

The Cyanosed Infant

The investigation of cyanosis includes:

- Chest X-ray.

Table 20.2 Investigation and diagnosis of causes of apnoea

Investigation	Diagnosis
Microbiological	
Blood culture	Infection
Suprapubic aspiration of urine	
Endotracheal secretions	
Lumbar puncture	
Haematological	
Full blood count	Anaemia
Coagulation	Infection
Biochemical	
C-reactive protein	Infection
Blood gases	
Electrolytes	
Glucose	Hypoglycaemia
Imaging	
Chest X-ray	Infection or aspiration
Cranial ultrasound	Intraventricular
Echocardiography	haemorrhage or increased intracranial pressure
Other	
Oesophageal pH studies	Reflux
Electrocardiogram (ECG)	Arrhythmia
Electroencephalogram (EEG)	Seizures

- Arterial blood gas and, if indicated, hyperoxia test.
- Blood cultures and C-reactive protein may be helpful.

It is important to determine clinically whether cyanosis is central or peripheral and to assess the peripheral circulation. Careful examination of the cardiovascular and respiratory systems will provide further clues to the final diagnosis. Infants who are centrally cyanosed require further investigation.

For the hyperoxia test, a preductal arterial specimen is taken from the right radial artery for blood gas analysis. If hypoxia is confirmed the analysis is repeated after 10–20 min in 100% oxygen. If the cyanosis is due to lung disease the pO_2 will invariably rise after oxygen administration and will usually reach 20 kPa. In cyanotic heart disease the pO_2 usually remains below 13.3 kPa. It is worth remembering that non-cardiac causes of cyanosis outnumber cardiac causes.

In respiratory disorders other signs are usually present. These include tachypnoea, grunting, and intercostal and sternal recession. In cardiovascular disease other signs may include heart murmur, tachycardia, heart failure, absent or diminished peripheral pulses, and gallop rhythm. A careful history and the investigations listed above will often discriminate between respiratory and cardiovascular disease. In the remaining cases, echocardiography and cardiac catheterization may be necessary.

Methaemoglobinaemia

Haemoglobin (oxygenated or deoxygenated) is usually in the ferrous state. Oxidation to the ferric state results in methaemoglobin which is non-functional and imparts a chocolate hue to the blood. Normal methaemoglobin levels are less than 2% of the blood. Several forms of hereditary methaemoglobinaemia exist.

Sudden Onset of Cyanosis in a Ventiliated Baby

Ventilate the baby using an AMBU bag or equivalent attached to an oxygen supply. Consider:

- Endotracheal tube displacement.
- Endotracheal tube occlusion.
- Pneumothorax (transilluminate).
- Pulmonary haemorrhage.
- Ventilator failure.
- Leak in ventilator circuit.

The Infant with Stridor

Investigation of stridor includes:

- Chest X-ray.
- Urea and electrolytes including calcium.
- Barium swallow.
- Laryngoscopy or flexible bronchoscopy.

Inspiratory stridor may cause considerable respiratory difficulty and respiratory failure may develop. Intubation or tracheostomy may be necessary. Stridor may be continuous or present only when the infant is agitated or distressed. Congenital laryngomalacia may produce intermittent stridor but has a benign course and resolves as the infant grows. If stridor is present at rest the infant requires further investigation.

Barium swallow will reveal indentation of the oesophagus in cases of vascular ring due to double aortic arch or anomalous origin of a major vessel. Direct laryngoscopy will confirm laryngo or tracheo-malacia and detect congenital paralysis of the vocal cords or haemangiomata of the cords.

Echocardiography and cineradiography may provide further information in cases where the diagnosis remains unclear. Although it is important to exclude hypocalcaemia, metabolic cause of stridor are rare. (See Table 20.3.)

BLOOD DISORDERS (see also Chapter 1)

Investigation of blood disorders includes:

- History with family profile.
- Full blood count (platelets and film).
- Prothrombin time (PT).
- Partial thromboplastin time (PTT), or equivalent.
- Thrombin time (TT).
- Plasma fibrinogen concentration.

Table 20.3 Causes of stridor in the newborn

Laryngomalacia
Tracheomalacia
Vascular ring
Subglottic stenosis
Laryngeal web
Vocal cord palsy
Vocal cord haemangioma
Hypocalcaemia

The infant with a bleeding disorder is likely either to be preterm or to have a temporary disorder due to either hypoxia or infection. Inherited disorders can often be suggested from the family history. It is essential to obtain cleanly collected venous blood in appropriate specimen containers. Coagulation parameters are gestational-age related (Table 20.4).

Bleeding disorders can be simply divided into three groups: those with thrombocytopenia alone; those with coagulation system abnormalities alone; and a large group in which there is disturbance of both. The latter group is likely to be due to disseminated intravascular coagulation.

Table 20.4 gives a list of commonly used haemostatic screening tests with normal values. A minimum profile would include platelet count, prothrombin time, partial thromboplastin time (or equivalent), and fibrinogen concentration. A blood film is also necessary to look for red cell fragments.

The commonest cause of thrombocytopenia is consumption coagulopathy, but if this is not the underlying cause and maternal drug ingestion has been excluded, mother's platelet count and platelet antibody status should be investigated to exclude auto and isoimmune thrombocytopenia. The mother herself may have had autoimmune thrombocytopenia but no longer have a low platelet count. If she is platelet antigen negative, she will have platelet antibodies and there will be iso immune neonatal thrombocytopenia. Rarely, thrombocytopenia is the first sign of bone marrow infiltration, and thus acute neonatal leukaemia, histiocytosis X and metastic neuroblastoma need to be considered and will require bone marrow examination and urinary catecholamine estimation.

Coagulation Defects

Apart from consumption coagulopathy the commonest cause of coagulation factor deficiencies is haemorrhagic disease of the newborn, and initial enquiries should

Table 20.4 Normal values in common haemostatic tests

Test	Preterm (30–36 weeks)	Term
PT (s)	13–23	13–17
PTT (s)	35–100	35–70
Thrombotest (%)	15–50	15–60
TT (s)	12–24	12–18
Platelet count ($\times 10^9$/l)	100–350	150–400
Fibrinogen concentration (g/l)	1.2–3.8	1.5–3.5

(See also Tables A1.13 and A1.14.)

Table 20.5 Causes of bleeding in newborns

Platelet related
Isoimmune neonatal (INT)
Autoimmune neonatal (ANT)
Infection
Drugs
Bone marrow defects
Platelet function disorders

Coagulation factor deficiencies
Hamorrhagic disease (vitamin K deficiency)
Maternal therapy: anticonvulsant; anticoagulant
Gastrointestinal and hepatic disorders
Inherited factor deficiencies, e.g. haemophilia A, von Willebrand's disease

Consumption coagulopathy (DIC)
Sepsis
Hypoxia

clarify whether the infant has received vitamin K or not (Table 20.5). It is worth recalling that one dose of oral vitamin K does not prevent the late variety of haemorrhagic disease. There will be a prolonged prothrombin time whilst other screening tests will be normal.

If the infant is well, isolated prolongation of the partial thromboplastin time raises the possibility of haemophilia A and other unusual coagulation factor deficiencies. Specific factor assays are occasionally necessary to establish diagnoses, such as factor XIII deficiency which usually presents with persisting oozing from the umbilical stump.

If major blood vessel thrombosis has occurred in either the mother or infant, levels of antithrombin III and protein C and S should be measured since their deficiency can cause bleeding and/or thrombosis in the newborn. Low levels of plasma fibrinogen are usually associated with severe intravascular coagulation, although occasionally either congenital hypofibrinogenaemia or afibrinogenaemia can occur.

If the screening tests are widely deranged, almost certainly the diagnosis will be disseminated intravascular coagulation from some major perinatal insult. In these circumstances, fibrin degradation products and D-dimers will be elevated.

The Pale Infant

Investigation includes:

- Full blood count (may need to be repeated 4–6 h later).

- Maternal blood group.
- Maternal blood for haemolysins.
- Infant's blood group and Coomb's test.
- Infant's blood and urine for virology including parvo-virus B19.

The history may provide the most likely diagnosis. Details of labour, including history of antepartum haemorrhage, rupture of the cord, placenta praevia or abruption, must be sought. A fetomaternal bleed may result in pallor in the infant with no obvious history or with a history of unexplained fetal distress in labour. Pallor may occur in the donor twin in cases of twin-to-twin transfusion.

A specimen should be obtained for full blood count. However, the result may be unremarkable and the investigation may have to be repeated after 4–6 h once there has been time for haemodilution. If the infant is anaemic and there is no history of blood loss, a Kleihauer test on maternal blood should be performed. This will detect the presence of fetal red blood cells in cases of fetomaternal haemorrhage.

All twins should have full blood counts performed shortly after delivery. Attention should be paid to the infant's and mother's blood group and the possibility of rhesus or ABO incompatibility considered. In unusual cases more detailed investigations may be required to exclude abnormalities of red cell enzymes or morphology.

Maternal autoimmune disease and congenital infections are rare causes of fetal anaemia. Preterm infants lose a relatively large amount of blood to the laboratory and all blood sampling in intensive care should be documented. Late anaemia may occur in vitamin E, copper or iron deficiency.

More detailed haematological investigations may be necessary and may include osmotic fragility on parental blood and estimation of G6PD or pyruvate kinase levels.

The Plethoric Infant

Investigation includes:

- Full blood count.
- Haematocrit.
- Monitor serum bilirubin (SBR) and blood glucose.

Plethoric infants (Table 20.6) may develop circulatory problems related to hyperviscosity and, if symptomatic, dilutional plasma exchange transfusion may be necessary.

Table 20.6 Causes of polycythaemia in the newborn

Placental insufficiency
Infant of diabetic mother
Thyrotoxicosis
Congenital adrenal hyperplasia
Maternal–fetal transfusion
Twin-to-twin transfusion
Excessive delay in cord clamping

THE JAUNDICED INFANT (see also Chapter 8)

Initial investigation involves:

- Serum bilirubin (total and unconjugated).
- Full blood count and film.
- Blood group and Coombs test – infant.
- Blood group and antibodies – mother.
- Urine – microscopy and chemical testing (reducing substances).

Subsequent investigation involves:

- Family history.
- Infection screen.
- Glucose-6-phosphate dehydrogenase (G6PD) level (male – Chinese, Eastern Mediterranean, tropical Africa, Middle East).
- T4 and TSH.
- Galactose-1-phosphate uridyl transferase.
- Stool colour.
- Bilirubinuria.
- Tests for conjugated hyperbilirubinaemia (see Chapter 8).

Perhaps the most helpful information in the planning of investigation of jaundice in the newborn infant is the age of onset and type of infant feeding. For most infants presenting with jaundice after the second day of life the only investigation required is measurement of the serum unconjugated and total bilirubin. In most units there is some form of chart in which the serum unconjugated bilirubin concentration is plotted against the age of the infant as an *aide mémoire* for treatment and investigation (Figure 20.1).

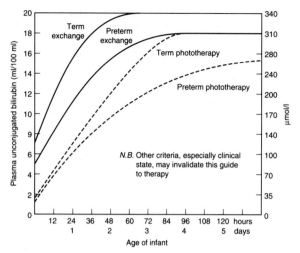

Figure 20.1   Chart of the criteria for exchange transfusion and phototherapy.

Breast feeding, because of either increased enterohepatic circulation or poor fluid intake, is a common factor in moderate jaundice. In infants who reach an action line before 48 h of age, maternal blood group and antibody measurement is mandatory, as is blood group, Coombs test, full blood count and serum bilirubin (unconjugated and total) for the infant. The urine should be checked for reducing substances with clinitest, and urine microscopy performed to help exclude a urinary tract infection. If clinitest is positive, red cell galactose-1-phosphate uridyl transferase should be measured to exclude galactosaemia.

In male children of Chinese, Eastern Mediterranean, tropical Africa and Middle Eastern descent, determination of G6PD level is also strongly recommended. Congenital spherocytosis can usually be excluded by examination of the blood film and by family history. Osmotic fragility investigations are inappropriate in the immediate newborn period. Pyruvate kinase deficiency is rare and requires specialized laboratory analysis.

In unusually prolonged jaundice, that is jaundice persisting after the 10th day of life, check stool colour, look for bilirubinuria and exclude hypothyroidism by assessment of thyroid function tests. At the same time, begin investigations to exclude congenital infections such as cytomegalovirus (throat swab, urine and IgM levels) (see Chapter 8).

It is assumed that the maternal syphilis serology and rubella status is known, but if this is missing, these investigations should be performed as a matter of some urgency, especially if there is hepatosplenomegaly.

The causes of unconjugated hyperbilirubinaemia are listed in Table 20.8.

Table 20.7   Causes of unconjugated hyperbilirubinaemia

Physiological jaundice
Haemolysis Blood group incompatibilities (ABO and rhesus) Trauma Polycythaemia Red cell enzyme defects (G6PD, PK, etc.) Red cell membrane defects (spherocytosis, etc.) Extravascular blood collections
Metabolic causes, e.g. galactosaemia
Endocrine causes, e.g. hypothyroidism
Sepsis

NEUROLOGICAL DISORDERS (see also Chapter 9)

Abnormal Movements

The Jittery Infant

Investigation involves:

- History and clinical examination, including maternal history.
- Blood glucose.
- Plasma calcium, phosphorus and magnesium.
- Urine toxicology screen.

Jitteriness must be distinguished from seizure movements because of its good prognosis and since anticonvulsant medication is unnecessary. Jittery movements have the quality of tremor, can be abolished by flexion of the limb and are usually provoked by external stimuli (e.g. noise). There are seldom other associated movements, e.g. nystagmus. Hypoglycaemia is probably the commonest cause whilst hypocalcaemia and hypoxia are less common. Drug withdrawal is an important cause in some communities (Table 20.8). A knowledge of the social aspects of the local community is therefore helpful. In many infants no cause is found, but since the biochemical disturbances are readily treatable they must be sought urgently. Recently hypoglycaemia has been redefined as a blood glucose of less than 2.2 mmol/l in the first

Table 20.8   Causes of jitteriness

Hypoglycaemia
Hypoxia
Hypocalcaemia
Drug withdrawal
Idiopathic

24 h of life and less than 2.2–2.8 mmol/l thereafter, in infants of any gestation or birthweight. This definition is widely accepted in the UK and a suspicious blood glucose of less than 2.5 mmol/l on a properly performed "stix" test mandates an urgent whole blood glucose by the laboratory. Samples must be collected in an appropriate fluoride container. Most infants with hypoglycaemia will be light for gestational age, or preterm infants with inadequate feeding regimes, whilst infants of diabetic mothers are at special risk.

However, sepsis, hypothermia and perinatal hypoxia need consideration and if recurrent, hyperinsulinism, adrenal and pituitary pathologies must be addressed (see Chapter 3). The combination of hypoglycaemia with metabolic acidosis alerts us to the possibilities of infection, hypoxia or errors of carbohydrate and amino acid metabolism.

In drug withdrawal there are often other features which include irritability, wakefulness, lacrimation, rhinorrhoea and diarrhoea. These signs may be preceded by apnoea or hypoventilation in the first hours of life. Toxicological analysis of fresh urine sample will confirm the suspicions raised by the maternal history.

The Infant with Seizures (see also Chapter 9)

Initial investigation involves:

- Birth and family history.
- Blood glucose.
- Plasma calcium, phosphate, and magnesium.
- Blood gas analysis.
- Plasma electrolytes.
- Infection screen.
- Ultrasound of head.

Subsequent investigation may include:

- Plasma ammonia, lactate and pyruvate.
- CSF
  (a) Microscopy, culture and viral samples.
  (b) Glucose, protein, glycine.
  (c) Lactate and pyruvate.
- Urine organic acids.
- Plasma and urine amino acids.
- EEG/Medilog.
- Trial of pyridoxine.
- CT scan.
- MRI scan.

As well as hypoglycaemia, a variety of conditions including hypoxic ischaemic damage, severe infection and

Table 20.9 Causes of seizures

Hypoglycaemia
Hypocalcaemia/magnesaemia
Hypoxic ischaemic encephalopathy
Meningitis/encephalitis/cerebral abscess
Hypo and hyper-natraemia
Urea cycle defects
Aminoacidaemias
Organic acidaemias
Pyridoxine dependency
Trauma/haemorrhage/infarction
Malformation
Familial

intracranial haemorrhage must be considered (see also Chapter 9) (Table 20.9). Hypocalcaemia, hypomagnesaemia, inborn errors of metabolism (including pyridoxine dependency), organic and amino acid disorders, urea cycle defects and, more rarely, the self-limiting "fifth-day fits" also occur. Seizure type may be a guide to the likely cause. Clonic seizures are more likely to be metabolic and multifocal seizures suggest hypocalcaemia. Tonic seizures are more likely to be due to structural abnormalities or hypoxic ischaemic damage. These are of more sinister importance and require more extensive investigation.

The family history will often suggest the possibility of drug withdrawal or familial neonatal seizures, the gene locus for which lies on chromosome 22.

Once the initial investigations have been carried out and the infant stabilized, we would proceed to perform a lumbar puncture unless the history clearly pointed to hypoxic ischaemic encephalopathy. In male infants particularly, a blood ammonia (collected and analysed within 30 min) is essential. The cranial ultrasound, as well as demonstating evidence of haemorrhage, infarction or midline shift, may also show poorly pulsating cerebral vessels. The timing of seizures after birth may also be helpful, those occurring earlier are more likely to be associated with hypoxic ischaemic encephalopathy, haemorrhage or congenital infection.

The classical form of hypocalcaemia has become rare since the phosphate content of formula milks was reduced. In our experience its occurrence should trigger a search for maternal problems such as grossly inadequate vitamin D intake and hyperparathyroidism. It is worth estimating the infant parathormone levels and the 1,25-dihydroxycholecalciferol levels of both infant and mother. Both hypo- and hyper-natraemia may be associated with seizures. The former may be found associated with hypoxic–ischaemic encephalopathy and sepsis, and is sometimes caused by inappropriate secretion of the antidiuretic hormone. The latter may occur from feeding inappropriately concentrated milks, parenteral fluids or from fluid deprivation. The seizures of pyridoxine dependency which may be due to the lack of γ-aminobutyric aid (GABA) synthesis may have been recognized *in utero*. Rapid response both clinically and on the EEG to intravenous pyridoxine is diagnostic.

Interpretation of the neonatal EEG is not easy and requires specialist experience. Interictal EEGs confirm an epileptic basis for abnormal movements in less than half of infants suspected of seizure, but serial or continuous EEG recordings and cerebral function monitoring may be more helpful. On the other hand, we find clinical assessment of seizures is often difficult, and it is of course impossible in paralysed infants. A negative interictal EEG does not exclude seizures. CT scans and MRI with expert interpretation will give additional information on lesions such as cerebral infarction, malformation and dysgenesis.

The Floppy Infant

Initial investigation involves:

- Assessment of gestational age.
- Family and birth history.
- Clinical examination, including search for associated anomalies.
- Blood glucose.
- Infection screen.
- Chest X-ray, chromosome analysis, cranial ultrasound.
- Metabolic screen (see below).

Subsequent investigation involves:

- Nerve conduction investigation.
- Electromyography (EMG).
- Creatine kinase.
- Muscle biopsy (open or needle).
- CSF (protein).
- Genetic ("biochemical") investigations.

Hypotonia can be due to a central disorder, anterior horn cell disease, peripheral neuropathy, neuromuscular junction defect, or disease of the peripheral muscle. Gestational age affects muscle tone and must be assessed early using a system such as the Dubowitz score. Evidence of decreased muscle bulk, diminished reflexes, and myotonia should be sought. Look for associated anomalies including dislocated hips, scoliosis, arthogryposis, high arched palate, and micrognathia. It is imperative to examine the parents, especially the mother, for myotonia and myasthenia and to obtain an extended family history.

Drug effects such as maternal ingestion of diazepam or lithium also require exclusion.

A central origin for hypotonia is more likely where there are dysmorphic features, normal reflexes and recoil strength, and altered consciousness. A neuromuscular origin is more likely when the above are absent. Antenatal hypotonia may have made the fetus more vulnerable to intrauterine hypoxia such that in the presence of hypoxic ischaemic challenge the features of hypotonia, and hence the underlying cause may be missed. Central hypotonia may also be due to metabolic disturbance, drug intoxication, or endocrine disorders (e.g. hypothyroidism), as well as intracranial infection and haemorrhage. Developmental abnormalities including Prader–Willi syndrome, oculocerebrorenal (Lowe's) syndrome, and cerebrohepatorenal (Zellweger) syndrome and other rare peroxisomal disorders may require investigation. Trauma to the spinal cord is rare, but usually apparent from the birth history.

Anterior horn cell diseases include Werdnig–Hoffmann disease (spinal muscular atrophy type I), type II glycogen storage disease (Pompe's) and neurogenic arthrogryposis multiplex congenita. In certain communities neonatal poliomyelitis may be implicated. The clinical clue to these disorders lies in the alertness of the infant and the presence of muscle fasciculation. The EMG and muscle biopsy findings are diagnostic. Peripheral nerve abnormalities are rare, but the diagnosis may be suggested by the presence of distal muscle wasting and weakness.

Myasthenia gravis (transient neonatal) acquired transplacentally from the mother is the most likely neuromuscular cause of floppiness. The delay in onset and variably of the degree of hypotonia may give a clue. In the permanent congenital variety the mother is not affected but other siblings may be (autosomal recessive). Infantile botulism and drugs such as aminoglycosides and high dose magnesium sulphate to mothers for eclampsia may, rarely, mimic myasthenia.

Muscle disorders include congenital myotonic dystrophy, congenital myopathies and congenital muscular dystrophy. The first two of these disorders are usually inherited in a dominant fashion, and the third recessively. In congenital myotonic dystrophy the affected parent is almost always the mother. The congenital myopathies include central core disease, nemaline and myotubular myopathies. The histological and electron microscopy changes observed on muscle biopsy are usually diagnostic. More recently a group of metabolic muscle disorders has been identified and a number of mitochondrial defects established. Carnitine and cytochrome *c* deficiency have been the most fully identified to date.

Once general causes (Table 20.10) have been excluded (hypoglycaemia, sepsis and hypoxia) the most valuable investigations are EMG and open muscle biopsy. Creatine kinase (CK) levels are usually uninformative since they are non-specifically elevated in the first 2–3 weeks of life. However, sequential estimations may demonstrate diagnostic patterns of elevation. Ultrasound imaging can be helpful in demonstrating abnormalities in muscle, but requires expert interpretation whilst cranial ultrasound and CT scan may demonstrate central abnormalities. The chest X-ray may show thinned ribs in neuromuscular disorders (Werdnig–Hoffmann) and cardiomegaly in metabolic myopathies. Although we usually delay muscle biopsy for several weeks after birth the characteristic histological and histochemical changes are present early in the congenital myopathies. The CSF protein is elevated in Krabbe's disease and other degenerative CNS disorders, but increasingly the key to many rarer disorders lies in molecular genetic techniques. The need for early referral of "difficult diagnostic problems" for specialist assessment by neurogenetic groups cannot be overstated. Only such teams have the facility to make specific diagnoses and give the counselling the family involved deserve.

Table 20.10 Causes of floppiness

	Family history	EMG	Muscle biopsy
Central e.g. hypoxic–ischaemic, drugs, Prader–Willi, Zellweger*	No	No	No
Anterior horn e.g. Werdnig–Hoffmann, Pompe's	Yes	Yes	Yes
Peripheral neuropathy e.g. neuronal–axonal disease, metabolic neuropathies	Often	Yes	Yes
Neuromuscular junction e.g. myasthenia gravis (transient)	Yes	(maternal antiacetylcholine antibodies)	
Muscle disease e.g. myotonic dystrophy, muscular dystrophy, congenital myopathies	Yes	Yes	Yes

*Zellweger syndrome is autosomal recessive and there may therefore be affected siblings.

The Infant with a Small Head

Investigation involves:

- History, including family history.
- Blood (IgM).
- Urine (viral culture).
- Throat swab (viral culture).
- Viral antibody titres (CMV, rubella, etc.).
- Toxoplasma antibody titres.
- Maternal phenylalanine concentration.
- Skull imaging (not ultrasound).
- Chromosomal analysis.

Microcephaly, a head circumference below the third centile, is frequently of indeterminate origin but may be associated with environmental factors such as congenital rubella infection, cytomegalovirus, varicella and toxoplasma infection (Table 20.11). Chromosome defects including trisomy 8, 13 and 22, deletions of 4p and 5p have all been associated with microcephaly. An autosomal recessive variety also occurs. Previous recessive microcephaly in the family will be obvious by measuring head size. We would initiate the above investigations and, if toxoplasma seemed likely, send CSF for serological analysis. The high risk of microcephaly in untreated maternal phenylketonuria cannot be overstressed. If available, access to a syndrome register may be of value especially in the presence of other malformations (see Chapter 19). Imaging techniques but not ultrasound may demonstrate intracerebral calcification in congenital CMV (periventricular) and toxoplasmosis.

The Child with a Large Head

Investigation involves:

- History.
- Measure parental head circumference.
- Cranial ultrasound.
- CT scan.

Table 20.11 Causes of microcephaly

Autosomal recessive

Chromosomal abnormality (trisomy 9, 13 or 22)

Environmental factors in pregnancy (CMV, rubella, toxoplasmosis)

Maternal phenylketonuria

Table 20.12   Causes of large head

Familial
Hydrocephalus: congenital; posthaemorrhagic
Agenesis of corpus callosum
Hydranencephaly
Metabolic disorders

Hydrocephalus is not the only cause of a large head (Table 20.12) in an infant and among the first investigations which should be performed is measurement of the parents' head size. Moulding of the skull can also lead to a large occipitofrontal circumference measurement, but this returns to normal after a few days.

If the head circumference is above the 90th centile, for the infant's gestational age and the sutures are widely separated there is a need for immediate cranial ultrasound. If this shows ventricular dilatation, consideration should be given to performing a CT scan which will usually clarify causes such as congenital malformation, for example Dandy–Walker cyst or Arnold–Chiari malformation. The rarer X-linked variety of aqueduct stenosis is associated with flexion and adduction defects of the thumbs. Agenesis of the corpus callosum can also be identified by ultrasound or CT scan, whilst hydranencephaly and congenital cerebral cysts can also present with a large head. As in microcephaly, a search of the literature through a syndrome register may well prove helpful. Rarely, hydrocephalus can be associated with metabolic disorders such as pyruvate dehydrogenase deficiency, and this is confirmed by measurements of plasma and CSF, pyruvate and lactate.

THE INFANT WITH SUSPECTED INFECTION

Investigation involves:

* Surface swabs (ear, umbilicus and gastric aspirate or throat swab if infant has been fed).
* Blood culture.
* Suprapubic aspiration of urine.
* Lumbar puncture.
* Blood, urine and throat swab for virology.

In the newborn period signs of infection are often non-specific. Close attention to maternal history is important. Vaginal discharge, pyrexia during labour, rupture of membranes for greater than 24 h or offensive liquor all suggest possible infection. Infection is a common cause of preterm labour. Signs of infection in the newborn include poor temperature control with hyper or hypothermia. The infant may fail to feed or be lethargic. Experienced nursing staff are often able to detect subtle changes in an infant's behaviour or handling and their advice should never be discounted. Early treatment of infection is important and may be life-saving. This is especially true in preterm infants. A high index of suspicion is appropriate.

MISCELLANEOUS DISORDERS

The Infant with an Abdominal Mass

Investigation may include:

* Abdominal X-ray.
* Abdominal ultrasound.
* Urea, electrolytes, and liver function tests; creatinine and creatinine clearance.
* α-Fetoprotein.
* Urinary homovanillic and vanillylmandelic acid.
* Urine culture.

An abdominal mass in infancy is most likely to be renal in origin, but may arise from the genital or gastrointestinal tracts, e.g., ovarian cysts or gastrointestinal duplication. Non-renal retroperitoneal masses include adrenal haemorrhage, neuroblastoma and teratoma. Liver or splenic masses are uncommon. Antenatal diagnosis of abdominal mass is possible using ultrasound.

Renal Mass

If the mass is of renal origin and obstruction is found on ultrasound, this must be relieved by insertion of a urinary catheter. Further investigation will include a cystogram and DMSA scan.

The Infant with Oliguria/Renal Failure (see also Chapter 6)

Investigation involves:

* Timed urine collection (chemical analysis, volume, electrolytes).
* Abdominal ultrasound.
* Blood urea, creatinine, electrolytes.

- Cystogram.
- DMSA scan.

Oliguria is defined as a urine output of less than 1 ml/kg per hour in an infant older than 24 h. It is often due to prerenal causes such as hypoxia, sepsis or hypotension but may be due to renal or postrenal causes (Table 20.13). It is important to initiate a method of urine collection and this will usually involve the use of an adhesive urine collection bag. In very immature infants, weighed cottonwool balls may be used and in a few circumstances a urethral catheter may be indicated. If possible the urine stream should be observed. In infants who appear otherwise well, abdominal ultrasound will demonstrate whether there is bladder enlargement and may demonstrate anatomical abnormality of the upper renal tract and the urethra. We would usually delay investigations for other abnormalities in the renal tract such as hydronephrosis for at least 48 h to obtain adequate imaging. If an obstruction exists, as well as making an assessment of renal function with plasma creatinine and urea, any urine passed should be analysed for electrolyte content in particular, sodium.

A cystogram is the next investigation indicated. Where there is evidence of a drainage problem, especially in the lower renal tract or bladder, a urethral catheter should be left *in situ* and the child treated with prophylactic antibiotics before referral to a surgeon.

If no lower tract obstructive lesion has been identified and there is no evidence of associated hypovolaemia, hypotension, or sepsis to cause pre renal failure, it should be assumed that the oliguria is due to a primary renal disorder and a DMSA scan is indicated. Where there has been haematuria, the possibility of renal venous thrombosis requires assessment and a Doppler scan of renal vessels can be diagnostic.

Table 20.13 Causes of oliguria/renal failure

Prerenal
Hypoxic/ischaemic
Sepsis
Dehydration

Renal
Renal anomaly: dysplastic; polycystic
Infection
Thrombosis: arterial venous
Tubular necrosis

Postrenal
Urethral obstruction
Ureteric abnormality
Bladder innervation abnormality

The Infant with Hydrops

Investigation involves:

- Full blood count and film.
- Group and Coomb's test.
- Haemoglobin electrophoresis.
- Bilirubin.
- Urea and eletrolytes.
- Liver function tests including protein and albumin.
- Urine analysis.
- Chromosome analysis.
- TORCH screen.
- Virology (parvovirus)
- Serology (leptospirosis).
- Chest X-ray (other imaging may be required later).
- ECG; echocardiography.

There are many causes of hydrops (Table 20.14), but as antenatal investigation becomes increasingly sophisticated, diagnosis and even treatment *in utero* is now possible. Fetal anomalies can frequently be diagnosed by antenatal ultrasound. Hydrops secondary to fetal anaemia caused by rhesus disease or parvovirus B19 can be treated by intrauterine intravascular transfusion. Resolution of hydrops may follow.

Haematological causes of hydrops are usually diagnosed antenatally and neonatal investigation is for confirmation. Anomalies of the cardiovascular, respiratory

Table 20.14 Causes of hydrops

Haematological
Rhesus disease
Thalassaemia
Fetal–maternal or twin-to-twin transfusion

Cardiovascular
Congenital anomalies
Tachy- and brady-arrhythmias

Chromosomal
Turner's syndrome
Trisomy 21, 18, 13

Infections
TORCH group
Parvovirus B19

Hypoproteinaemia
Congenital nephrotic syndrome
Congenital hepatitis

Anomalies
Respiratory, e.g. chylothorax, diaphragmatic hernia
Gastrointestinal, e.g. atresia, volvulus

and gastrointestinal tract will require appropriate imaging. Chromosomal abnormalities are frequently found, especially Turner's syndrome and the common trisomies. Congenital infection must be excluded. Further investigation may include ultrasound of the chest and abdomen for evidence of ascitic fluid, and contrast studies for atresia or volvulus. Many other conditions are associated with hydrops without an obvious causal relationship. Reference to major textbooks may be essential.

The Vomiting Infant

Investigation involves:

Biochemical
- Urea and electrolytes and glucose.
- Blood gas.

Microbiological
- Urine analysis and culture.
- Blood culture.

Imaging
- Chest X-ray (with nasogastric tube).
- Abdominal X-rays.
- Abdominal ultrasound.
- Contrast studies.

Vomiting is common in the first week of life due to immaturity of the co-ordination of the gastrointestinal tract. Vomiting may be a sign of obstruction of the gastrointestinal tract. A history of polyhydramnios would lead to suspicion of high gut obstruction especially oesophageal atresia. Antenatal ultrasound may have shown the "double-bubble" appearance of duodenal atresia. In infants with polyhydramnios, a large radio-opaque gastric tube should be passed and acid response on litmus paper obtained to exclude oesophageal atresia. If the tube cannot be passed an X-ray will confirm the position of the atresia. In this situation if gas is present in the stomach, a tracheo-oesophageal fistula exists. These investigations should be carried out before the first feed.

If the obstruction is high then the vomiting may appear after the first feed. Investigation is tailored to the clinical history and findings on examination. If vomiting is less immediate and more copious abdominal X-ray and ultrasound may be helpful in diagnosis of duodenal or jejunal atresia. Bilious vomiting suggests an obstruction distal to the ampulla of Vater. Vomiting may be a non-specific sign of infection.

Failure to tolerate feeds, especially in the preterm infant, may be an early sign of necrotizing enterocolitis.

Table 20.15   Causes of vomiting

Infection
Obstruction/atresia
Ileus
Necrotizing enterocolitis
Raised intracranial pressure
Biochemical or metabolic disturbance

Abdominal distention may occur with obstruction or with necrotizing enterocolitis. Hirschsprung's disease, meconium ileus and herniae should be considered (Table 20.15).

The Infant with Diarrhoea (see also Chapter 7)

Investigation involves:

- Stool culture and virology.
- Blood culture.
- Abdominal X-rays.
- Urea and electrolytes.
- Full blood count and coagulation.
- Stool biochemical analysis: reducing substances; electrolyte composition.

Diarrhoea in infancy will quickly lead to biochemical imbalance. Loose stools with blood indicate necrotizing enterocolitis, until proven otherwise. Rare causes of diarrhoea include congenital enteropathy, chloridorrhoea and thyrotoxicosis (Table 20.16). Infants receiving phototherapy often have explosive green stools.

Table 20.16   Causes of diarrhoea

Gastroenteritis
Necrotizing enterocolitis
Drugs
Phototherapy
Chloridorrhoea
Thyrotoxicosis

The Infant with Delayed Passage of Meconium

Investigation involves:

- Examination of the perineum to ensure that the anus is patent.

Table 20.17   Causes of delayed passage of meconium

Imperforate anus
Meconium plug syndrome
Meconium ileus (cystic fibrosis)
Hirschsprung's disease
Low gut atresia
Hypothyroidism

- Abdominal X-rays.
- Barium enema.
- Immunoreactive trypsin.
- Thyroid function tests.
- Rectal biopsy.

Preterm infants often have delayed passage of meconium (Table 20.17). This may be due to delay in establishing enteral feeds or delay in propulsive gut activity. In term infants meconium is usually passed within the first 24 h of life. Investigation should be guided by the clinical history and examination findings. A meconium plug may occur in the preterm, in infants of diabetic mothers, and in those with Hirschsprung's disease. Ten per cent of children with cystic fibrosis present with a meconium ileus. This may result in ischaemia, perforation, and peritonitis. An abdominal X-ray may show radiological densities and a granular appearance within the gut lumen. Serum immunoreactive trypsin may be elevated. Hirschsprung's disease may present with delayed passage of meconium and abdominal distention. Rectal examination may be helpful and barium enema show dilated gut proximal to a narrowed distal segment. Rectal biopsy will confirm the diagnosis. Low gut atresia may present with delayed passage of meconium. Hypothyroidism should be considered.

The Infant with Metabolic Acidosis (see also Chapter 5)

Investigation involves:

- Blood gas analysis.
- Blood urea, creatinine and electrolytes, glucose, ammonia.
- Urine:
  pH, electrolytes, ketones
  Amino acids
  Organic acids.
- Plasma lactate and pyruvate.
- Plasma amino acids.

As a general guide, a base deficit of greater than 8 mmol/l is abnormal and in such a case we would investigate. If the blood analysed was collected by the capillary method it is important to confirm that the limb was well perfused and that a good flow of blood was obtained before further investigations are initiated. If in doubt, a further free-flowing capillary sample, or preferably an arterial sample, should be obtained.

Hypoxia is the most likely cause (Table 20.18) of metabolic acidosis in the newborn and in most cases there will be an associated respiratory acidosis. If however, the respiratory component hs been corrected the metabolic acidosis may persist for some time. A diagnosis of hypoxia can usually be confirmed from the history and from knowledge of the infant's condition at birth. Hypovolaemia and hypotension are also important causes of metabolic acidosis to be considered and excluded by examination.

In simple terms, metabolic acidosis may be due to under excretion or over production of acid. Under excretion is due to either glomerular dysfunction (with a raised urea and creatinine) or tubular disease. The clue to tubular disease would be the presence of a raised plasma chloride, a normal amino acid pattern and absence of ketones in the urine. In renal tubular acidosis there is an alkaline urine (pH > 6, irrespective of the blood standard bicarbonate concentration) and a low urinary sodium to potassium ratio and mild hypokalaemia (see Chapter 6).

Overproduction of acid is usually associated with a normal or low plasma chloride and an unexplained anion gap. In most inborn errors of metabolism particularly of the amino acid variety there will be features such as coma and seizures and there is an abnormal plasma amino acid screen and ketonuria. In galactosaemia there are reducing substances in the urine. Family history and consanguinity are important indicators.

If none of these diagnoses seems appropriate a lactic acidosis may be the underlying cause. In consultation with the laboratory, blood should be taken for plasma lactate levels (normally less than 1.4 mmol/l). (See Chapter 4.)

In the infant with metabolic alkalosis, the most common cause is metabolic compensation for a raised pCO$_2$ or inappropriate use of alkali. Other less common causes are excessive vomiting, chloride losing diarrhoea

Table 20.18   Causes of metabolic acidosis

Hypoxia
Hypotension
Renal disorders: glomerular; tubular
Inborn errors: e.g. amino acid disorders, urea cycle
  disorders
Lactic acidosis

and Barter's syndrome; biochemistry will show an associated hyponatraemia, hypochloraemia and hypokalaemia.

Since many causes of metabolic acidosis have a genetic basis, when death is inevitable the following samples should be collected, with parental consent and with the co-operation of biochemical, pathology and genetic departments:

- Plasma – separated and stored at $-70°C$.
- White cells – stored at $-70°C$.
- Urine – stored at $-70°C$.
- CSF – stored at $-70°C$.
- Skin biopsy – in tissue culture medium.
- Liver biopsy (needle or open):
  Histology – stored in formalin
  Electron microscopy – stored in gluteraldehyde
  Genetics/biochemistry – stored at $-70°C$.
- Muscle biopsy – stored at $-70°C$.

An early autopsy is essential and we find that most parents recognize the need to give consent before the infant's death. Communication with laboratory colleagues is the key to a successful investigation.

The Baby with Ambiguous Genitalia (see also Chapter 3)

Investigation involves:

- Chromosomal analysis: by the fastest reliable method. Bone marrow examination will provide results within hours and lymphocyte culture within 2 days.
- Imaging: ultrasound of the pelvis; cystogram.
- Laboratory investigation: urea and electrolytes; 17-hydroxyprogesterone (interference from maternal and placental steroids may occur if samples are taken within 24 h of birth); urinary steroid profile.

If the gender of the infant is not obvious (Table 20.19) this must be explained to the parents. Part of this early investigation includes careful questioning of the parents: for example, history of maternal exposure to androgens or a family tree with an unexpected number of women who have been infertile and amenorrhoeic.

Careful clinical examination of the external genitalia and measurement of the blood pressure followed by early and urgent investigation is essential. Phenotypic sex may differ from chromosomal sex and the differentiation of an incompletely developed male and a virilized female may take a few days.

Since congenital adrenal hyperplasia is the most life-

Table 20.19   Causes of ambiguous genitalia

Chromosomes XX
Either female pseudohermaphrodite or true hermaphrodite
Virilizing congenital adrenal hyperplasia
Exogenous androgens

Chromosomes XY
Male pseudohermaphrodite
Enzyme block in testis
Target organ failure (testicular feminization)

Chromosomes XO XY/XO
True hermaphrodite
Mixed or dysgenetic gonads

threatening cause, once these investigations have been carried out treatment of the patient with hydrocortisone and fludrocortisone may be commenced, without jeopardizing the diagnosis. In rare cases, biopsy of the gonad or surgical exploration may be required.

The Infant with Thyroid Disease (see also Chapter 3)

Investigation involves:

- Biochemical: Thyroid function tests (reduced T4 and raised TSH).
- Imaging: bone age; radioisotope scan.

Hypothyroidism

Hypothyroidism occurs in approximately 1 in 3500 births (Table 20.20). Females are more commonly affected. The infant may be post mature and of large size. The posterior fontanelle may be wide, umbilical hernia and goitre may be present. Within the first few weeks, feeding may be poor. The infant may have prolonged jaundice and become constipated. The Guthrie test card provides a screening test for all infants. In those with abnormal Guthrie or clinical suspicion of thyroid disease, thyroid function tests are carried out. The diagnosis may

Table 20.20   Causes of hypothyroidism

	Prevalence (%)
Athyreosis	15
Thyroid ectopia	43
Dyshormonogenesis	22
Atrophic congenital hypothyroidism	20

be more precise if a radioisotope scan is carried out, but this can usually be delayed until 12–18 months when reassessment is necessary.

Although bone age estimation using hand and wrist X-ray adds nothing to the diagnosis, films of the small bones of the foot and of the distal femoral epiphyses may give information regarding the duration and the severity of the disease. Infants with low T4 and raised TSH may not have permanent hypothyroidism. Transplacental transfer of maternal blocking antibodies may have a transient effect on the infant. It is important therefore to reassess infants at age 12–18 months.

Hyperthyroidism

Investigation involves:

- Thyroid function tests.
- Thyroid receptor antibodies (TRABs): maternal; infant.

Most neonatal cases are as a result of maternal Graves' disease and transplacental transfer of thyroid stimulating immunoglobulin. Maternal TRAB and infant TRAB can be measured.

The disease is transient but may require treatment with carbimazole for a period of months. Rarely, a dominantly inherited form of Graves' disease may occur and definitive therapy is ultimately required.

ACKNOWLEDGEMENT

The authors wish to thank Mrs Karyn Cooper for assistance in preparing the manuscript for this chapter.

REFERENCES

Nathan DG, Oski FA (1992) *Haematology of Infancy and Childhood*. WB Saunders, New York.
Roberton NRC (1992) *Textbook of Neonatology*. Churchill Livingstone, Edinburgh.
Volpe JJ (1987) *Neurology of the Newborn*. WB Saunders, Philadelphia.

Index